This book belongs to:

_____

If found, please contact:

_____

_____

D1788626

A Personal Acupuncture Handbook

For questions, comments, or suggestions go to:

www.acupuncturebookstore.com

WARNING:

This book is created as a handbook for students and practitioners of Traditional Chinese Medicine (TCM). No one other than students or practitioners of acupuncture or TCM should be using this book. Acupuncture should only be used by individuals who have received training. The practice of acupuncture without a license is prohibited by law.

ISBN 0-9722153-0-1

A PERSONAL ACUPUNCTURE HANDBOOK

Create Your Own Textbook of Acupuncture Points

By Jennifer Sobel

Illustrations by David Knox

To order, visit:

www.acupuncturebookstore.com

Dedicated to
ParamahansaYogananda
with love and gratitude.

HOW TO USE THIS BOOK

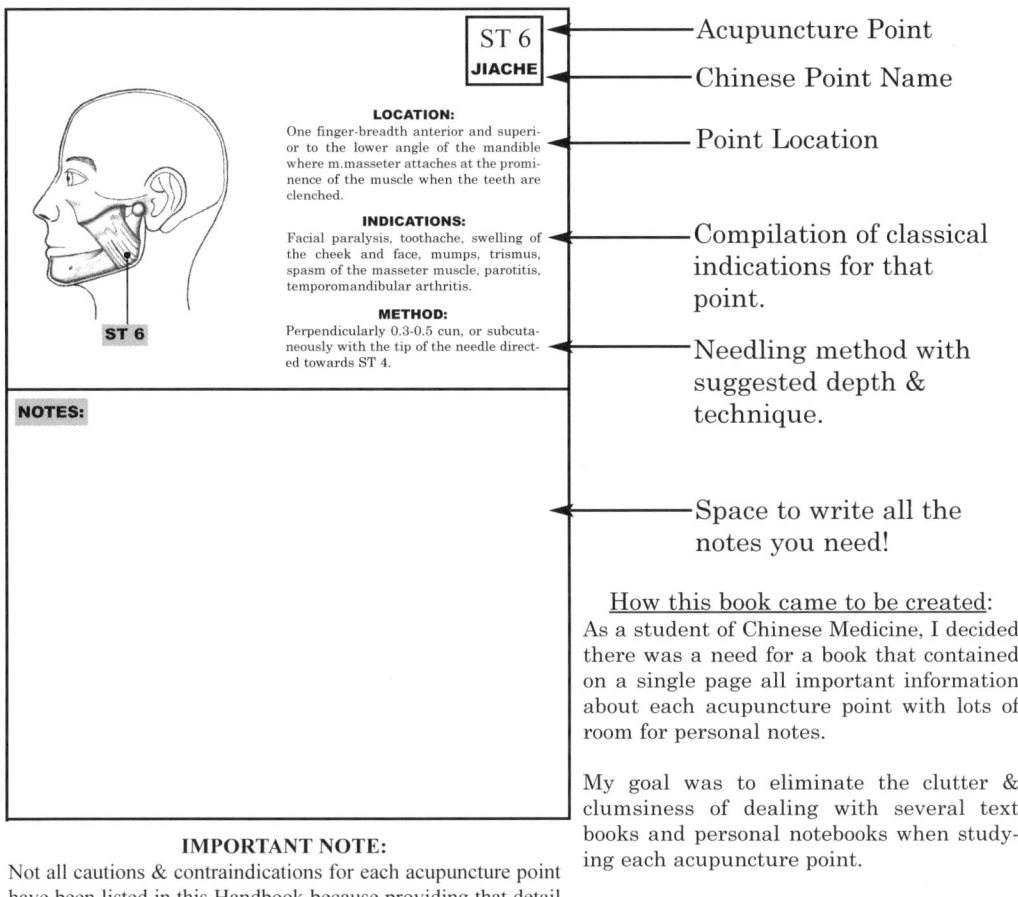

ST 6 ◄─────── Acupuncture Point

JIACHE ◄─────── Chinese Point Name

Point Location ◄───────

LOCATION:
One finger-breadth anterior and superior or to the lower angle of the mandible where m.masseter attaches at the prominence of the muscle when the teeth are clenched.

INDICATIONS:
Facial paralysis, toothache, swelling of the cheek and face, mumps, trismus, spasm of the masseter muscle, parotitis, temporomandibular arthritis. ◄─────── Compilation of classical indications for that point.

METHOD:
Perpendicularly 0.3-0.5 cun, or subcutaneously with the tip of the needle directed towards ST 4. ◄─────── Needling method with suggested depth & technique.

ST 6

NOTES:

◄─────── Space to write all the notes you need!

How this book came to be created:
As a student of Chinese Medicine, I decided there was a need for a book that contained on a single page all important information about each acupuncture point with lots of room for personal notes.

My goal was to eliminate the clutter & clumsiness of dealing with several text books and personal notebooks when studying each acupuncture point.

IMPORTANT NOTE:
Not all cautions & contraindications for each acupuncture point have been listed in this Handbook because providing that detail of information is not the function of this book. This book is designed so that you, the student and/or practitioner, can compile that information yourself from TCM instructional sources, including Chinese medicine textbooks and acupuncture instructors.

My desire for such a single resource went unsatisfied until I created this book. It has become a handbook that can be personalized by the student and practitioner alike, providing usefulness for an entire career.

Suggestions for getting the most out of this book:

● Write small. You'll be adding notes for years to come.

● Each "notes" section is useful for: referencing information from other texts, classes, clinical experience, seminars, and so forth.

● When making your own notes, consider color coding your pens to match the major texts from which you will be taking notes.

● Extra "note" pages have been provided for your use at the end of each channel, as well as at the end of the book.

TABLE OF CONTENTS

LUNG CHANNEL

LUNG MERIDIAN OF HAND TAI-YIN

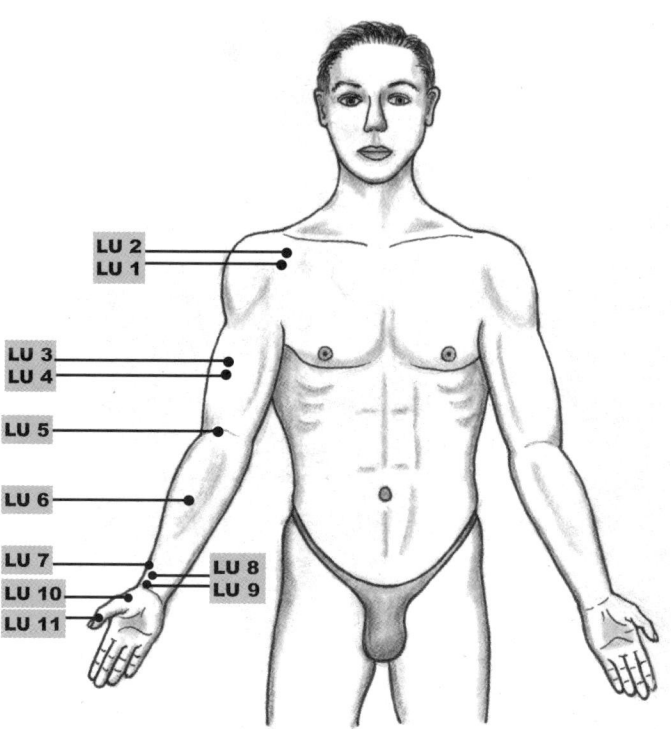

THERAPEUTIC INDICATIONS

- Diseases of the throat, chest, lung, and other diseases of areas the meridian supplies.

CHANNEL/ORGAN RELATIONSHIPS

- This channel is associated with the Lung and connects with the Large Intestine.

- It crosses the diaphragm and also connects with the Stomach and Kidneys.

PATHOLOGY

Channel: Fever and sensitivity to cold, hemoptysis, cough, asthma, nasal congestion, chest fullness, congested and sore throat, headache, pain in the chest, shoulder, back, supraclavicular fossa, and along the anterior border of the medial aspect of the arm.

Organ: Asthma, coughing, shortness of breath, chest fullness, dry throat, changes in the color of urine, irritability, bloody sputum, hot palms.

LUNG MERIDIAN OF HAND TAI-YIN

GENERAL PATHWAY	•Begins in the middle jiao & descends to meet the Large Intestine. •Returns upward connecting with the Stomach, passes through the diaphragm, and enters the Lung, its pertaining organ. •From the Lung and throat, it emerges from LU 1. •Descends along medial aspect of upper arm, passing in front of the Heart and Pericardium channels. •Continues downward along anterior border of radial side of medial forearm and enters the radial artery. •Passing through the thenar eminence, it ends at the medial side of the tip of the thumb (LU 11). **BRANCH:** •A branch emerges from LU 7 and connects with LI 1 and the Large Intestine channel.
CONNECTING CHANNEL	•Arises from LU 7 and connects to the Large Intestine meridian. **BRANCH:** A branch follows the Lung meridian into the palm of the hand and spreads through the thenar eminence.
DIVERGENT CHANNEL	•Derives from the Lung meridian at the axilla. •Runs anterior to the Pericardium meridian into the chest. •Connects with the Lung and then disperses in the Large Intestine. **BRANCH:** A branch extends upward from the lung, emerges at the supraclavicular fossa, ascends across the throat and converges with the Large Intestine meridian.
MUSCULAR REGION	•Arises from the tip of the thumb (LU 11) and binds at the thenar eminence. •Follows the radial pulse, ascends along the forearm, and binds at the elbow. •Ascends along medial aspect of arm and enters the chest below the axilla. •Emerging from ST 12, it travels to LI 15. •Above, it connects with the supraclavicular fossa, and below with the chest, dispersing over the diaphragm and converging again at the lowest rib.

FRONT MU POINT OF THE LUNG

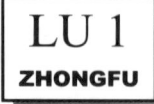

LU 1
ZHONGFU

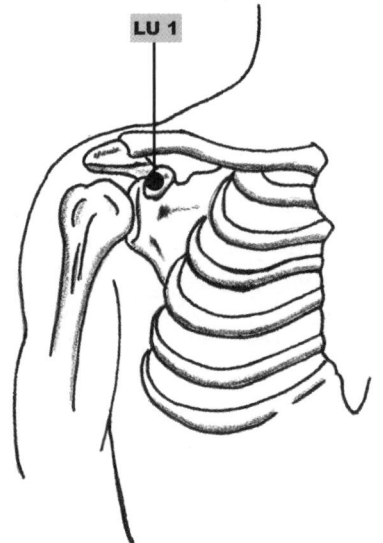

LOCATION:
Laterosuperior to the sternum at the lateral side of the first intercostal space, 6 cun lateral to the Ren meridian.

INDICATIONS:
Cough, asthma, pain in the chest, shoulder, and back, fullness of the chest, bronchitis, pneumonia, pulmonary tuberculosis.

METHOD:
Obliquely 0.5-0.8 cun towards the lateral aspect of the chest. Never puncture deeply towards medial aspect.

NOTES:

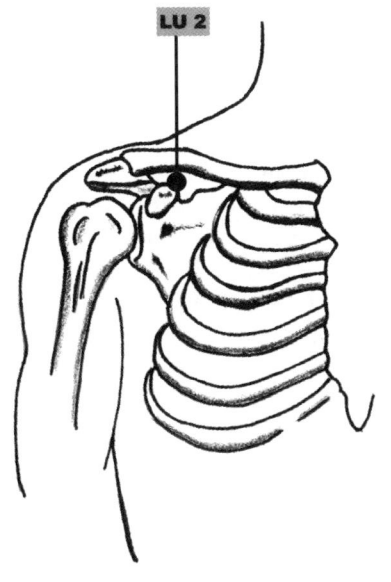

LU 2

LU 2
YUNMEN

LOCATION:
In the depression below the acromial extremity of the clavicle, 6 cun lateral to the Ren Meridian.

INDICATIONS:
Cough, asthma, chest pain, fullness or depression, perifocal inflammation of the shoulder joint, pain in the arm.

METHOD:
Obliquely 0.5-0.8 cun towards lateral aspect of the chest. Never puncture deeply towards the medial aspect.

NOTES:

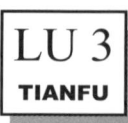

LU 3
TIANFU

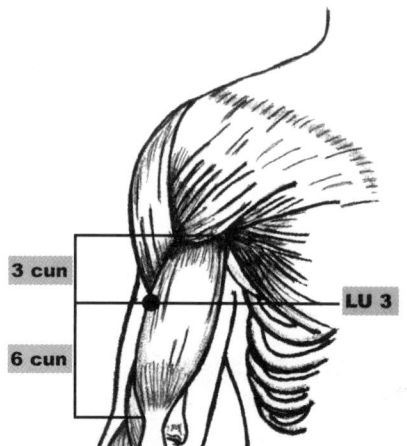

3 cun

LU 3

6 cun

LOCATION:
On the medial aspect of the upper arm, 3 cun below the end of the axillary fold, on the radial side of m.biceps brachii.

INDICATIONS:
Asthma, epistaxis, pain in the medial aspect of the upper arm, bronchitis.

METHOD:
Perpendicularly 0.5-1.0 cun.

NOTES:

6

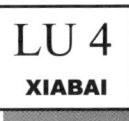

LU 4
XIABAI

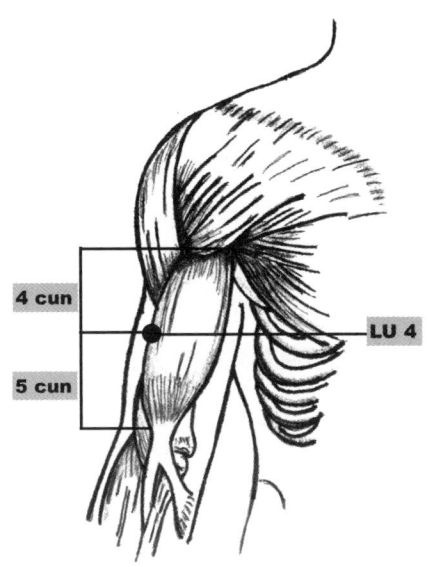

4 cun

LU 4

5 cun

LOCATION:
On the medial aspect of the upper arm, 1 cun below Lung 3, on the radial side of m.biceps brachii.

INDICATIONS:
Cough, fullness in the chest, pain in the medial aspect of the upper arm, asthma, bronchitis, nosebleed.

METHOD:
Perpendicular 0.5-1.0 cun.

NOTES:

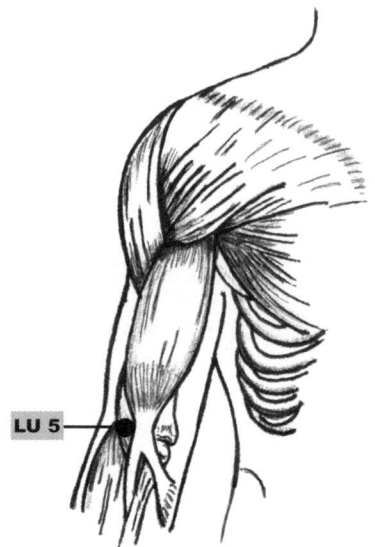

LU 5

LOCATION:
On the cubital crease, on the radial side of the tendon of m. biceps brachii. This point is located with the elbow slightly flexed.

INDICATIONS:
Cough, hemoptysis, afternoon fever, asthma, sore throat, fullness in the chest, infantile convulsions, spasmodic pain of the elbow and arm, mastitis, pneumonia, bronchitis, pleurisy, swelling & pain in the throat, erysipelas.

METHOD:
Perpendicularly 0.5-1.0 cun.

NOTES:

XI-CLEFT POINT

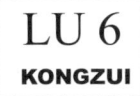

LU 6
KONGZUI

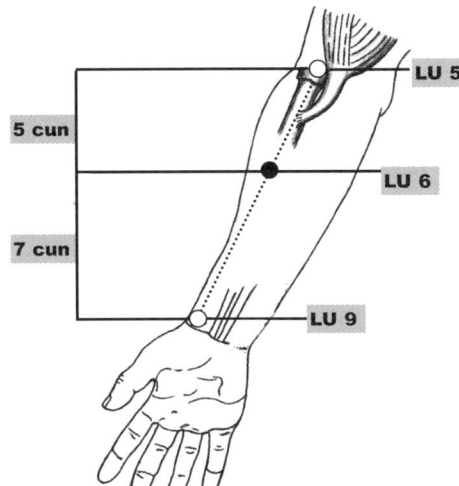

5 cun

7 cun

LU 5

LU 6

LU 9

LOCATION:
On the palmar aspect of the forearm, on the line joining Lung 9 and Lung 5, 7 cun above the transverse crease of the wrist.

INDICATIONS:
Cough, pain in the chest, asthma, hemoptysis, sore throat, spasmodic pain of the elbow and arm, pneumonia, tonsillitis.

METHOD:
Perpendicularly 0.5-1.0 cun.

NOTES:

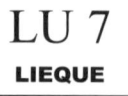
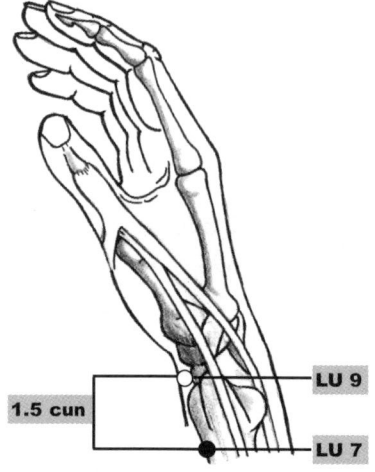

LU 9

1.5 cun

LU 7

LOCATION:
Superior to the styloid process of the radius, 1.5 cun above the transverse crease of the wrist.

INDICATIONS:
Headache, migraine, neck rigidity, cough, asthma, sore throat, facial paralysis, toothache, pain, weakness, and diseases of the wrist joint, urticaria.

METHOD:
Puncture 0.3-0.5 cun obliquely upward.

NOTES:

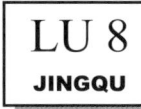
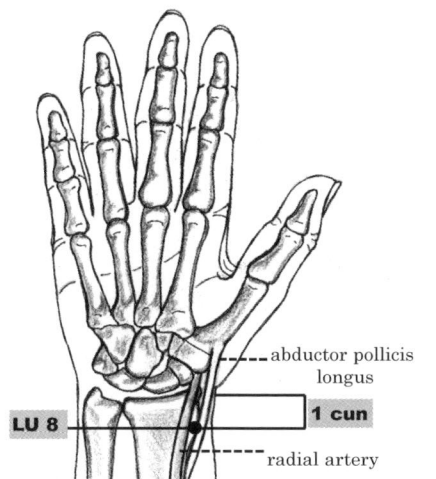

abductor pollicis longus

LU 8

1 cun

radial artery

LOCATION:
1 cun above the transverse crease of the wrist in the depression on the lateral side of the radial artery.

INDICATIONS:
Cough, asthma, fever, pain in the chest, sore throat, pain in the wrist, bronchitis.

METHOD:
Perpendicularly 0.1-0.3 cun. Avoid puncturing the radial artery.

NOTES:

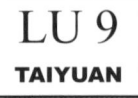

LU 9
TAIYUAN

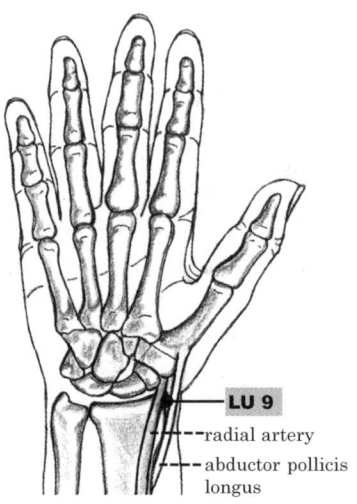

LU 9
radial artery
abductor pollicis
longus

LOCATION:
At the radial end of the transverse crease of the wrist, in the depression on the lateral side of the radial artery.

INDICATIONS:
Cough, asthma, hemoptysis, sore throat, palpitation, pain in the chest, wrist, and arm, bronchitis, pertussis, influenza, pulmonary tuberculosis, pain in the chest, diseases affecting radial side of the wrist joint.

METHOD:
Perpendicularly 0.2-0.3 cun. Avoid puncturing the radial artery.

NOTES:

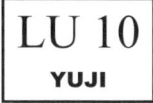
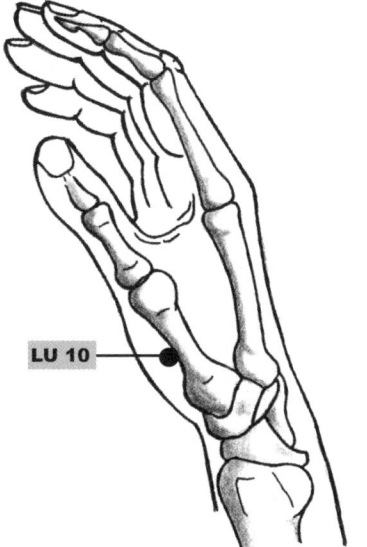

LU 10

LOCATION:
On the radial aspect of the midpoint of the first metacarpal bone, on the junction of the red & white skin (e.g. the junction of the dorsum and palm of the hand.)

INDICATIONS:
Cough, hemoptysis, sore throat, loss of voice, fever, feverish sensation in the palm, laryngopharyngitis, tonsillitis, hoarseness, asthma, infantile malnutrition syndrome.

METHOD:
Perpendicularly 0.5-0.8 cun.

NOTES:

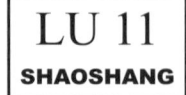
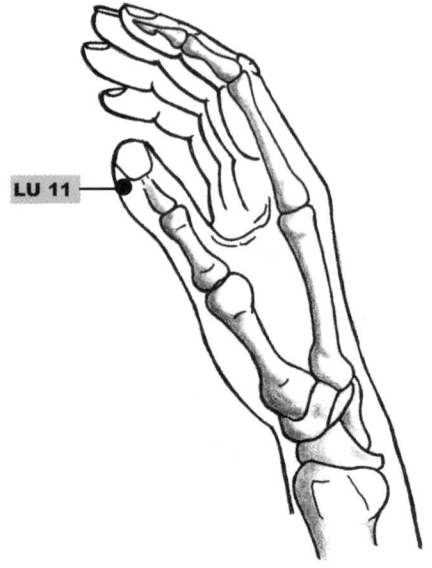

LU 11

LOCATION:
On the radial side of the thumb, about 0.1 cun posterior to the corner of the nail.

INDICATIONS:
Sore throat, cough, asthma, epistaxis, fever, loss of consciousness, mania, spasmodic pain of the thumb, tonsillitis, parotitis, common cold, pneumonia, stroke, infantile indigestion, psychosis.

METHOD:
Puncture 0.1 cun, or prick to cause bleeding.

NOTES:

NOTES

LARGE INTESTINE
CHANNEL

LARGE INTESTINE MERIDIAN OF HAND YANG-MING

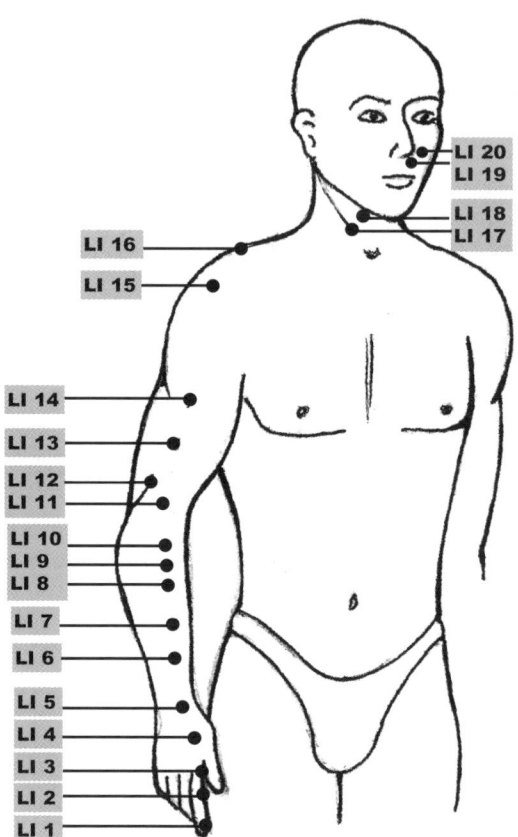

THERAPEUTIC INDICATIONS

• Diseases of the head & face, five sense organs, pharynx & larynx, febrile diseases, and other diseases of the areas the meridian supplies.

CHANNEL/ORGAN RELATIONSHIPS

• This channel is associated with the Large Intestine and connects with the Lung.

• It also joins directly with the Stomach.

PATHOLOGY

Channel: Fever, dry mouth, thirst, congested and sore throat, epistaxis, watery nasal discharge, toothache, abdominal pain, borborygmus, diarrhea, dysentery, red & painful eyes, swelling of the neck, pain in the neck, anterior part of shoulder, anterior border of lateral aspect of upper limb, and motor impairment of the fingers.

Organ: Abdominal pain, borborygmus, loose stool, occasionally with shortness of breath and belching.

GENERAL PATHWAY	●Begins at the tip of the index finger (LI 1), & runs upward along the radial side of the index finger, passing through the interspace of the 1st & 2nd metacarpal bones. ●It then passes between tendons extensor pollicis longus and brevis at the wrist. ●Following the lateral anterior aspect of the forearm, it reaches the lateral side of the elbow. ●It then ascends the lateral anterior aspect of the upper arm to the shoulder joint (LI 15). ●Then, along the anterior border of the acromion, it goes up to C7 (DU 14) and descends to the supraclavicular fossa to connect with the lung. ●Finally, it passes through the diaphragm and enters the Large Intestine. **BRANCHES:** ●A branch separates from the main channel at the supraclavicular fossa, moves upward through the neck, crosses the cheek and enters the gums of the lower teeth. ●From here, it curves around the lip and intersects the same channel coming from the opposite side of the body at the philtrum. The branch finally terminates at the side of the nose.
CONNECTING CHANNEL	●After separating from the primary channel at LI 6 on the wrist, this channel joins the Lung channel 3 cun above the wrist. **BRANCH 1:** A branch follows the arm to the shoulder, crosses the jaw and extends to the teeth. **BRANCH 2:** A branch separates at the jaw and enters the ear region to join the Chong.
DIVERGENT CHANNEL	●After deriving from the LI channel on the hand, it continues upward across the arm & shoulder to the breast. **BRANCH 1:** A branch diverges at the top of the shoulder, enters the spine at the nape of the neck, and runs downward to connect with the Large Intestine and the Lung. **BRANCH 2:** A branch ascends from the shoulder along the throat, emerging at the supraclavicular fossa where it rejoins the Large Intestine meridian.
MUSCULAR REGION	●Begins at the tip of the index finger & connects at the dorsum of the wrist. ●From here, it ascends across the forearm, & connects at the lateral aspect of the elbow before continuing up the arm, where it connects at the shoulder (LI 15). ●It proceeds from the top of the shoulder to the neck, where a branch separates and connects at the side of the nose. ●Continuing upward, it runs anterior to the Small Intestine Muscle channel and crossses over the head, connecting at the mandible on the opposite side of the face. **BRANCH:** A branch encircles the scapula & attaches to the spine.

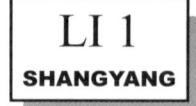

LI 1
SHANGYANG

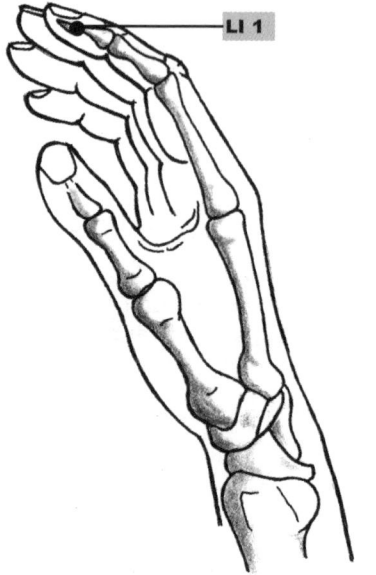

LI 1

LOCATION:
On the radial side of the index finger, about 0.1 cun posterior to the corner of the nail.

INDICATIONS:
Toothache, sore throat, swelling of the submandibular region, numbness of the fingers, febrile diseases with anhidrosis, loss of consciousness, apoplectic coma, high fever, deafness.

METHOD:
Puncture 0.1 cun, or prick the point to cause bleeding.

NOTES:

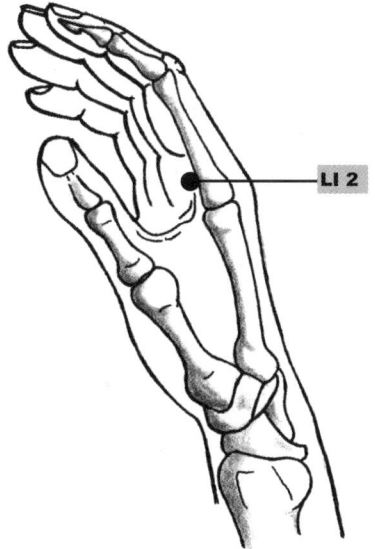

LI 2

LOCATION:
On the radial side of the index finger, distal to the metacarpal-phalangeal joint, at the junction of the red & white skin. The point is located with the finger slightly flexed.

INDICATIONS:
Blurring of vision, epistaxis, toothache, sore throat, febrile diseases, facial paralysis, trigeminal neuralgia.

METHOD:
Perpendicularly 0.2-0.3 cun.

NOTES:

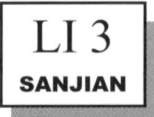
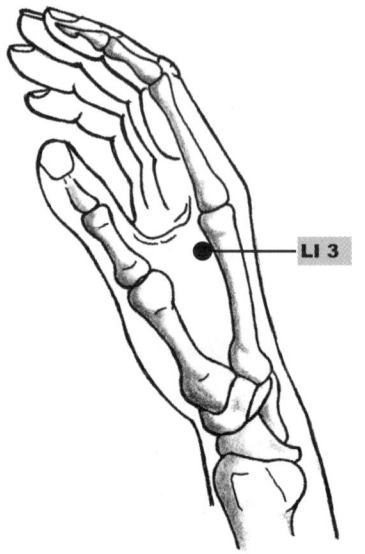

LI 3

LOCATION:
When a loose fist is made, the point is on the radial side of the index finger, in the depression proximal to the head of the second metacarpal bone.

INDICATIONS:
Toothache, opthalmalgia, sore throat, redness and swelling of fingers and the dorsum of the hand, malaria, painful eyes, trigeminal neuralgia.

METHOD:
Perpendicularly 0.5-0.8 cun.

NOTES:

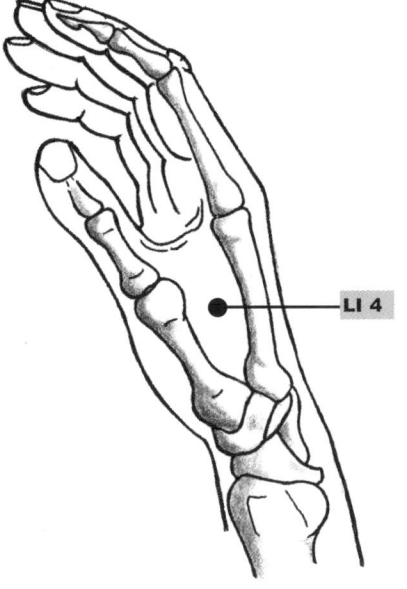

LI 4

LOCATION:
On the dorsum of the hand, between the 1st and 2nd metacarpal bones, approximately in the middle of the 2nd metacarpal bone on the radial side.

INDICATIONS:
Headache, neck pain, redness, swelling and pain of the eye, epistaxis, nasal obstruction, rhinnorhea, toothache, deafness, swelling of the face, sore throat, parotitis, trismus, facial paralysis, febrile diseases with anhidrosis, hidrosis, abdominal pain, dysentery, constipation, amenorrhea, delayed labor, infantile convulsion, pain, weakness and motor impairment of the upper limbs, hemiplegia, diseases of the sensory organs.

METHOD:
Perpendicularly 0.5-1.0 cun. Acupuncture & moxa contraindicated in pregnancy.

NOTES:

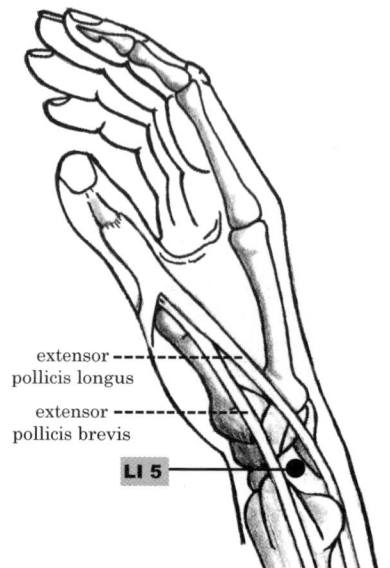

extensor
pollicis longus

extensor
pollicis brevis

LI 5

LOCATION:
On the radial side of the wrist. When the thumb is tilted upward, it is in the depression between the tendons of m.extensor pollicis longus and brevis.

INDICATIONS:
Headache, redness, pain and swelling of the eye, toothache, sore throat, diseases of the soft tissues of the wrist joint, opthalmalgia, headache, tinnitus, deafness, infantile indigestion.

METHOD:
Perpendicularly 0.3-0.5 cun.

NOTES:

LUO-CONNECTING POINT

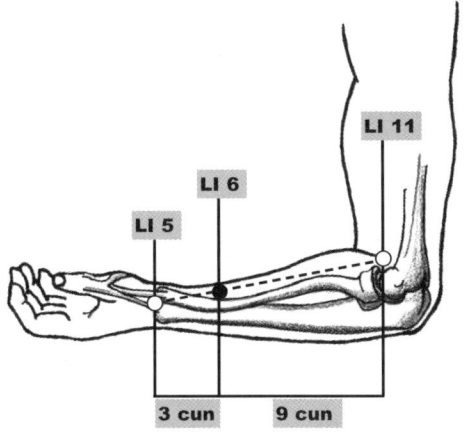

LOCATION:
With the elbow flexed and the radial side of the arm upward, the point is on the line joining LI 5 and LI 11, 3 cun above LI 5.

INDICATIONS:
Redness of the eye, tinnitus, deafness, epistaxis, aching of the hand and arm, sore throat, edema, facial paralysis, tonsillitis, neuralgia of the forearm.

METHOD:
Perpendicularly or obliquely 0.5-0.8 cun.

NOTES:

XI-CLEFT POINT

LI 7
WENLIU

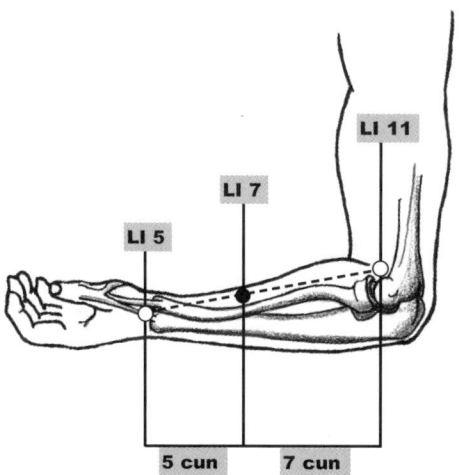

LOCATION:
With the elbow flexed and the radial side of the arm upward, the point is on the line joining LI 5 and LI 11, 5 cun above LI 5.

INDICATIONS:
Headache, swelling of the face, sore throat, borborygmus, abdominal pain, aching of the shoulder and arm, stomatitis, parotitis, glossitis, facial paralysis.

METHOD:
Perpendicularly 0.5-1.0 cun.

NOTES:

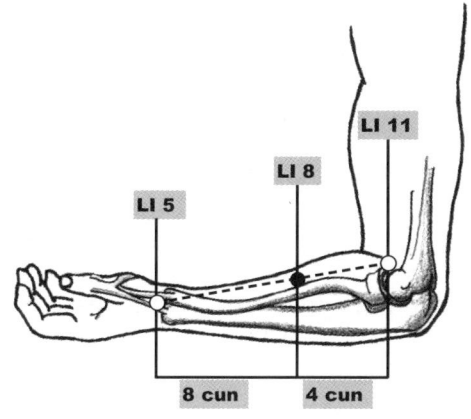

LOCATION:
On the line joining LI 5 and LI 11, 4 cun below LI 11.

INDICATIONS:
Abdominal pain, borborygmus, pain in the elbow and arm, motor impairment of the upper limbs, headache, painful eyes, vertigo, mastitis.

METHOD:
Perpendicularly 0.5-1.0 cun.

NOTES:

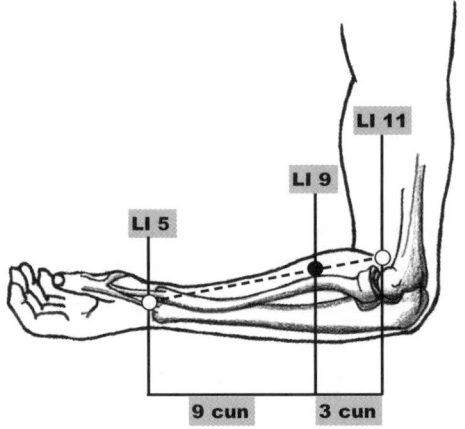

LOCATION:
On the line joining LI 5 and LI 11, 3 cun below LI 11.

INDICATIONS:
Aching of the shoulder and arm, motor impairment of the upper limbs, numbness of the hand and arm, borborygmus, abdominal pain, numbness of the arms & legs, hemiplegia, sprain, intestinal noises, abdominal pain.

METHOD:
Perpendicularly 0.5-1.0 cun.

NOTES:

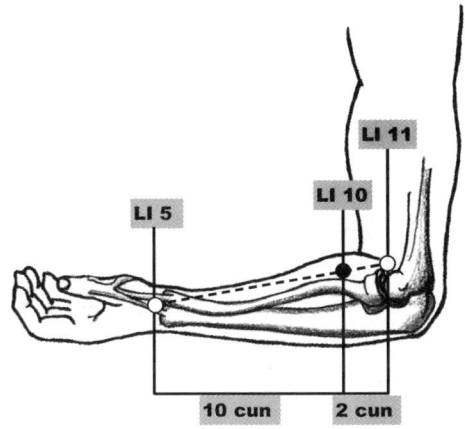

LOCATION:
On the line joining LI 5 and LI 11, 2 cun below LI 11.

INDICATIONS:
Abdominal pain, diarrhea, toothache, swelling of the cheek, motor impairment of the upper limbs, pain in the shoulder and back, ulcer, indigestion.

METHOD:
Perpendicularly 0.8-1.2 cun.

NOTES:

29

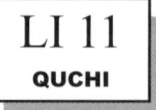
LOCATION:

When the elbow is flexed, the point is in the depression at the lateral end of the transverse cubital crease, midway between LU 5 and the lateral epicondyle of the humerus.

INDICATIONS:

Sore throat, toothache, redness and pain of the eye, scrofula, urticaria, motor impairment of the upper extremities, abdominal pain, vomiting, diarrhea, febrile diseases, arthritic pain in the upper limb, paralysis, hemiplegia, hypertension, high fever, measles, anemia, allergies, goiter, skin diseases.

METHOD:

Perpendicularly 1.0-1.5 cun.

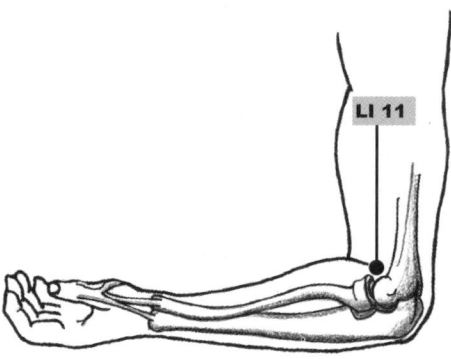

LI 11

NOTES:

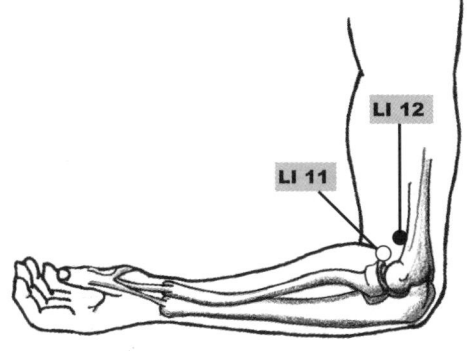

LOCATION:
When the elbow is flexed, the point is superior to the lateral epicondyle of the humerus, about 1 cun superolateral to LI 11, on the medial border of the humerus.

INDICATIONS:
Pain, numbness, and contracture of the elbow and arm, inflammation of the lateral epicondyle of the humerus.

METHOD:
Perpendicularly 0.5-1.0 cun.

NOTES:

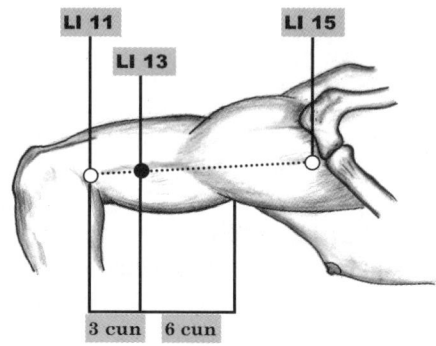

LOCATION:

Superior to the lateral epicondyle of the humerus, on the line joining LI 11 and LI 15, 3 cun above LI 11.

INDICATIONS:

Contracture and pain of the elbow and arm, scrofula, peritonitis, pneumonia, coughing blood.

METHOD:

Perpendicularly 0.5-1.0 cun.

NOTES:

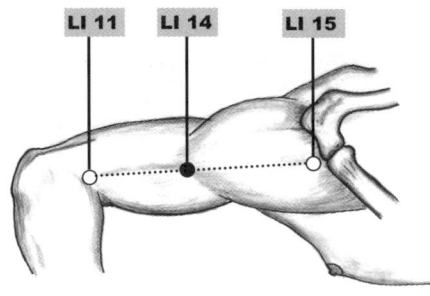

LI 11   LI 14   LI 15

LOCATION:
On the line joining LI 11 and LI 15, 7 cun above LI 11, on the radial side of the humerus, superior to the lower end of m.deltoideus.

INDICATIONS:
Pain in the shoulder and arm, rigidity of the neck, scrofula, eye diseases, paralysis of the upper limb.

METHOD:
Perpendicularly or obliquely upward 0.8-1.5 cun.

NOTES:

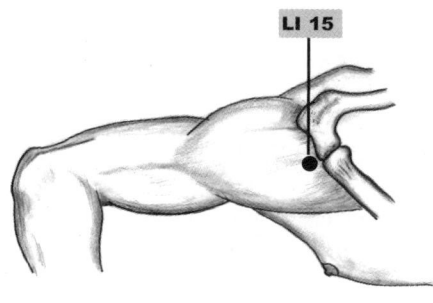

LI 15

LI 15

JIANYU

LOCATION:

Antero-inferior to the acromion, on the upper portion of m.deltoideus. When the arm is in full abduction, the point is in the depression appearing at the anterior border of the acromioclavicular joint.

INDICATIONS:

Pain in the shoulder and arm, motor impairment of the upper extremities, rubella, scrofula, perifocal inflammation of the shoulder joint, excess sweating, hemiplegia, hypertension.

METHOD:

Perpendicularly or obliquely 0.8-1.5 cun.

NOTES:

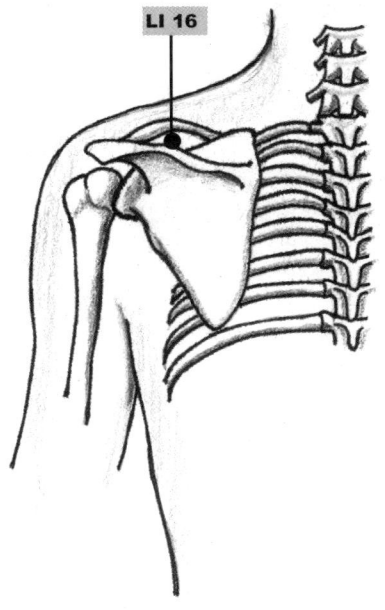

LI 16

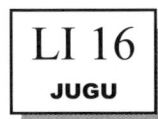
LOCATION:

In the upper aspect of the shoulder, in the depression between the acromial extremity of the clavicle and the scapular spine.

INDICATIONS:

Pain and motor impairment of the upper extremities, pain in the shoulder and back, diseases of the shoulder joint & soft tissues of the shoulder, spitting blood, scrofula.

METHOD:

Perpendicularly 0.5-0.7 cun.

NOTES:

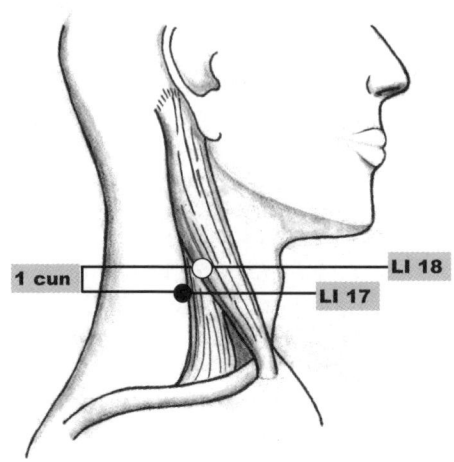

LOCATION:
On the lateral side of the neck, 1 cun below LI 18, on the posterior border of m.sternocleidomastoideus.

INDICATIONS:
Sudden loss of voice, sore throat, scrofula, goiter, paralysis of the hyoglossus muscles, tonsillitis, laryngitis.

METHOD:
Perpendicularly 0.3-0.5 cun.

NOTES:

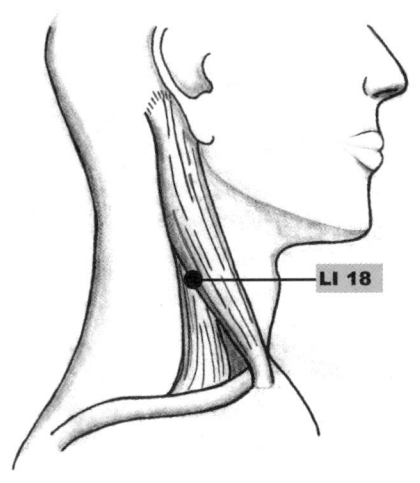

LI 18

LOCATION:
On the lateral side of the neck, level with the tip of the Adam's apple, between the sternal head and clavicular head of m.sternocleidomastoideus.

INDICATIONS:
Cough, asthma, sore throat, sudden loss of voice, scrofula, goiter, wheezing, excessive mucus, hoarse voice, distention, difficulty swallowing.

METHOD:
Perpendicularly 0.3-0.5 cun.

NOTES:

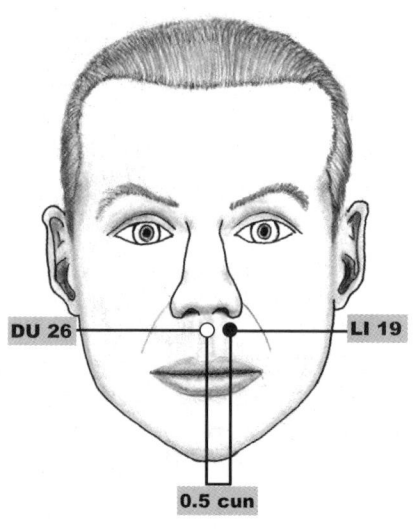

DU 26   LI 19

0.5 cun

LOCATION:
Right below the lateral margin of the nostril, 0.5 cun lateral to DU 26.

INDICATIONS:
Nasal obstruction, epistaxis, deviation of the mouth, rhinitis, facial paralysis.

METHOD:
Obliquely 0.2-0.3 cun.

NOTES:

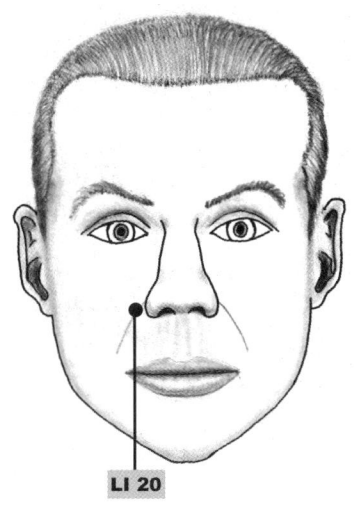

LI 20

LOCATION:
In the nasolabial groove, at the level of the midpoint of the lateral border of ala nasi.

INDICATIONS:
Nasal obstruction, hyposmia, epistaxis, rhinnorhea, deviation of the mouth, itching and swelling of the face, rhinitis, nasosinusitis, facial paralysis, roundworm in the bile duct.

METHOD:
Obliquely or subcutaneously 0.3-0.5 cun.

NOTES:

NOTES

NOTES

STOMACH CHANNEL

STOMACH MERIDIAN OF FOOT YANG-MING

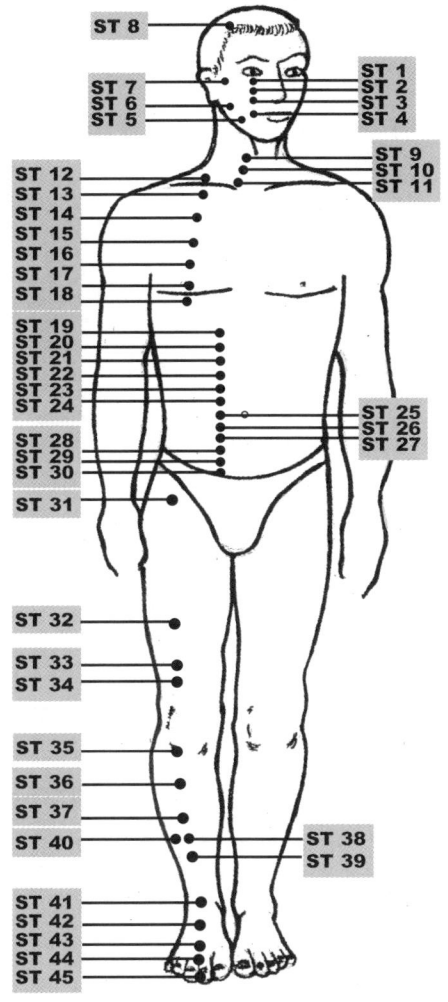

ST 8
ST 7
ST 6
ST 5
ST 1
ST 2
ST 3
ST 4
ST 9
ST 10
ST 11
ST 12
ST 13
ST 14
ST 15
ST 16
ST 17
ST 18
ST 19
ST 20
ST 21
ST 22
ST 23
ST 24
ST 25
ST 26
ST 27
ST 28
ST 29
ST 30
ST 31
ST 32
ST 33
ST 34
ST 35
ST 36
ST 37
ST 40
ST 38
ST 39
ST 41
ST 42
ST 43
ST 44
ST 45

CHANNEL/ORGAN RELATIONSHIPS

- This channel is associated with the Stomach & connects with the Spleen.

- It also joins directly with the Heart, Large Intestine, and Small Intestine.

THERAPEUTIC INDICATIONS

- GI diseases, disorders of the head, face, eye, nose, mouth & tooth, mental disorders, and other diseases in areas the meridian supplies.

PATHOLOGY

Channel: High fever, tidal fever, flushed face, sweating, mania, occasionally sensitivity to cold, pain in the eyes, dry nostrils, epistaxis, fever blisters, sore or congested throat, borborygmus, abdominal distention, epigastric pain, edema, vomiting, hunger, swelling on the neck, facial paralysis, deviation of the mouth, pain in the chest, abdomen, and lateral aspect of the lower limbs.

Organ: Constant hunger, yellow urine, abdominal distention, edema or sensation of fullness, seizures, discomfort when reclining.

GENERAL PATHWAY	●Begins at the lateral side of the nose, & ascends to the inner canthus where it meets the Bladder channel at UB 1. ●Descends along the lateral side of the nose, enters the upper gum & joins the DU channel at the philtrum (DU 24). ●Circling back around the lips, it meets the Ren channel at the mental labial groove on the chin (Ren 24). ●From here, it follows the angle of the jaw and runs upward in front of the ear & connects with GB 3. ●It proceeds along the hairline until it intersects the GB channel at GB 6. ●Finally, it follows the hairline to join the DU channel at DU 24. **BRANCHES:** ●**BRANCH 1:** A branch separates from the main channel on the lower jaw, descends along the throat, & enters the supraclavicular fossa. It then moves to the upper back where it meets the DU channel at DU 14. It proceeds downward across the diaphragm, intersecting the Ren channel internally at Ren 13 and Ren 12, before entering the Stomach & Spleen organs. ●**BRANCH 2:** A vertical branch descends from the supraclavicular fossa along the mammillary line, passing beside the umbilicus & through the lower abdomen to the inguinal region. ●**BRANCH 3:** A branch begins at the pylorus & descends internally to the inguinal region where it joins with BRANCH 2. From here, the channel crosses to ST 31 on the thigh, & descends to the patella. It then moves along the lateral side of the tibia to the dorsum of the foot, terminating at the lateral side of the tip of the 2nd toe. ●**BRANCH 4:** A parallel branch separates from the main channel at ST 36 & terminates at the lateral side of the middle toe. ●**BRANCH 5:** A branch separates on the dorsum of the foot at ST 42 & terminates at the medial side of the big toe, where it connects with the Spleen channel at SP 1.
CONNECTING CHANNEL	●After separating from the main channel at ST 40, this channel connects with the Spleen channel. ●**BRANCH 1:** A branch follows the lateral margin of the tibia upward across the thigh and trunk to the top of head, where it converges with the other Yang channels. ●**BRANCH 2:** A branch separates in the neck and connects with the throat.
DIVERGENT CHANNEL	●After diverging from the main channel on the thigh, it then enters the abdomen, connects with the Stomach, and then disperses through the Spleen. ●From there, it ascends across the Heart and follows the esophagus until it reaches the mouth. ●It continues upward beside the nose and connects with the eye before rejoining the Stomach channel.
MUSCULAR REGION	●Originating at the 2nd, 4th, and middle toes, it crosses the dorsum of the foot and slants upward along the lateral aspect of the leg, joining at the knee. ●From here, the channel crosses the hip and lower ribs before circling behind the body to connect with the spine. ●From the knee, the channel ascends across the thigh & connects again in the pelvic region where it joins with the reproductive organs. ●Continuing upward across the abdomen & chest, the channel connects with the clavicle then extends up the neck & around the mouth, connecting at the side of the nose. Above, it joins with the UB muscle channel to form a muscular net around the eye. **BRANCHES:** ●**BRANCH 1:** A branch separates from the first branch above the ankle and follows the tibia to the knee. ●**BRANCH 2:** A sub-branch crosses to the head of the fibula, where it joins the GB channel. ●**BRANCH 3:** A sub-branch separates at the jaw & traverses the face, connecting in front of the ear.

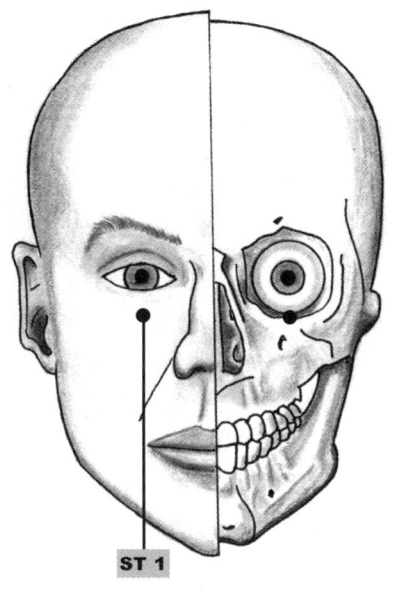

ST 1

LOCATION:

With the eyes looking straight forward, the point is directly below the pupil, between the eyeball and the infraorbital ridge.

INDICATIONS:

Redness, swelling and pain of the eye, lacrimation, night blindness, twitching of the eyelids, facial paralysis, acute & chronic conjunctivitis, myopia, hypermetropia, astigmatism, esotropia, colorblindness, glaucoma, inflammation or atrophy of the optic nerve, cataract, keratitis, retinitis pigmentosa.

METHOD:

Push the eyeball upward with the left thumb and puncture perpendicularly and slowly 0.5-1.0 cun along the infraorbital ridge. It is not advisable to manipulate the needle with large amplitude.

NOTES:

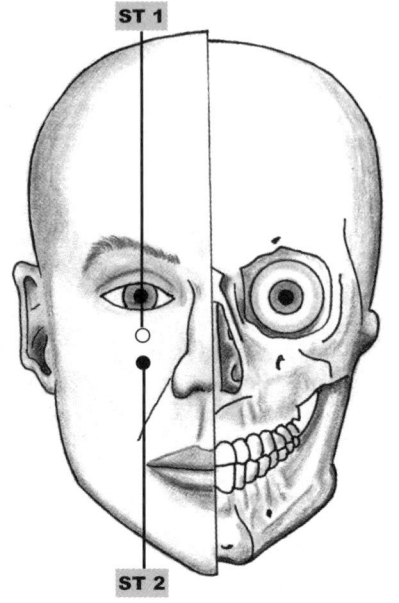

ST 1

ST 2

LOCATION:
Below ST 1, in the depression at the infraorbital foramen.

INDICATIONS:
Redness, pain and twitching of the eye, facial paralysis or spasm, twitching of the eyelids, pain in the face, trigeminal neuralgia, keratitis, myopia, sinusitis, roundworms in the bile duct, allergic facial swelling.

METHOD:
Perpendicularly 0.2-0.3 cun. It is not advisable to puncture deeply.

NOTES:

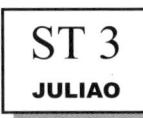

ST 3
JULIAO

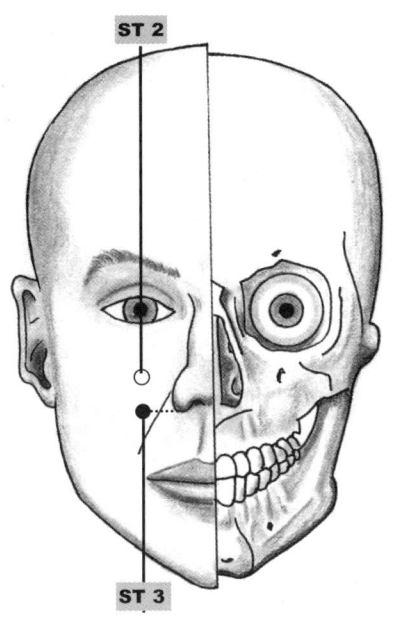

ST 2

ST 3

LOCATION:
Directly below ST 2, at the level of the lower border of ala nasi, on the lateral side of the nasolabial groove.

INDICATIONS:
Facial paralysis, twitching of the eyelids, epistaxis, toothache, swelling of the lips and cheek, rhinitis, trigeminal neuralgia.

METHOD:
Perpendicularly 0.3-0.5 cun.

NOTES:

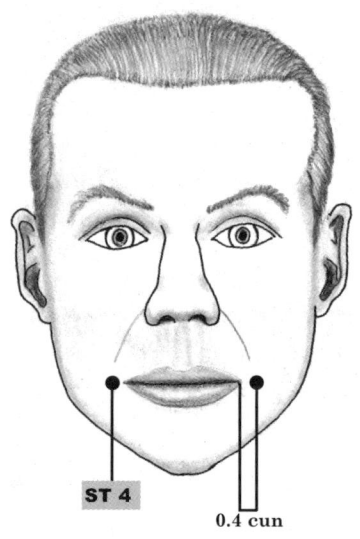

ST 4

0.4 cun

LOCATION:
0.4 cun lateral to the corner of the mouth.

INDICATIONS:
Deviation of the mouth, excessive saliva-tion, twitching or spasm of the eyelids, facial paralysis, trigeminal neuralgia.

METHOD:
Puncture subcutaneously 1.0-1.5 cun with the tip of the needle directed towards ST 6.

NOTES:

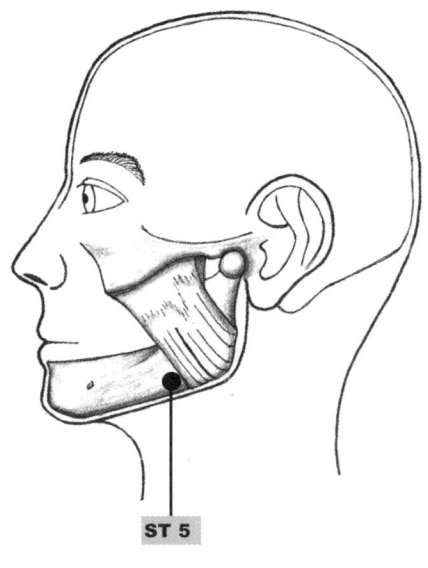

ST 5

LOCATION:
Anterior to the angle of the mandible, on the anterior border of the attached portion of m.masseter, in the groove-like depression appearing when the cheek is bulged.

INDICATIONS:
Facial paralysis, trismus, swelling of the cheek, pain in the face, toothache, "lockjaw", parotitis.

METHOD:
Avoid puncturing the artery. Puncture obliquely 0.3-0.5 cun.

NOTES:

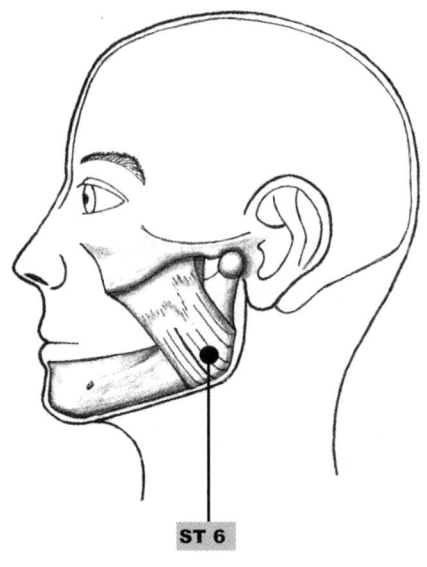

ST 6

LOCATION:
One finger-breadth anterior and superior to the lower angle of the mandible where m.masseter attaches at the prominence of the muscle when the teeth are clenched.

INDICATIONS:
Facial paralysis, toothache, swelling of the cheek and face, mumps, trismus, spasm of the masseter muscle, parotitis, temporo-mandibular arthritis.

METHOD:
Perpendicularly 0.3-0.5 cun, or subcutaneously with the tip of the needle directed towards ST 4.

NOTES:

50

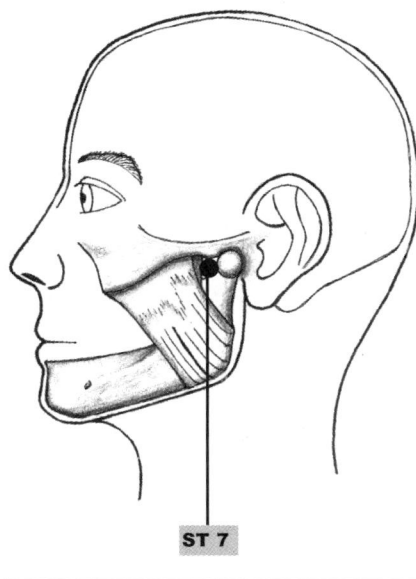

ST 7

LOCATION:
At the lower border of the zygomatic arch, in the depression anterior to the condyloid process of the mandible. This point is located with the mouth closed.

INDICATIONS:
Deafness, tinnitus, otorrhea, toothache, facial paralysis, pain of the face, motor impairment of the jaw, trigeminal neuralgia, otitis media, deaf-mutism, spasm of the masseter muscle, temporomandibular arthritis.

METHOD:
Perpendicularly 0.3-0.5 cun.

NOTES:

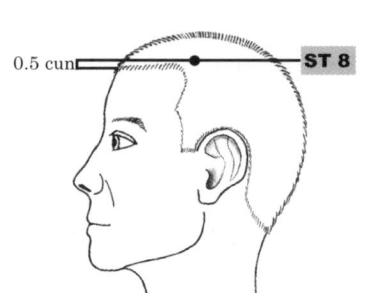

LOCATION:
0.5 cun within the anterior hairline at the corner of the forehead, 4.5 cun lateral to DU 24.

INDICATIONS:
Headache, blurry vision, ophthalmalgia, lacrimation, migraine headache, psychosis, facial paralysis.

METHOD:
Puncture 0.5-1.0 subcutaneously.

NOTES:

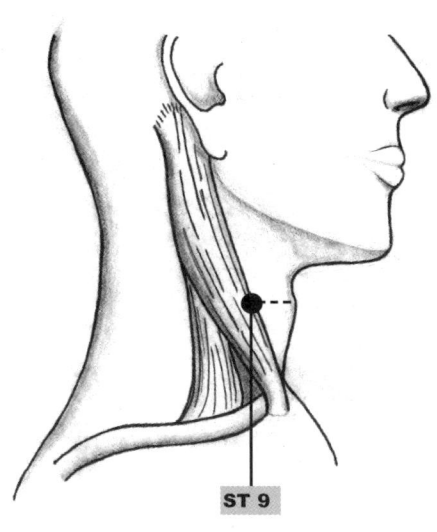

ST 9

LOCATION:
Level with the tip of the Adam's apple, just on the course of the common carotid artery, on the anterior border of m. sternocleidomastoideus.

INDICATIONS:
Sore throat, asthma, goiter, dizziness, flushing of the face, distension in the throat, speech impediment, high or low blood pressure.

METHOD:
Avoid puncturing the common carotid artery, puncture perpendicularly 0.3-0.5 cun.

NOTES:

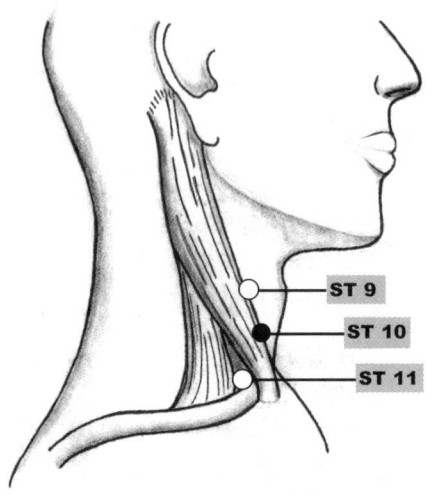

LOCATION:
At the midpoint of the line joining ST 9 and ST 11, on the anterior border of m. sternocleidomastoideus.

INDICATIONS:
Sore throat, asthma, cough, diseases of the vocal cords, goiter.

METHOD:
Perpendicularly 0.3-0.5 cun. Avoid the common carotid artery.

NOTES:

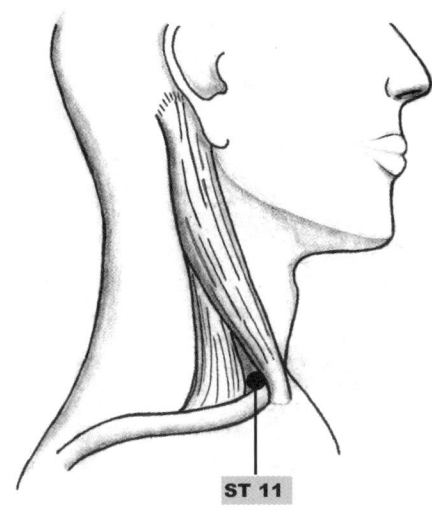

ST 11

LOCATION:

At the superior border of the sternal extremity of the clavicle, between the sternal head and clavicular head of m. sternocleidomastoideus.

INDICATIONS:

Sore throat, pain and rigidity of the neck, asthma, hiccup, goiter, pharyngitis, scrofula.

METHOD:

Perpendicularly 0.3-0.5 cun.

NOTES:

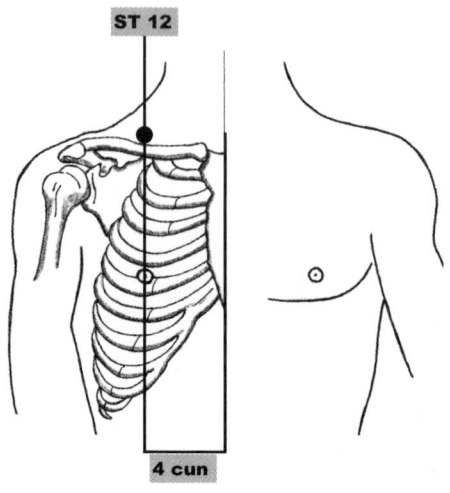

LOCATION:
In the midpoint of the supraclavicular fossa, 4 cun lateral to the Ren meridian.

INDICATIONS:
Cough, asthma, sore throat, pain in the supraclavicular fossa, hiccups, intercostal neuralgia.

METHOD:
Avoid puncturing the artery. Puncture perpendicularly 0.3-0.5 cun. Deep puncture is not advisable.

NOTES:

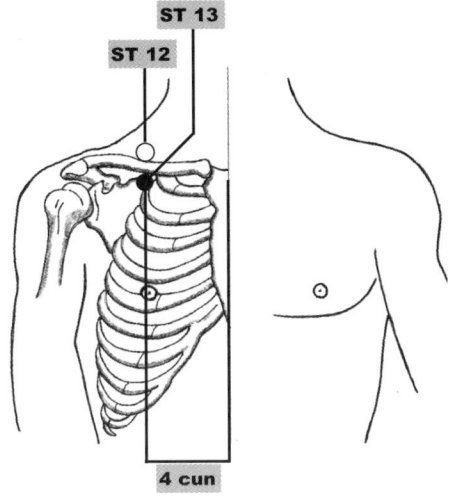

LOCATION:
At the lower border of the middle of the clavicle, 4 cun lateral to the Ren meridian.

INDICATIONS:
Fullness in the chest, asthma, cough, hiccup, pain in the chest and hypochondrium, bronchitis, intercostal neuralgia.

METHOD:
Puncture obliquely 0.3-0.5 cun.

NOTES:

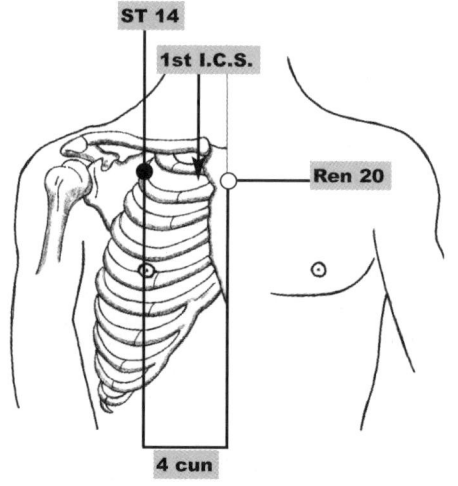

ST 14
1st I.C.S.
Ren 20
4 cun

LOCATION:
In the 1st intercostal space, 4 cun lateral to the Ren meridian.

INDICATIONS:
Sensation of fullness and pain in the chest, cough, bronchitis, intercostal neuralgia.

METHOD:
Obliquely 0.3-0.5 cun.

NOTES:

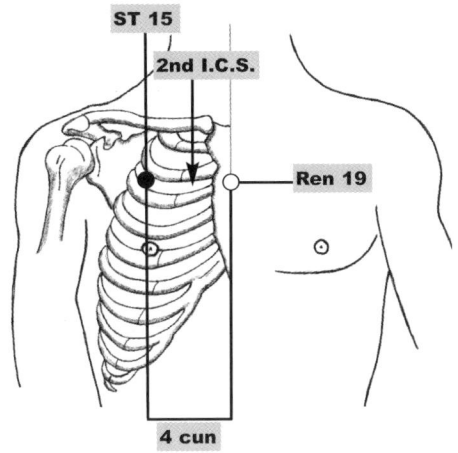

LOCATION:
In the 2nd intercostal space, 4 cun lateral to the Ren meridian.

INDICATIONS:
Fullness and pain in the chest and costal region, cough, asthma, mastitis, bronchitis, intercostal neuralgia.

METHOD:
Obliquely 0.3-0.5 cun.

NOTES:

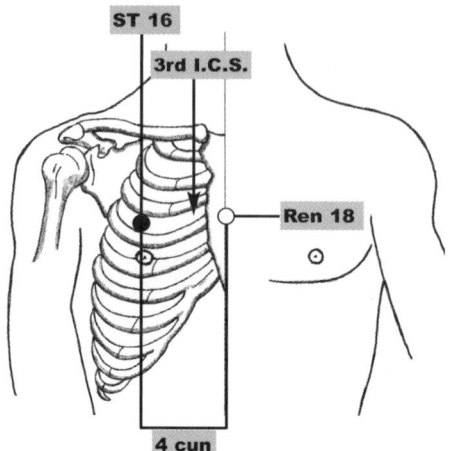

LOCATION:
In the 3rd intercostal space, 4 cun lateral to the Ren meridian.

INDICATIONS:
Fullness and pain in the chest and hypochondrium, cough, asthma, mastitis, bronchitis, intercostal neuralgia, intestinal noises and diarrhea.

METHOD:
Obliquely 0.3-0.5 cun.

NOTES:

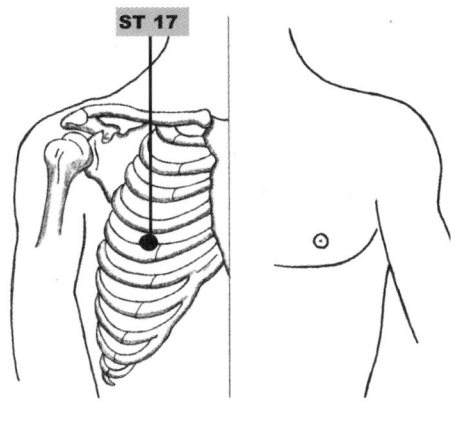

ST 17

LOCATION:
In the 4th intercostal space, in the center of the nipple.

INDICATIONS:
This point serves only as a landmark for locating points on the chest and abdomen.

METHOD:
Acupuncture and moxibustion on this point are contraindicated.

NOTES:

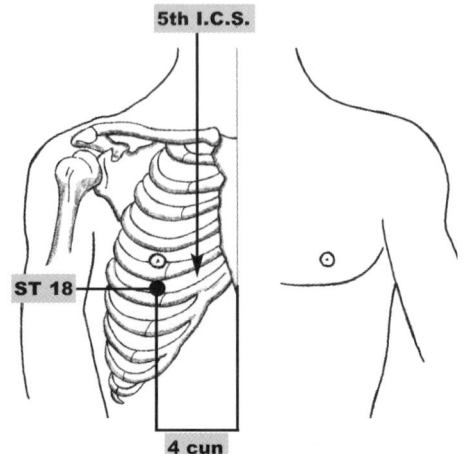

5th I.C.S.

ST 18

4 cun

LOCATION:
In the 5th intercostal space, directly below the nipple.

INDICATIONS:
Pain in the chest, cough, asthma, mastitis, insufficient lactation, bronchitis.

METHOD:
Obliquely 0.3-0.5 cun.

NOTES:

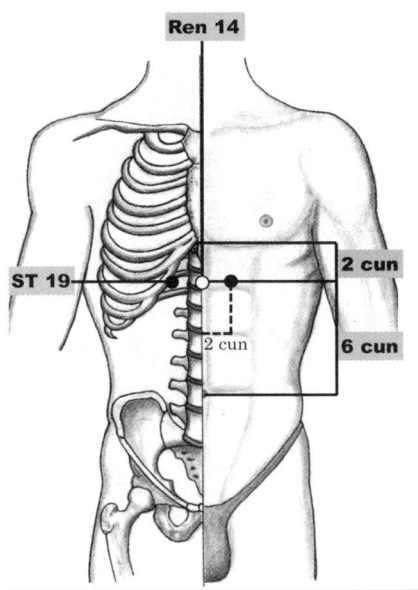

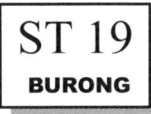

LOCATION:
6 cun above the umbilicus, 2 cun lateral to Ren 14.

INDICATIONS:
Abdominal distention, vomiting, gastric pain, anorexia, stomachache, gastrectasis, intercostal neuralgia.

METHOD:
Perpendicularly 0.5-0.8 cun.

NOTES:

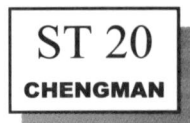

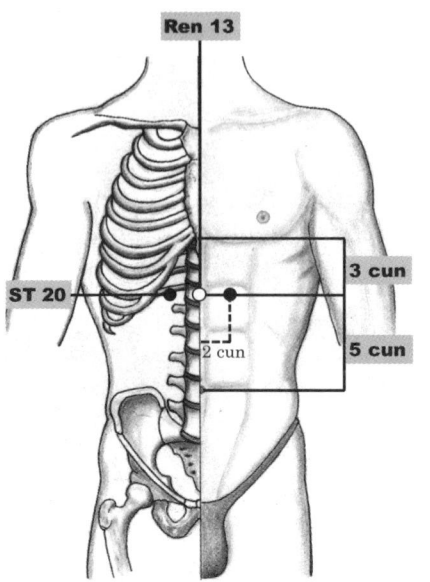

Ren 13

ST 20

3 cun

2 cun

5 cun

LOCATION:
5 cun above the umbilicus, 2 cun lateral to Ren 13.

INDICATIONS:
Gastric pain, abdominal distention, vomiting, anorexia, stomachache, acute & chronic gastritis, intestinal noises, colic, indigestion.

METHOD:
Perpendicularly 0.5-1.0 cun.

NOTES:

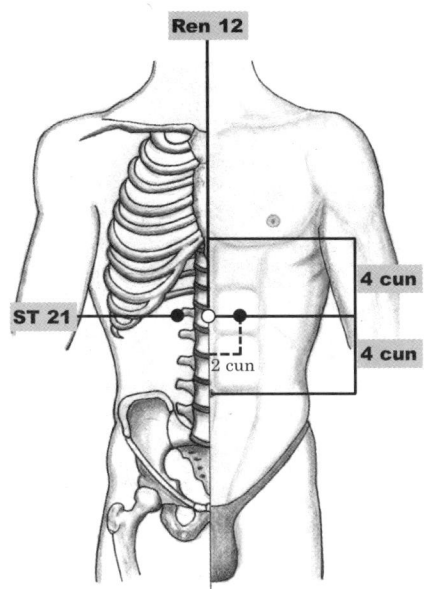

LOCATION:
4 cun above the umbilicus, 2 cun lateral to Ren 12.

INDICATIONS:
Gastric pain, vomiting, anorexia, abdominal distention, diarrhea, stomachache, stomach ulcers, acute & chronic gastritis, nervous dysfunction of the stomach.

METHOD:
Perpendicularly 0.8-1.0 cun.

NOTES:

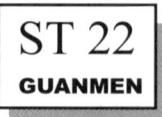

ST 22
GUANMEN

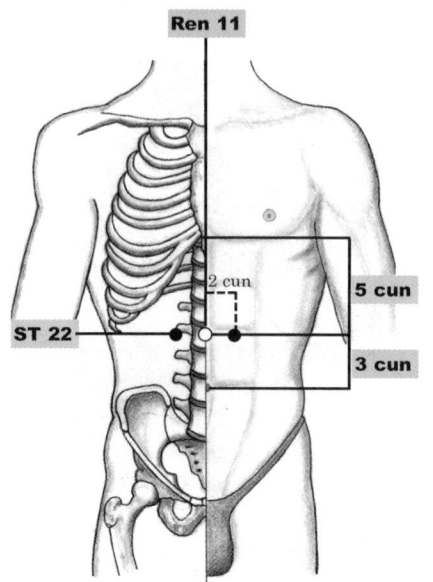

Ren 11

2 cun

5 cun

ST 22

3 cun

LOCATION:
3 cun above the umbilicus, 2 cun lateral to Ren 11.

INDICATIONS:
Abdominal distention and pain, anorexia, borborygmus, diarrhea, edema, intestinal noises.

METHOD:
Perpendicularly 0.8-1.0 cun.

NOTES:

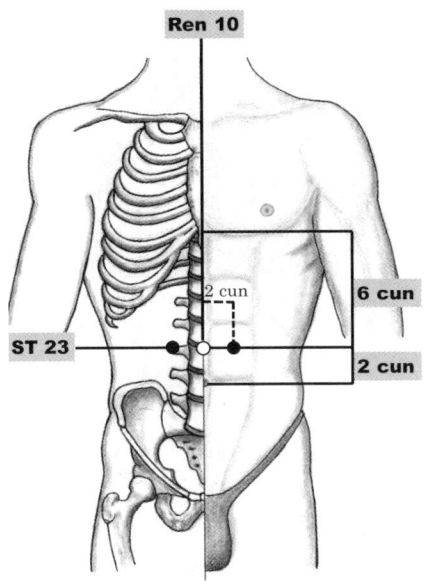

LOCATION:
2 cun above the umbilicus, 2 cun lateral to Ren 10.

INDICATIONS:
Gastric pain, irritability, mania, indigestion, stomachache, intestinal pain, hernia, beriberi, enuresis, insanity.

METHOD:
Perpendicularly 0.7-1.0 cun.

NOTES:

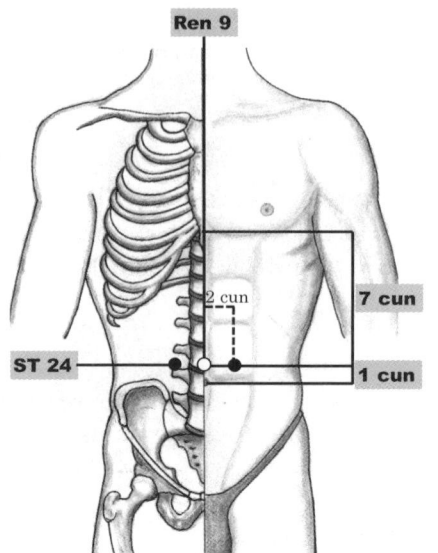

LOCATION:
1 cun above the umbilicus, 2 cun lateral to Ren 9.

INDICATIONS:
Gastric pain, vomiting, mania, acute & chronic gastritis, insanity.

METHOD:
Perpendicularly 0.7-1.0 cun.

NOTES:

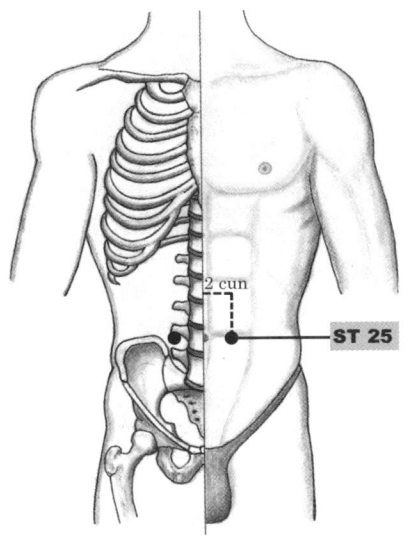

2 cun

ST 25

LOCATION:
2 cun lateral to the center of the umbilicus.

INDICATIONS:
Abdominal pain and distention, borborygmus, pain around the umbilicus, constipation, diarrhea, dysentery, irregular menstruation, edema, acute & chronic gastritis or enteritis, intestinal paralysis, peritonitis, roundworm in intestinal tract, endometritis, low back pain.

METHOD:
Perpendicularly 0.7-1.2 cun.

NOTES:

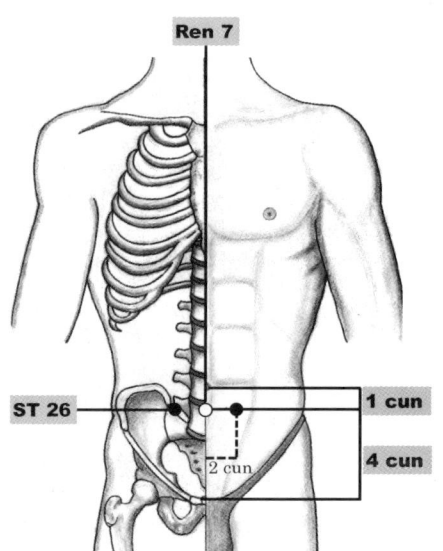

Ren 7

ST 26

1 cun

2 cun

4 cun

LOCATION:
1 cun below the umbilicus, 2 cun lateral to Ren 7.

INDICATIONS:
Abdominal pain, hernia, dysmennorhea.

METHOD:
Perpendicularly 0.7-1.2 cun.

NOTES:

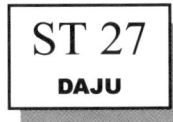

ST 27
DAJU

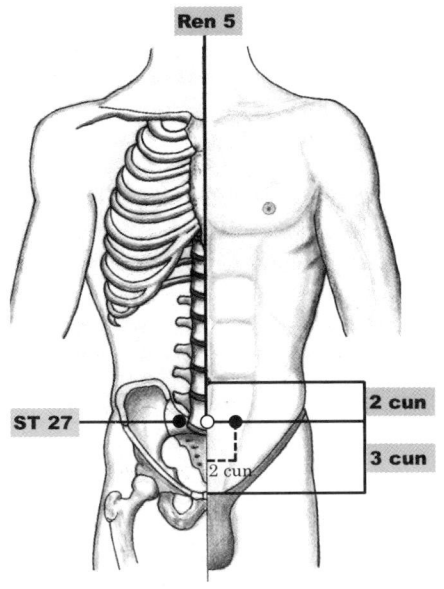

Ren 5

ST 27

2 cun

2 cun

3 cun

LOCATION:
2 cun below the umbilicus, 2 cun lateral to Ren 5.

INDICATIONS:
Lower abdominal distention, dysuria, hernia, premature ejaculation, abdominal pain, intestinal obstruction, retention of urine, cystitis, spermatorhea.

METHOD:
Perpendicularly 0.7-1.2 cun.

NOTES:

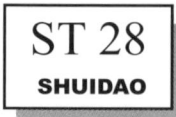

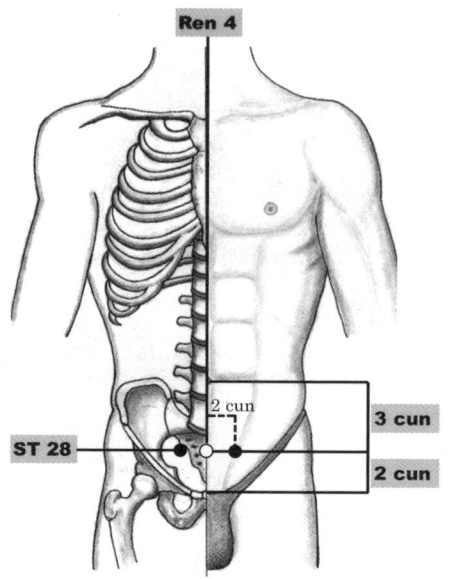

Ren 4

2 cun

3 cun

2 cun

ST 28

LOCATION:
3 cun below the umbilicus, 2 cun lateral to Ren 4.

INDICATIONS:
Lower abdominal distention, retention of urine, edema, hernia, dysmenorrhea, sterility, nephritis, cystitis, ascites, orchitis.

METHOD:
Perpendicularly 0.7-1.2 cun.

NOTES:

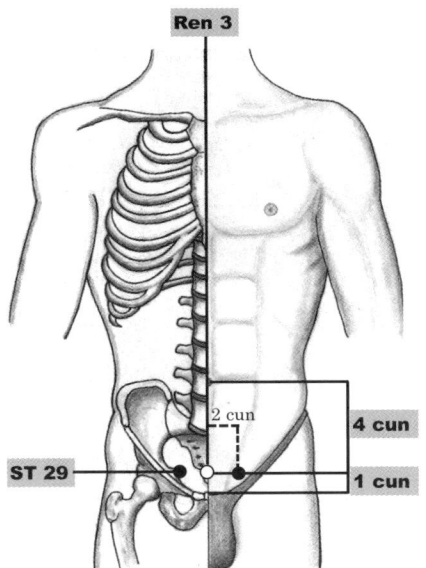

Ren 3

ST 29

2 cun

4 cun

1 cun

LOCATION:
4 cun below the umbilicus, 2 cun lateral to Ren 3.

INDICATIONS:
Abdominal pain, hernia, dysmennorhea, irregular menstruation, amenorrhea, leukorrhea, prolapse of the uterus, inflammation of the adnexa, endometritis, orchitis.

METHOD:
Perpendicularly 0.7-1.2 cun.

NOTES:

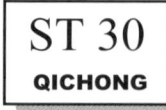

ST 30
QICHONG

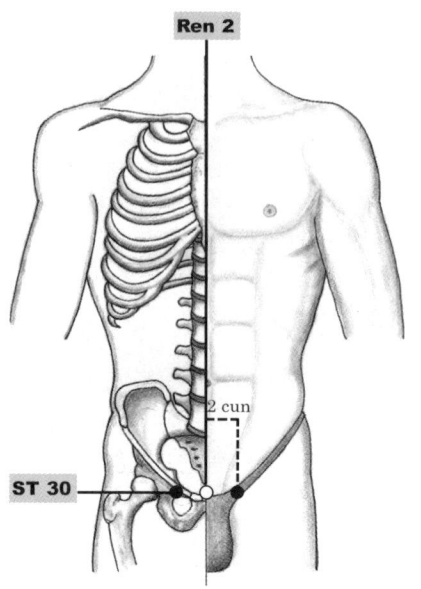

Ren 2

2 cun

ST 30

LOCATION:
5 cun below the umbilicus, 2 cun lateral to Ren 2.

INDICATIONS:
Abdominal pain, borborygmus, hernia, swelling and pain of the external genitalia, impotence, dysmennorhea, irregular menstruation, diseases of the reproductive organs.

METHOD:
Perpendicularly 0.5-1.0 cun.

NOTES:

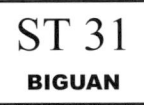
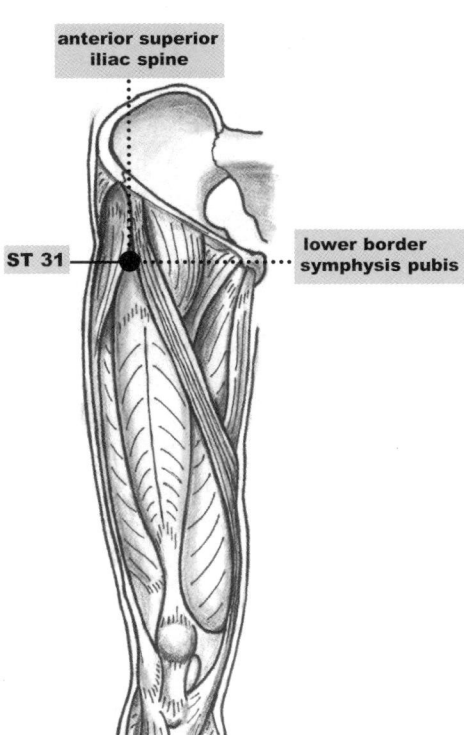

anterior superior
iliac spine

ST 31

lower border
symphysis pubis

LOCATION:

At the crossing point of the line drawn direct-ly down from the anterior superior iliac spine and the line level with the lower border of the symphysis pubis, in the depression on the lat-eral side of m.sartorius when the thigh is flexed.

INDICATIONS:

Abdominal pain, borborygmus, hernia, swelling and pain of the external genitalia, impotence, dysmennorhea, irregular menstru-ation, paralysis of the lower limb, lym-phadenitis of the inguinal lymph glands, arthritis of the knee, low back pain.

METHOD:

Perpendicularly 0.5-1.0 cun.

NOTES:

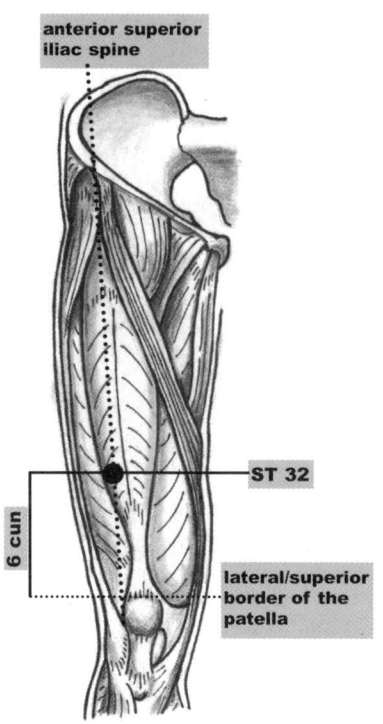

anterior superior
iliac spine

ST 32

6 cun

lateral/superior
border of the
patella

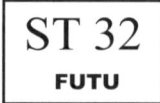

ST 32
FUTU

LOCATION:
On the line connecting the anterior superior iliac spine and the lateral border of the patella, 6 cun above the laterosuperior border of the patella, in m. rectus femoris.

INDICATIONS:
Pain in the lumbar and iliac region, coldness of the knee, paralysis or motor impairment and pain of the lower extremities, beriberi, arthritis of the knee, urticaria.

METHOD:
Perpendicularly 1.0-1.5 cun.

NOTES:

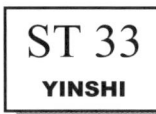

ST 33
YINSHI

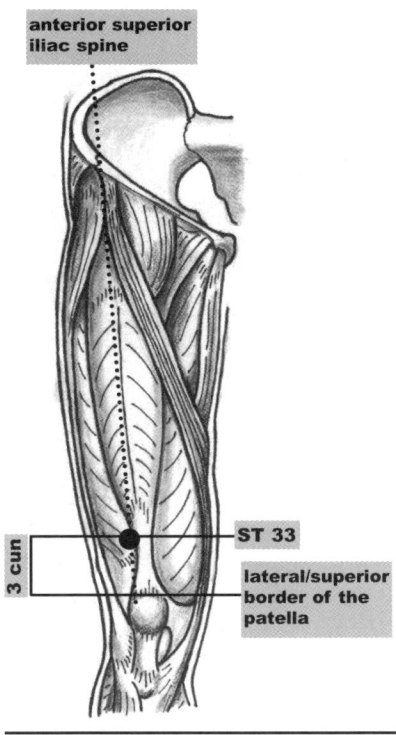

anterior superior
iliac spine

3 cun

ST 33

lateral/superior
border of the
patella

LOCATION:
When the knee is flexed, the point is 3 cun above the laterosuperior border of the patella, on the line joining the laterosuperior border of the patella and the anterior superior iliac spine.

INDICATIONS:
Numbness, soreness, motor impairment of the leg and knee, motor impairment or paralysis of the lower extremities, arthritis of the knee.

METHOD:
Perpendicularly 0.7-1.0 cun.

NOTES:

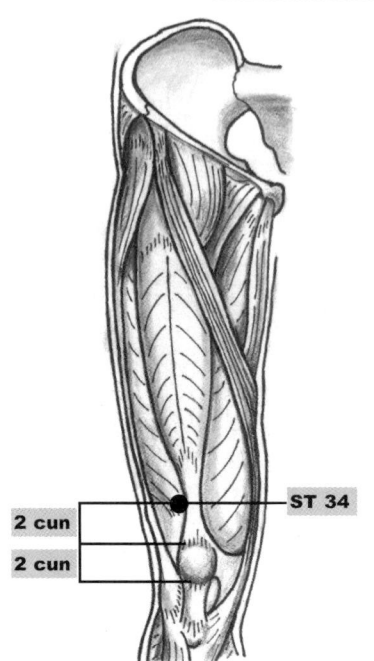

2 cun

2 cun

ST 34

LOCATION:
When the knee is flexed, the point is 2 cun above the laterosuperior border of the patella.

INDICATIONS:
Pain and numbness of the knee, gastric pain, gastritis, mastitis, motor impairment of the lower extremities, diarrhea, diseases of the knee & surrounding soft tissues.

METHOD:
Perpendicularly 0.5-1.0 cun.

NOTES:

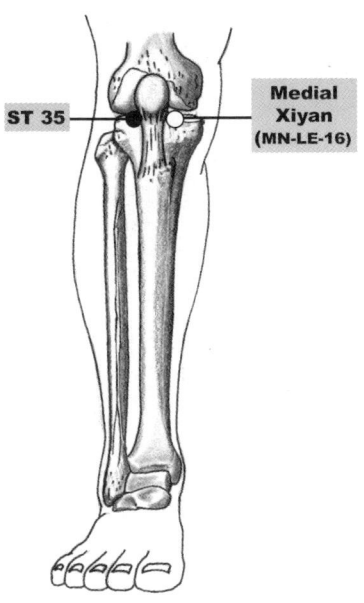

ST 35
ST 35
Medial
Xiyan
(MN-LE-16)

LOCATION:
When the knee is flexed, the point is at the lower border of the patella, in the depresion lateral to the patellar ligament.

INDICATIONS:
Pain, numbness, and motor impairment of the knee, diseases of the knee & surrounding soft tissue, beriberi.

METHOD:
Perpendicularly 0.7-1.0 cun.

NOTES:

HE-SEA & EARTH POINT
LOWER HE-SEA FOR THE STOMACH
COMMAND POINT FOR THE ABDOMEN

ST 36
ZUSANLI

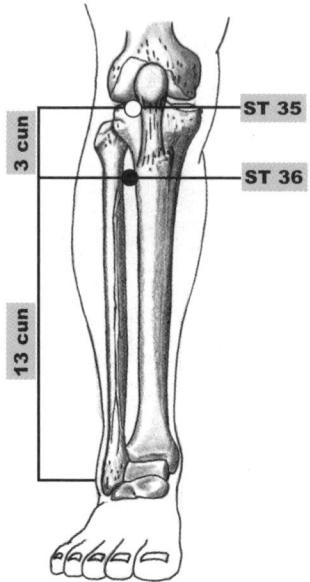

LOCATION:
3 cun below ST 35, one finger-breadth from the anterior crest of the tibia, in m. tibialis anterior.

INDICATIONS:
Gastric pain, acute & chronic gastritis, vomiting, ulcers, hiccup, abdominal distention, borborygmus, diarrhea, dysentery, constipation, mastitis, acute & chronic enteritis, acute pancreatitis, aching of the knee joint and leg, beriberi, edema, cough, asthma, emaciation due to general deficiency, indigestion, apoplexy, hemiplegia, dizziness, insomnia, mania, shock, general weakness, anemia, hypertension, allergies, jaundice, seizures, enuresis, reproductive system diseases, neurasthenia.

METHOD:
Perpendicularly 0.5-1.2 cun.

NOTES:

ST 37
SHANGJUXU

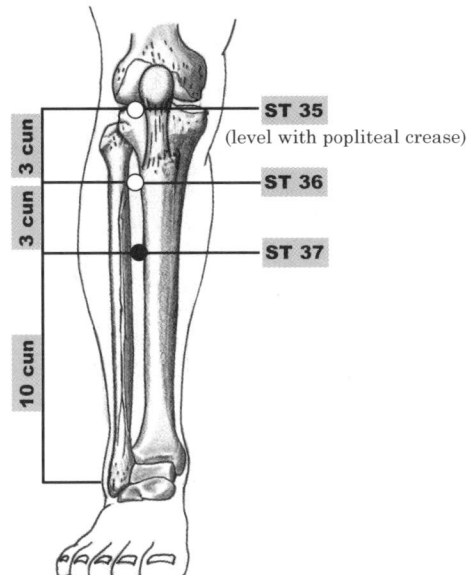

ST 35
(level with popliteal crease)

ST 36

ST 37

3 cun

3 cun

3 cun

10 cun

LOCATION:
3 cun below ST 36, one finger-breadth from the anterior crest of the tibia, in m.tibialis anterior.

INDICATIONS:
Abdominal pain and distention, borborygmus, diarrhea, dysentery, constipation, enteritis, paralysis due to stroke, beriberi, appendicitis, gastritis, hemiplegia.

METHOD:
Perpendicularly 0.5-1.2 cun.

NOTES:

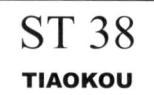

ST 38
TIAOKOU

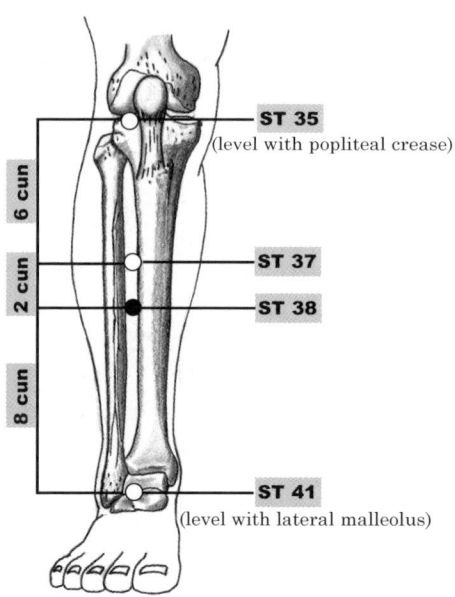

ST 35
(level with popliteal crease)

6 cun

2 cun

ST 37

ST 38

8 cun

ST 41
(level with lateral malleolus)

LOCATION:
2 cun below ST 37, midway between ST 35 and ST 41. Or, 8 cun below the knee.

INDICATIONS:
Numbness, soreness and pain of the knee and leg, arthritis of the knee, paralysis of the lower limb, weakness and motor impairment of the foot, pain and motor impairment of the shoulder, perifocal inflammation of the shoulder, abdominal pain, stomachache, enteritis.

METHOD:
Perpendicularly 0.5-1.0 cun.

NOTES:

82

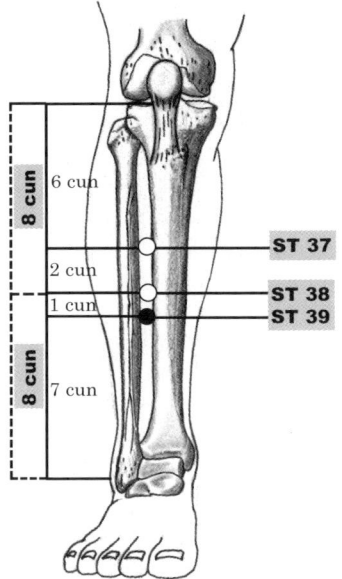

LOCATION:
3 cun below ST 37, one finger-breadth from the anterior crest of the tibia, in m.tibialis anterior.

INDICATIONS:
Lower abdominal pain, acute or chronic enteritis, hepatitis, backache referring to the testis, mastitis, numbness and paralysis of the lower extremities.

METHOD:
Perpendicularly 0.5-1.0 cun.

NOTES:

ST 40
FENGLONG

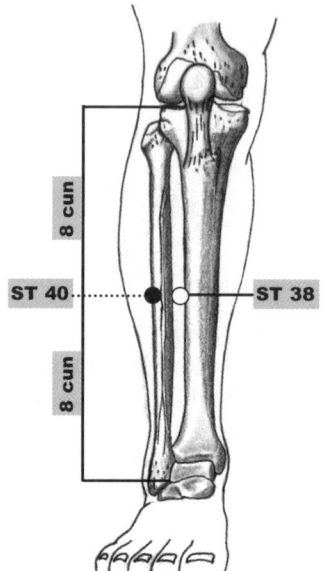

LOCATION:

8 cun superior to the external malleolus, about one finger-breadth lateral to ST 38.

INDICATIONS:

Headache, dizziness and vertigo, cough, asthma, excessive sputum, pain in the chest, constipation, mania, epilepsy, muscular atrophy, motor impairment, pain, swelling or paralysis of the lower extremities, beriberi, amennorhea, abnormal uterine bleeding.

METHOD:

Perpendicularly 0.5-1.0 cun.

NOTES:

ST 41
JIEXI

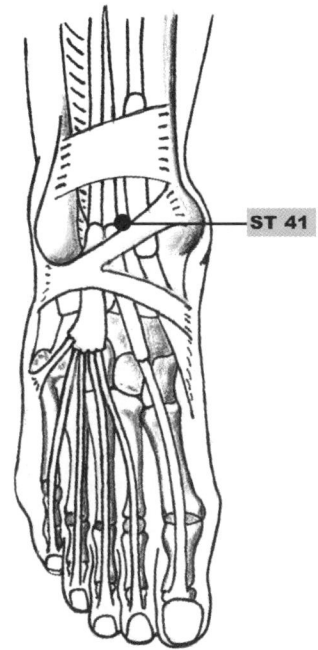

ST 41

LOCATION:

On the dorsum of the foot, at the midpoint of the transverse crease of the ankle joint, in the depression between the tendons of m.extensor digitorum longus and hallucis longus.

INDICATIONS:

Pain & diseases of the ankle & surrounding soft tissues, muscular atrophy, motor impairment, pain and paralysis of the lower extremities, epilepsy, headache, dizziness and vertigo, abdominal distention, constipation, nephritis, enteritis, drop foot.

METHOD:

Perpendicularly 0.5-0.7 cun.

NOTES:

ST 42
CHONGYANG

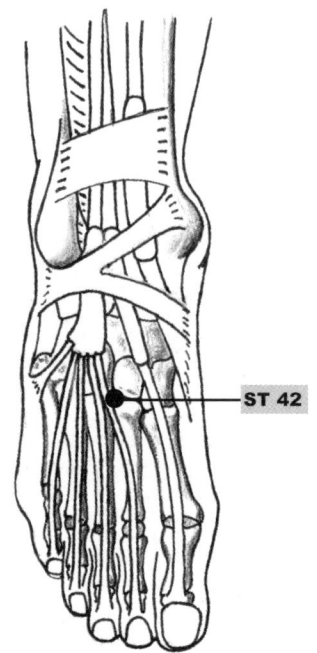

ST 42

LOCATION:
Distal to ST 41, at the highest point of the dorsum of the foot, in the depression between the second and third metatarsal bones and the cuneiform bone.

INDICATIONS:
Pain of the upper teeth, redness, pain, and swelling of the dorsum of the foot, facial paralysis, muscular atrophy and motor impairment of the foot, headache, malaria, insanity, fever, no strength in the arms or legs.

METHOD:
Perpendicularly 0.3-0.5 cun. Avoid puncturing the artery.

NOTES:

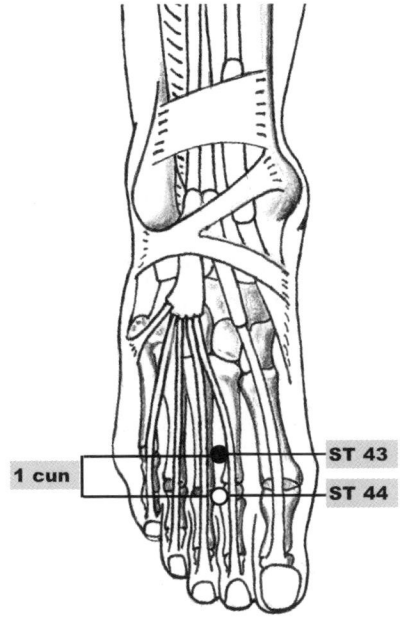

1 cun

ST 43
ST 44

LOCATION:
In the depression distal to the junction of the second and third metatarsal bones.

INDICATIONS:
Facial or general edema, abdominal pain, borborygmus, swelling and pain of the dorsum of the foot, conjunctivitis, hysteria.

METHOD:
Perpendicularly 0.3-0.5 cun.

NOTES:

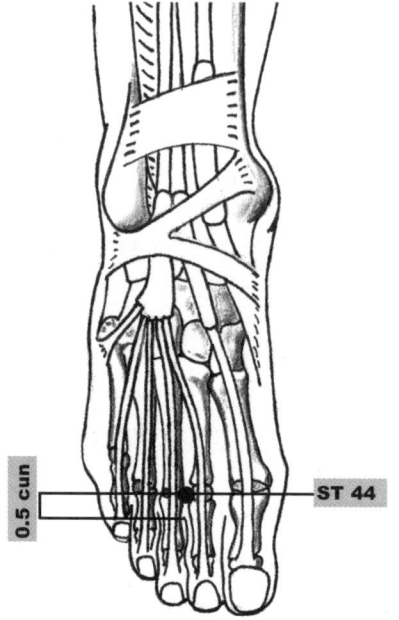

0.5 cun

ST 44

LOCATION:
Proximal to the web margin between the second and third toes, in the depression distal and lateral to the second metatarsodigital joint.

INDICATIONS:
Toothache, pain in the face, trigeminal neuralgia, tonsillitis, deviation of the mouth, sore throat, epistaxis, gastric pain, stomach ache, acute & chronic enteritis, acid regurgitation, abdominal distention, pain of intestinal hernia, beriberi, diarrhea, dysentery, constipation, swelling and pain of the dorsum of the foot, febrile disease.

METHOD:
Perpendicularly 0.3-0.5 cun.

NOTES:

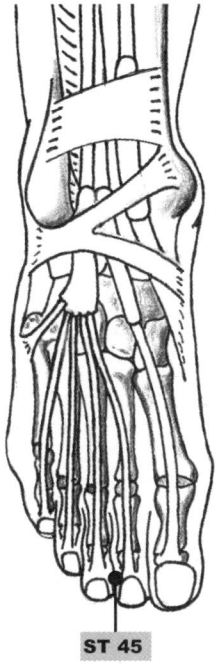

ST 45

LOCATION:
On the lateral side of the 2nd toe, 0.1 cun posterior to the corner of the nail.

INDICATIONS:
Facial swelling, deviation of the mouth, epistaxis, toothache, sore throat and hoarse voice, tonsillitis, abdominal distention, indigestion, coldness in the leg and foot, febrile diseases, hepatitis, dream-disturbed sleep, mania, hysteria, ischemia of the brain, neurasthenia.

METHOD:
Puncture subcutaneously 0.1 cun.

NOTES:

NOTES

NOTES

91

SPLEEN CHANNEL

SPLEEN MERIDIAN OF FOOT TAI-YIN

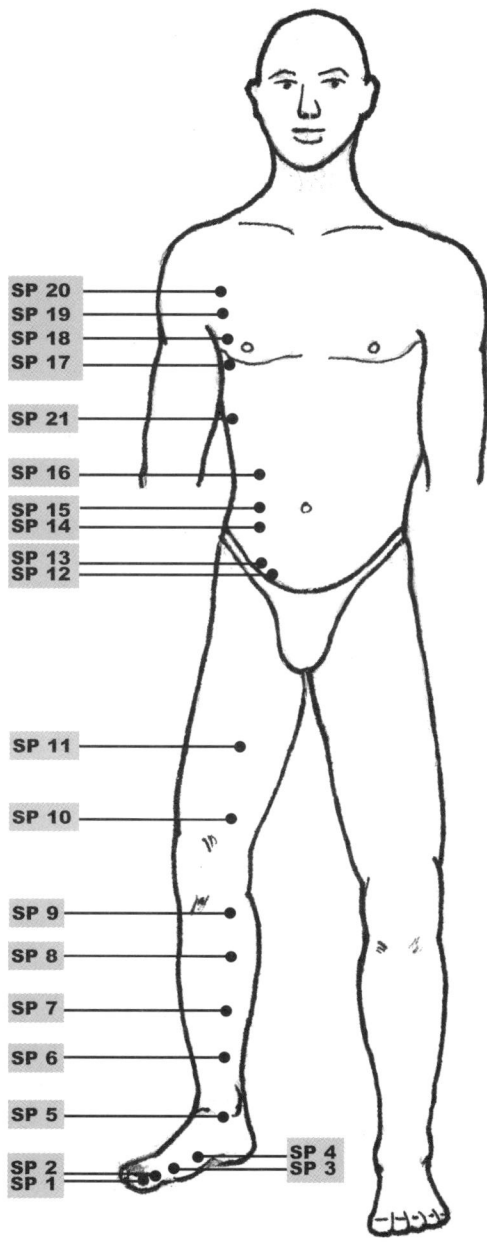

SP 20
SP 19
SP 18
SP 17

SP 21

SP 16

SP 15
SP 14

SP 13
SP 12

SP 11

SP 10

SP 9

SP 8

SP 7

SP 6

SP 5

SP 2
SP 1

SP 4
SP 3

THERAPEUTIC INDICATIONS

- Spleen & stomach diseases, gynecological, urinary, & genital problems, and other diseases of areas this meridian supplies.

CHANNEL/ORGAN RELATIONSHIPS

- This channel is associated with the Spleen & connects with the Stomach.

- It also directly joins with the Heart, Lungs, and Intestines.

PATHOLOGY

Channel: Heaviness in the body or head, general feverishness, fatigued limbs and emaciated muscles, belching, vomiting, epigastric pain, abdominal distention, loose stools, jaundice, lassitude, stiffness and pain at the root of the tongue, swelling and coldness along the medial aspect of the leg & knee, edema in foot or leg.

Organ: Abdominal pain, fullness or distention, diarrhea, constipation, incomplete digestion of food, borborgymus, vomiting, hard masses in the abdomen, reduced appetite, jaundice.

SPLEEN MERIDIAN OF FOOT TAI-YIN

GENERAL PATHWAY	●Begins on the medial side of the big toe & follows the border between the dark & light skin of the medial aspect of the foot. ●It then passes in front of the medial malleolus and up the leg, along the posterior side of the tibia, crossing, and then travelling anterior to, the Liver channel. ●Crossing over the medial aspect of the knee, it continues upward along the anterior medial aspect of the thigh and into the abdomen. ●At this point, after crossing the Ren channel at points Ren 3 and Ren 4, the channel enters the Spleen organ and communicates with the Stomach. ●It then ascends across the diaphragm & intersects the GB channel at GB 24 and the Liver channel at LIV 14. ●Continuing upward beside the esophagus, it crosses the Lung channel at LU 1 and finally reaches the root of the tongue, dispersing over its lower surface.
CONNECTING CHANNEL	●After separating from the main channel at SP 4 on the instep of the foot, this channel connects with the Stomach channel. **BRANCHES:** ●A branch ascends to the abdomen and connects with the Stomach and Intestines.
DIVERGENT CHANNEL	●After separating from the main channel on the thigh, this channel converges with the Divergent channel of the Stomach and proceeds upward to the throat, after which it enters the tongue.
MUSCULAR REGION	●This channel originates on the medial side of the big toe & ascends across the foot, connecting with the medial malleolus. ●It then proceeds upward and connects with the medial side of the knee, then traverses the medial aspect of the thigh to connect with the hip before joining with the reproductive organs. ●After crossing the abdomen and connecting with the umbilicus, the channel enters the abdominal cavity, connects with the ribs and then disperses through the chest. ●An internal branch adheres to the spine.
MAJOR CONNECTING CHANNEL OF THE SPLEEN	●Beginning from SP 21, it emerges at 3 cun below GB 22 and spreads through the chest & hypochondriac region, gathering blood all over the body.

SP 1
YINBAI

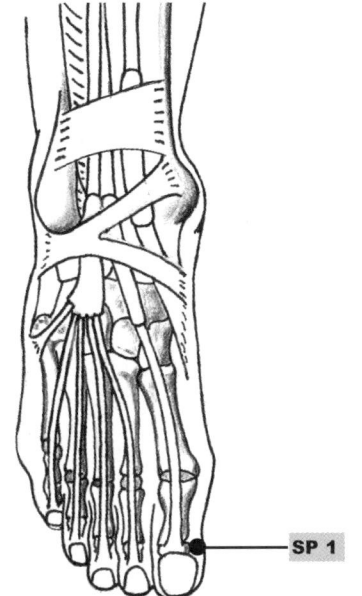

SP 1

LOCATION:
On the medial side of the great toe, 0.1 cun posterior to the corner of the nail.

INDICATIONS:
Abdominal pain or distention, bloody stools, bleeding of the digestive tract, menorrhagia, uterine bleeding, mental disorders, dream-disturbed sleep, convulsion.

METHOD:
Puncture subcutaneously 0.1 cun.

NOTES:

95

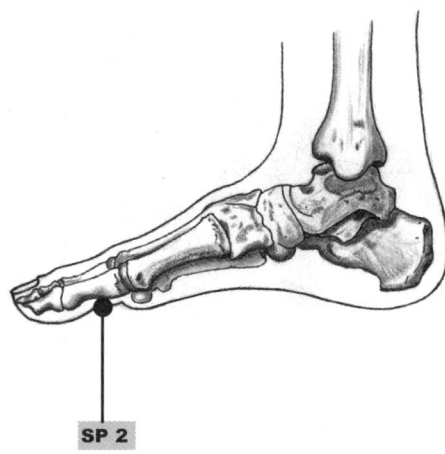

SP 2

LOCATION:
On the medial side of the great toe, distal and inferior to the first metatarsodigital joint, at the junction of the red and white skin.

INDICATIONS:
Abdominal distention or diarrhea, gastric pain, edema of the limbs, constipation, febrile diseases with anhidrosis, fever, apoplectic coma.

METHOD:
Perpendicularly 0.1-0.3 cun.

NOTES:

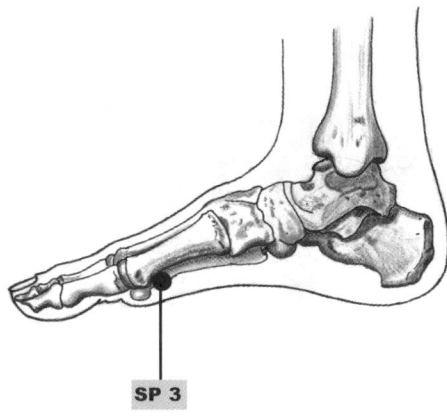

SP 3

LOCATION:
Proximal and inferior to the head of the first metatarsal bone, at the junction of the red and white skin.

INDICATIONS:
Gastric pain, abdominal distention, constipation, dysentery, vomiting, diarrhea, borborygmus, stomach ache, edema, acute gastroenteritis, sluggishness, beriberi, headache.

METHOD:
Perpendicularly 0.3-0.5 cun.

NOTES:

LUO-CONNECTING POINT
CONFLUENT POINT FOR THE CHONG

SP 4
GONGSUN

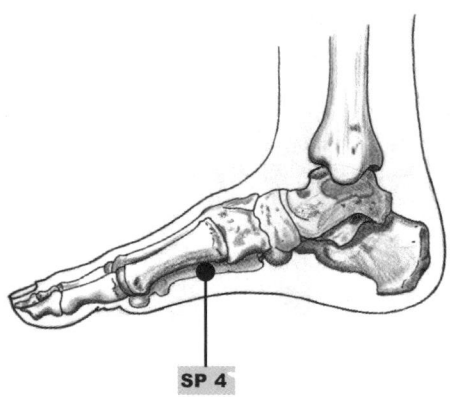

SP 4

LOCATION:
In the depression distal and inferior to the base of the first metatarsal bone, at the junction of the red and white skin.

INDICATIONS:
Gastric pain, vomiting, abdominal pain and distention, acute & chronic enteritis, vomiting, diarrhea, dysentery, borborygmus, endometritis, irregular menstruation, foot & ankle pain.

METHOD:
Perpendicularly 0.5-0.8 cun.

NOTES:

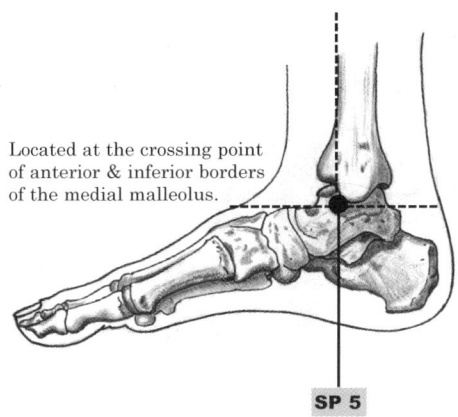

Located at the crossing point of anterior & inferior borders of the medial malleolus.

SP 5

LOCATION:
In the depression distal and inferior to the medial malleolus, midway between the tuberosity of the navicular bone and the tip of the medial malleolus.

INDICATIONS:
Abdominal distention, constipation, diarrhea, borborygmus, indigestion, beri beri, gastritis, enteritis, edema, pain and rigidity of the tongue, pain in the foot and ankle, diseases of the ankle & surrounding soft tissues, hemorrhoids.

METHOD:
Perpendicularly 0.2-0.3 cun.

NOTES:

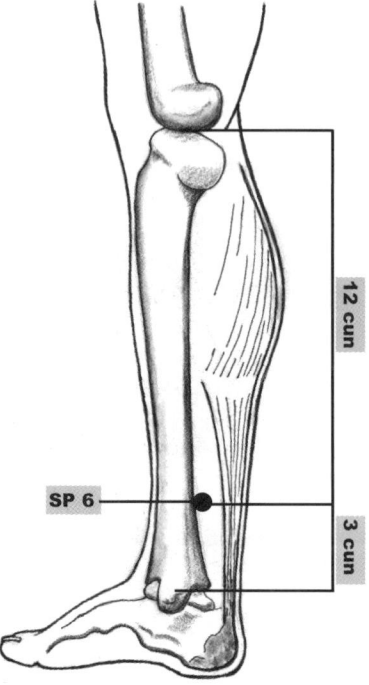

12 cun

SP 6

3 cun

LOCATION:
3 cun directly above the tip of the medial malleolus, on the posterior border of the medial aspect of the tibia.

INDICATIONS:
Abdominal pain, borborygmus, abdominal distention or pain, diarrhea, dysmenorrhea, irregular menstruation, uterine bleeding, morbid leukorrhea, prolapse of the uterus, diseases of the reproductive system, sterility, delayed labor, nocturnal emission, impotence, enuresis, dysuria, incontinence, edema, hernia, pain in the external genitalia, muscular atrophy, hemiplegia, motor impairment, paralysis and pain of the lower extremities, headache, dizziness and vertigo, insomnia, neurasthenia, neurodermatitis, eczema, urticaria.

METHOD:
Perpendicularly 0.5-1.0 cun. Contraindicated during pregnancy.

NOTES:

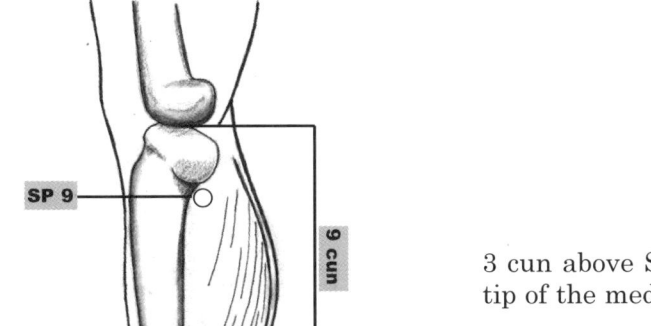

LOCATION:
3 cun above SP 6 on the line joining the tip of the medial malleolus and SP 9.

INDICATIONS:
Abdominal distention, borborygmus, coldness, numbness and paralysis of the knee and leg, urinary tract infection.

METHOD:
Perpendicularly 0.5-1.0 cun.

NOTES:

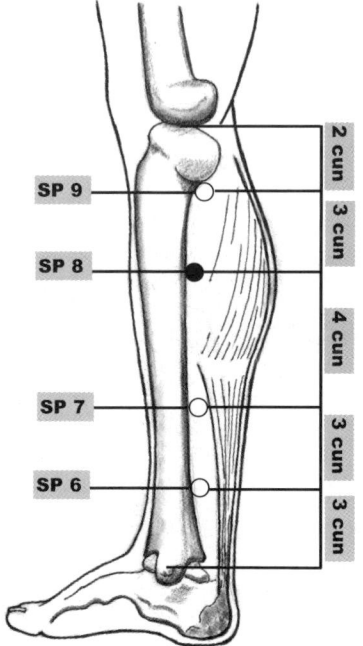

SP 9
SP 8
SP 7
SP 6

2 cun
3 cun
4 cun
3 cun
3 cun

LOCATION:
3 cun below SP 9, on the line connecting SP 9 and the medial malleolus.

INDICATIONS:
Abdominal pain and distention, diarrhea, edema, dysuria, nocturnal emission, irregular menstruation, dysmenorrhea, abnormal uterine bleeding.

METHOD:
Perpendicularly 0.5-1.0 cun.

NOTES:

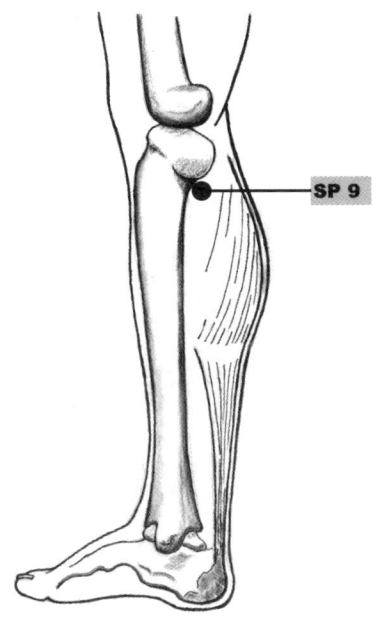

SP 9

LOCATION:

On the lower border of the medial condyle of the tibia, in the depression on the medial border of the tibia.

INDICATIONS:

Abdominal pain and distention, diarrhea, enteritis, dysentery, edema, ascites, jaundice, dysuria, enuresis, incontinence of urine, retention of urine, urinary tract infection, pain in the external genitalia, dysmenorrhea, irregular menstruation, nocturnal emission, impotence, nephritis, beri beri, pain in the knee.

METHOD:

Perpendicularly 0.5-1.0 cun.

NOTES:

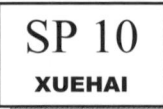

SP 10
XUEHAI

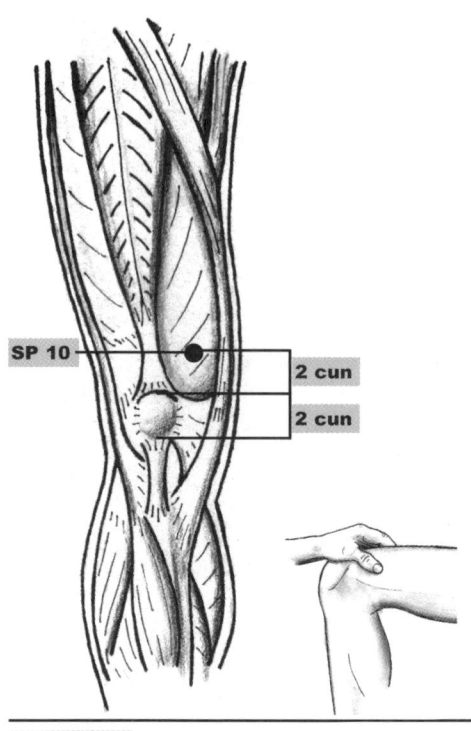

SP 10

2 cun

2 cun

LOCATION:
When the knee is flexed, the point is 2 cun above the mediosuperior border of the patella, on the bulge of the medial portion of m.quadriceps femoris.

INDICATIONS:
Irregular menstruation, dysmenorrhea, uterine bleeding, amenorrhea, urticaria, eczema, erysipelas, pain in the medial aspect of the thigh, pruritis, neurodermatitis, anemia.

METHOD:
Perpendicularly 0.5-1.2 cun.

NOTES:

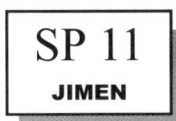

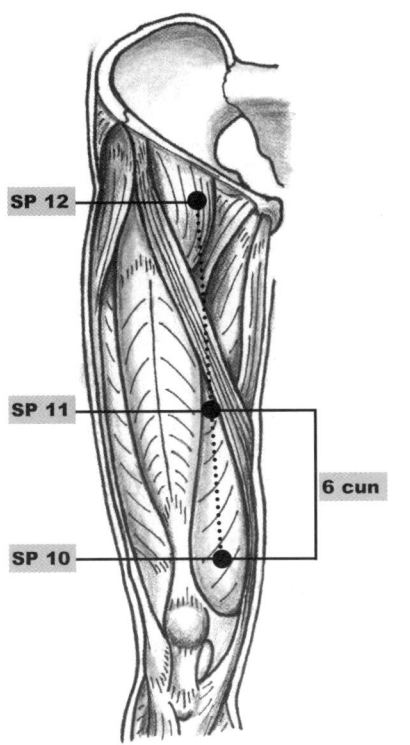

SP 12

SP 11

SP 10

6 cun

LOCATION:
6 cun above SP 10, on the line drawn from SP 10 to SP 12.

INDICATIONS:
Dysuria, enuresis, urethritis, pain and swelling in the inguinal region, inguinal lymphadenitis, muscular atrophy, motor impairment, pain and paralysis of the lower extremities.

METHOD:
Perpendicularly 0.5-1.0 cun

NOTES:

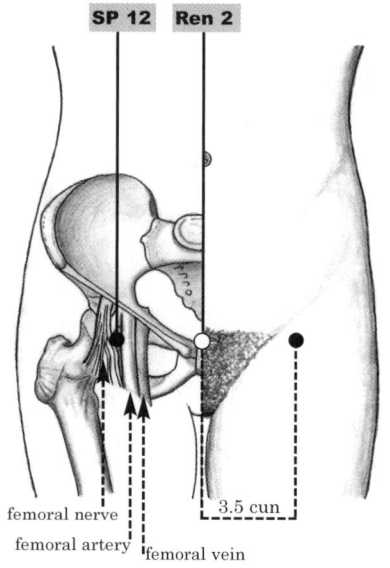

SP 12
Ren 2

femoral nerve
femoral artery
femoral vein
3.5 cun

SP 12
CHONGMEN

LOCATION:
Superior to the lateral end of the inguinal groove, on the lateral side of the femoral artery, at the level of the upper border of symphysis pubis, 3.5 cun lateral to Ren 2.

INDICATIONS:
Abdominal pain, hernia, dysuria, urinary retention, endometritis, orchitis.

METHOD:
Avoid puncturing the artery. Puncture perpendicularly 0.5-1.0 cun.

NOTES:

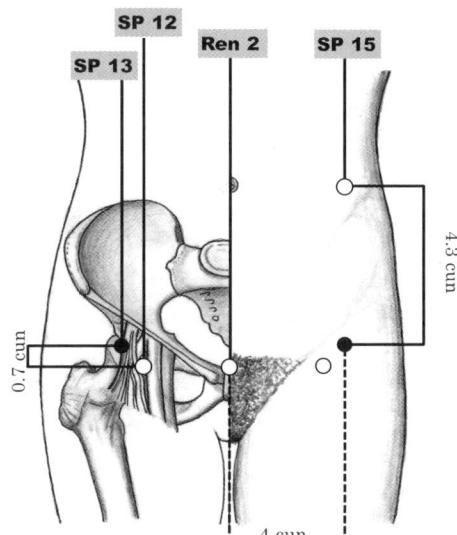

SP 12
Ren 2
SP 15
SP 13

0.7 cun
4.3 cun
4 cun

LOCATION:
0.7 laterosuperior to SP 12, 4 cun lateral to the Ren meridian.

INDICATIONS:
Lower abdominal pain, hernia, inguinal lymphadenitis, adnexitis, appendicitis.

METHOD:
Perpendicularly 0.5-1.0 cun.

NOTES:

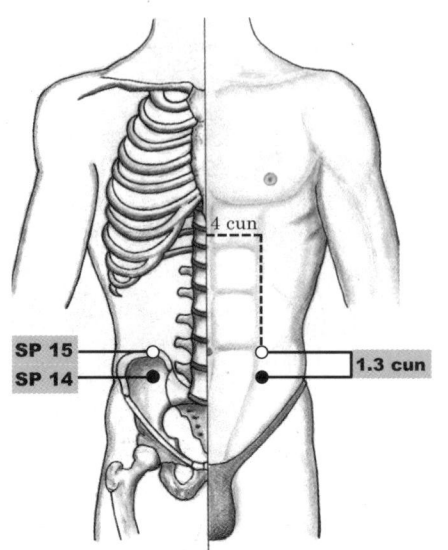

LOCATION:
1.3 cun below Sp 15, 4 cun lateral to the Ren meridian, on the lateral side of m.rectus abdominis.

INDICATIONS:
Pain around the umbilical region, abdominal distention, hernia, diarrhea, constipation.

METHOD:
Perpendicularly 0.5-1.0 cun.

NOTES:

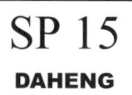

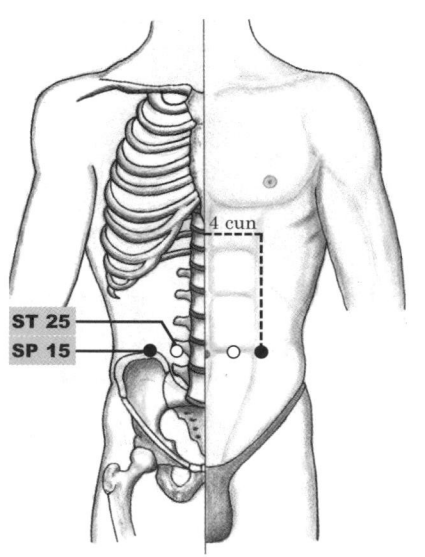

4 cun

ST 25

SP 15

LOCATION:
4 cun lateral to the center of the umbilicus, lateral to m.rectus abdominis.

INDICATIONS:
Abdominal pain and distention, diarrhea, dysentery, constipation, intestinal paralysis, parasitic worms in the intestines.

METHOD:
Perpendicularly 0.7-1.2 cun.

NOTES:

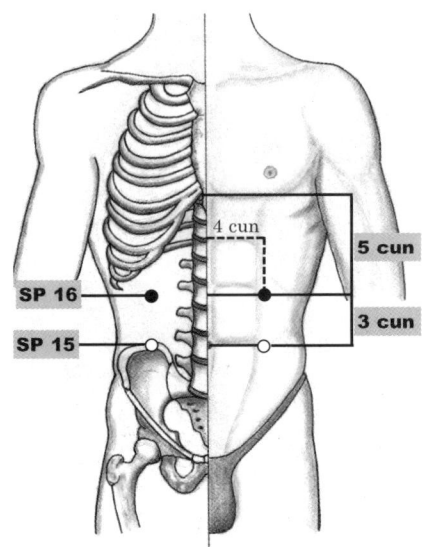

SP 16
FUAI

SP 16

SP 15

4 cun

5 cun

3 cun

LOCATION:
3 cun above SP 15, 4 cun lateral to Ren 11.

INDICATIONS:
Abdominal pain, pain in the region of the umbilicus, indigestion, constipation, dysentery.

METHOD:
Perpendicularly 0.5-1.0 cun.

NOTES:

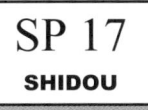

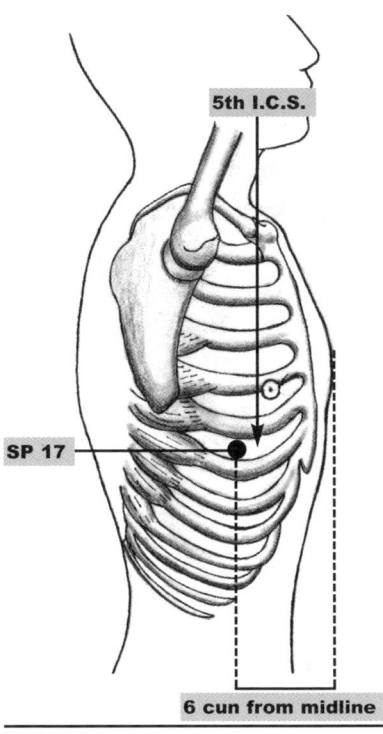

5th I.C.S.

SP 17

6 cun from midline

LOCATION:

In the fifth intercostal space, 6 cun lateral to the Ren meridian.

INDICATIONS:

Fullness and pain in the chest and hypochondriac region, intercostal neuralgia, ascites, retention of urine, gastritis.

METHOD:

Obliquely 0.3-0.5 cun.

NOTES:

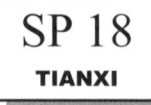

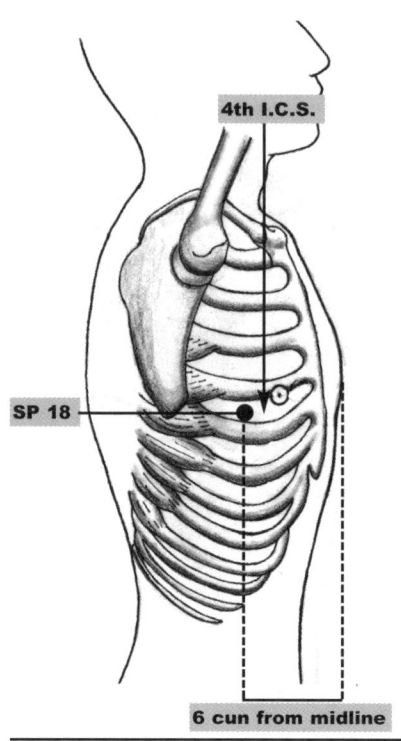

4th I.C.S.

SP 18

6 cun from midline

LOCATION:
In the fourth intercostal space, 6 cun lateral to the Ren meridian.

INDICATIONS:
Fullness and pain in the chest and hypochondrium, cough, bronchitis, asthma, hiccup, mastitis, insufficient lactation.

METHOD:
Obliquely 0.3-0.5 cun.

NOTES:

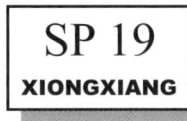
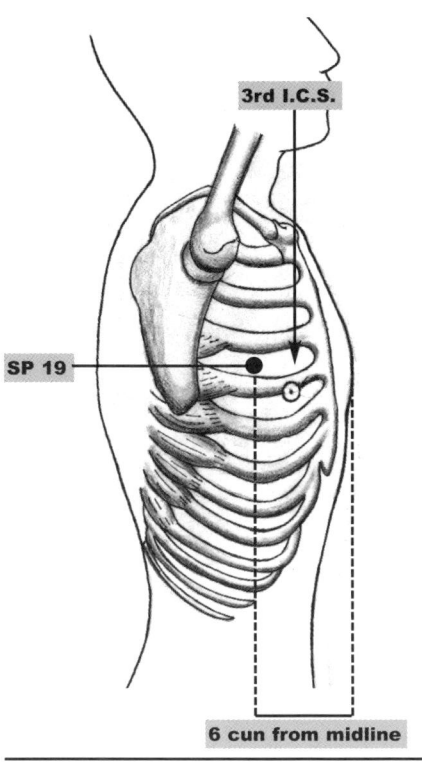

3rd I.C.S.

SP 19

6 cun from midline

LOCATION:
In the third intercostal space, 6 cun lateral to the Ren meridian.

INDICATIONS:
Fullness and pain in the chest and hypochondriac region, intercostal neuralgia.

METHOD:
Obliquely 0.3-0.5 cun.

NOTES:

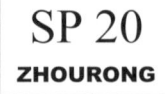

SP 20
ZHOURONG

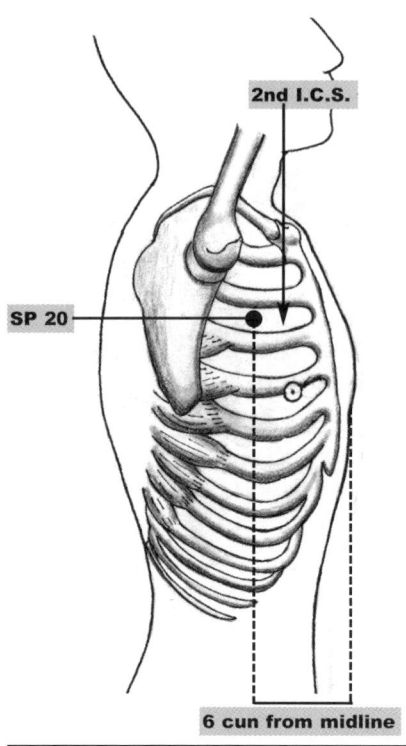

2nd I.C.S.

SP 20

6 cun from midline

LOCATION:
In the second intercostal space, 6 cun lateral to the Ren meridian.

INDICATIONS:
Fullness in the chest and hypochondriac region, intercostal neuralgia, pleurisy, pulmonary empyema, bronchiectasis, cough, hiccup.

METHOD:
Obliquely 0.3-0.5 cun.

NOTES:

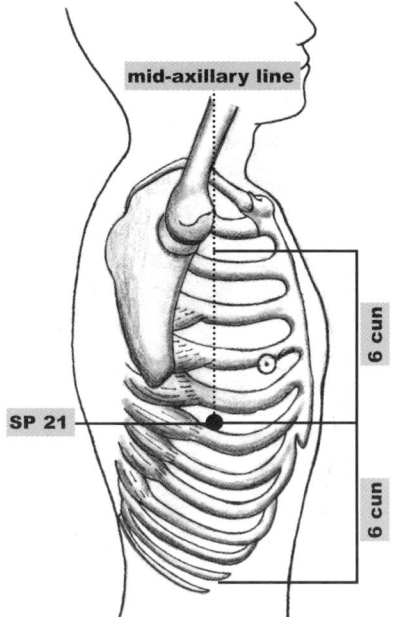

mid-axillary line

6 cun

6 cun

SP 21

LOCATION:
On the mid-axillary line, 6 cun below the axilla, midway between the axilla and the free end of the eleventh rib.

INDICATIONS:
Pain in the chest and hypochondriac region, intercostal neuralgia, asthma, general aching and weakness of the body.

METHOD:
Obliquely 0.3-0.5 cun.

NOTES:

NOTES

NOTES

HEART CHANNEL

HEART MERIDIAN OF HAND SHAO-YIN

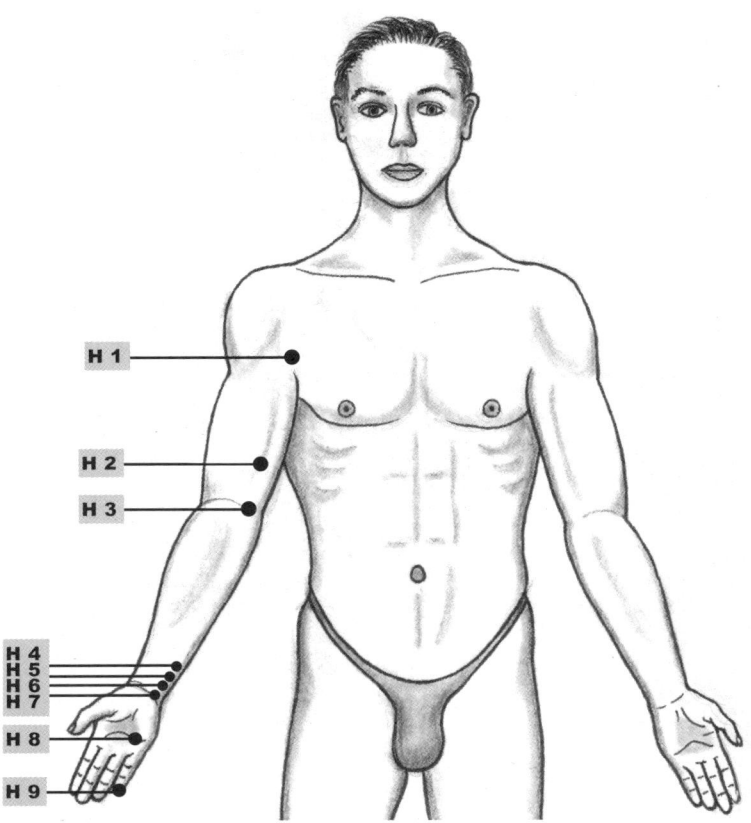

H 1
H 2
H 3
H 4
H 5
H 6
H 7
H 8
H 9

THERAPEUTIC INDICATIONS

- Diseases of the heart & chest, mental disorders, and other diseases of areas this meridian supplies.

CHANNEL/ORGAN RELATIONSHIPS

- This channel is associated with the Heart & connects with the Small Intestine.

- It also directly joins to the Lung & Kidneys.

PATHOLOGY

Channel: Cardiac pain, palpitations, hypochondriac pain, insomnia, night sweats, general feverishness, headache, pain in the eyes, dry throat, thirst, hot or painful palms, coldness in the palms and soles of the feet, pain along the scapula and medial aspect of the upper arm.

Organ: Mental disorders, shortness of breath, vertigo, irritability, pain or fullness in chest, ribs, or below ribs, discomfort when reclining.

119

HEART MERIDIAN OF HAND SHAO-YIN

GENERAL PATHWAY	•Beginning in the Heart organ, it emerges through the blood vessel system surrounding the Heart, and travels downward across the diaphragm where it connects with the Small Intestine. •From below the axilla (where Branch #2 ends) the channel descends along the medial border of the anterior aspect of the upper arm, behind the Lung and Pericardium channels, to the antecubital fossa, where it continues downward to the pisiform region proximal to the palm. •It then enters the palm and follows the medial side of the little finger to the finger tip. **BRANCHES:** •**BRANCH 1:** A branch of the main channel separates in the Heart and ascends alongside the esophagus to the face where it joins the tissues surrounding the eye. •**BRANCH 2:** Another branch goes directly from the Heart to the Lung, then goes downward to emerge below the axilla.
CONNECTING CHANNEL	•After separating from the main channel at H5 on the wrist, this channel joins the Small Intestine channel. •At about 1.5 cun above the transverse crease of the wrist, the channel again separates from the Small Intestine channel and follows the Heart channel to the Heart organ. •It then goes to the base of the tongue and connects with the eye.
DIVERGENT CHANNEL	•After diverging from the main channel in the axillary fossa, it then enters the chest and connects with the Heart. •It then ascends across the throat & emerges on the face, joining the Small Intestine channel at the inner canthus.
MUSCULAR REGION	•This channel originates on the medial aspect of the little finger, connects first with the pisiform bone of the hand, and again at the medial aspect of the elbow. •Then, the channel proceeds upward & enters the chest cavity below the axilla. •It crosses the Lung muscle channel in the breast region, and connects in the chest. •Descending across the diaphragm, the channel connects at the umbilicus.

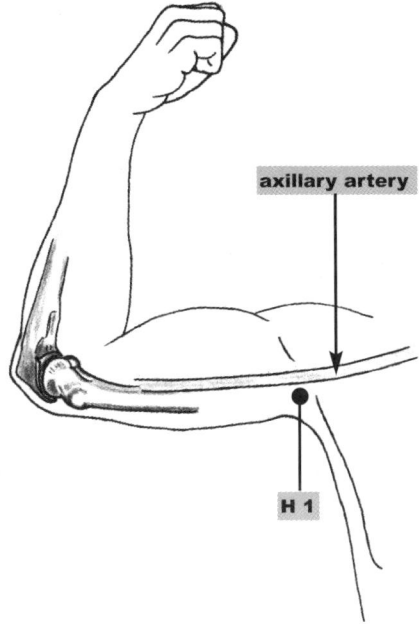

LOCATION:
When the upper arm is abducted, the point is in the center of the axilla, on the medial side of the axillary artery.

INDICATIONS:
Pain in the costal and cardiac regions, angina pectoris, intercostal neuralgia, scrofula, cold pain of the elbow and arm, perifocal inflammation of the shoulder joint, dryness of the throat.

METHOD:
Avoid puncturing the axillary artery. Puncture perpendicularly 0.5-1.0 cun.

NOTES:

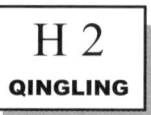

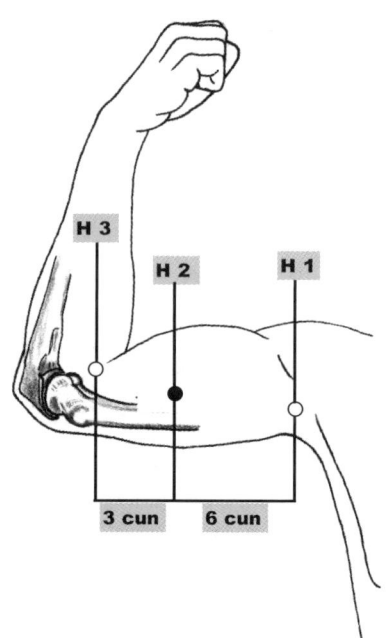

H 3

H 2

H 1

3 cun   6 cun

LOCATION:
When the elbow is flexed, the point is 3 cun above the medial end of the transverse cubital crease (H 3), in the groove medial to m. biceps brachii.

INDICATIONS:
Pain in the cardiac and hypochondriac regions, shoulder, and arm, costalgia, icteric sclera.

METHOD:
Perpendicularly 0.3-0.5 cun.

NOTES:

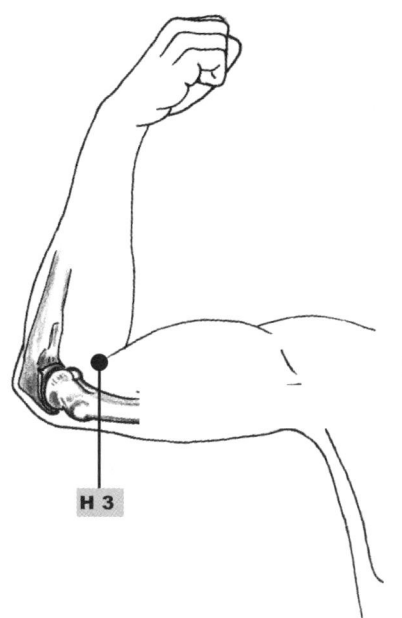

H 3

LOCATION:
When the elbow is flexed into a right angle, the point is in the depression between the medial end of the transverse cubital crease and the medial epicondyle of the humerus.

INDICATIONS:
Cardiac pain, spasmodic pain and numbness of the hand and arm, ulnar nerve neuralgia, diseases of the elbow, tremor of the hand, scrofula, lymphadenitis, pain in the axilla and hypochondriac region, intercostal neuralgia, neurasthenia, psychosis.

METHOD:
Perpendicularly 0.5-1.0 cun.

NOTES:

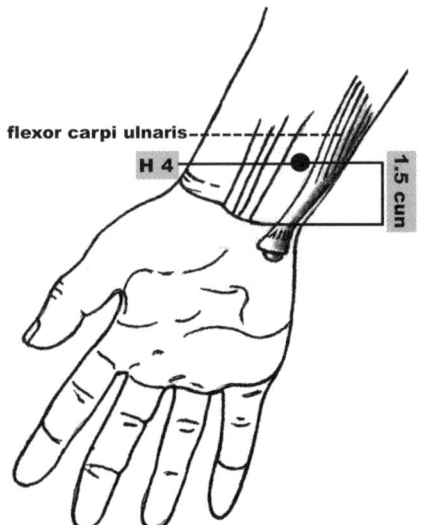

flexor carpi ulnaris

H 4

1.5 cun

LOCATION:

When the palm faces upward, the point is on the radial side of the tendon of m. flexor carpi ulnaris, 1.5 cun above the transverse crease of the wrist.

INDICATIONS:

Cardiac pain, chest pain, spasmodic pain of the elbow and arm, neuralgia of ulnar nerve, sudden loss of voice, psychosis, hysteria.

METHOD:

Perpendicularly 0.3-0.5 cun.

NOTES:

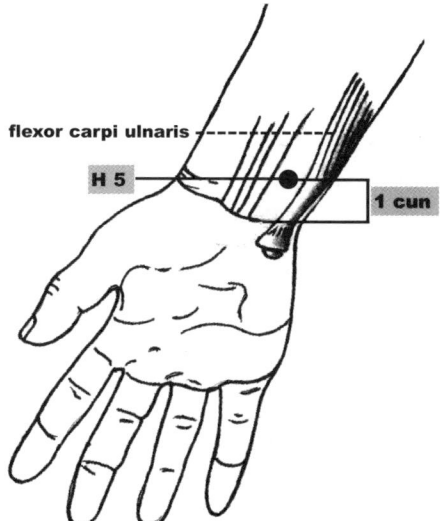

flexor carpi ulnaris

H 5

1 cun

LOCATION:
When the palm faces upward, the point is on the radial side of the tendon of m. flexor carpi ulnaris, 1 cun above the transverse crease of the wrist.

INDICATIONS:
Palpitation, chest pain, bradycardia, cough, asthma, neurasthenia, dizziness, blurring of vision, sore throat, sudden loss of voice, aphasia with stiffness of the tongue, psychosis, pain in the wrist and elbow.

METHOD:
Perpendicularly 0.3-0.5 cun.

NOTES:

XI-CLEFT POINT

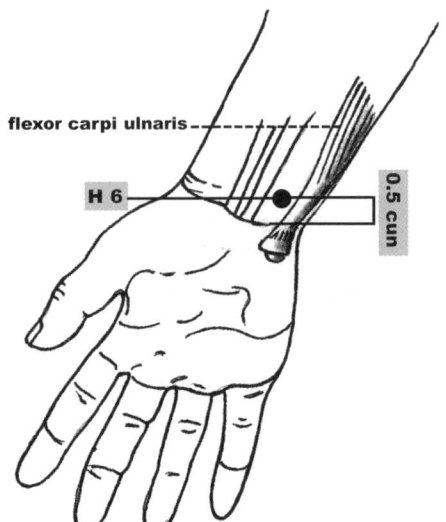

flexor carpi ulnaris

H 6

0.5 cun

LOCATION:
When the palm faces upward, the point is on the radial side of the tendon of m.flexor carpi ulnaris, 0.5 cun above the transverse crease of the wrist.

INDICATIONS:
Cardiac pain, palpitation, hysteria, night sweating, hemoptysis, epistaxis, pulmonary tuberculosis, sudden loss of voice, neurasthenia.

METHOD:
Perpendicularly 0.3-0.5 cun.

NOTES:

126

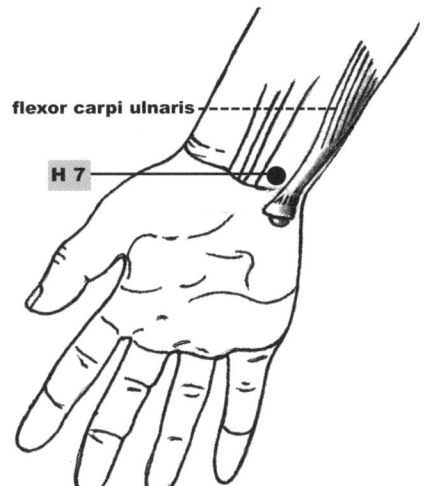

flexor carpi ulnaris

H 7

LOCATION:
At the ulnar end of the transverse crease of the wrist, in the depression on the radial side of the tendon of m.flexor carpi ulnaris.

INDICATIONS:
Cardiac pain, heart disease, angina pectoris, irritability, palpitation, hysteria, mental illness, amnesia, insomnia, mania, neurasthenia, epilepsy, dementia, absentmindedness, excessive dreaming, pain in the hypochondriac region, feverish sensation in the palm, yellowish sclera, paralysis of the hypoglossus muscle.

METHOD:
Perpendicularly 0.3-0.5 cun.

NOTES:

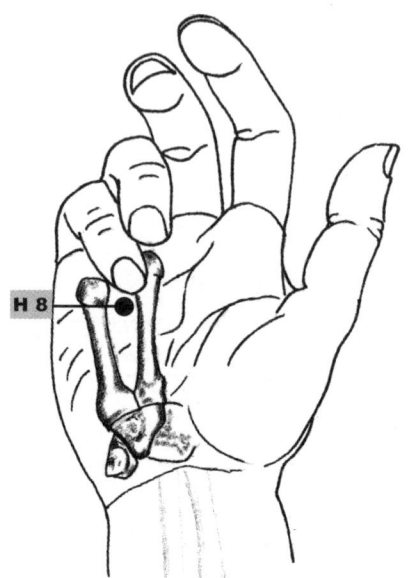

H 8

LOCATION:
When the palm faces upward, the point is between the fourth and fifth metacarpal bones. When a fist is made, the point is where the tip of the little finger rests.

INDICATIONS:
Palpitation, pain in the chest, cardiac arrhythmia, angina pectoris, rheumatic heart disease, spasmodic pain of the little finger, feverish sensation in the palm, enuresis, dysuria, pruritus of the external genitalia, hysteria.

METHOD:
Perpendicularly 0.3-0.5 cun.

NOTES:

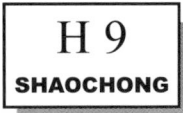

H 9
SHAOCHONG

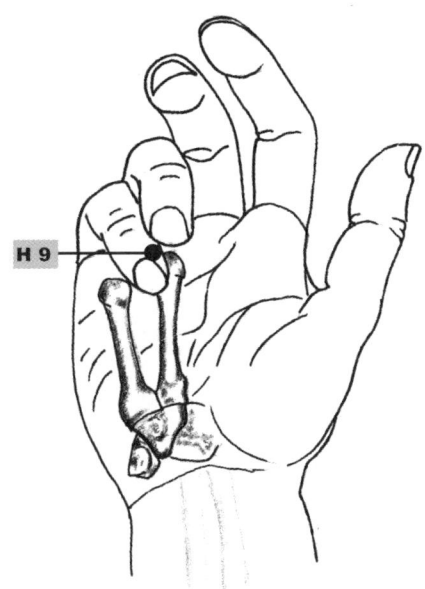

H 9

LOCATION:
On the radial side of the little finger, 0.1 cun posterior to the corner of the nail.

INDICATIONS:
Palpitation, cardiac pain, pain in the chest and hypochondriac regions, mania, hysteria, febrile diseases, loss of consciousness, apoplectic coma, infantile convulsions.

METHOD:
Puncture subcutaneously 0.1 cun, or prick with a three-edged needle to cause bleeding.

NOTES:

NOTES

SMALL INTESTINE CHANNEL

SMALL INTESTINE MERIDIAN OF HAND TAI-YANG

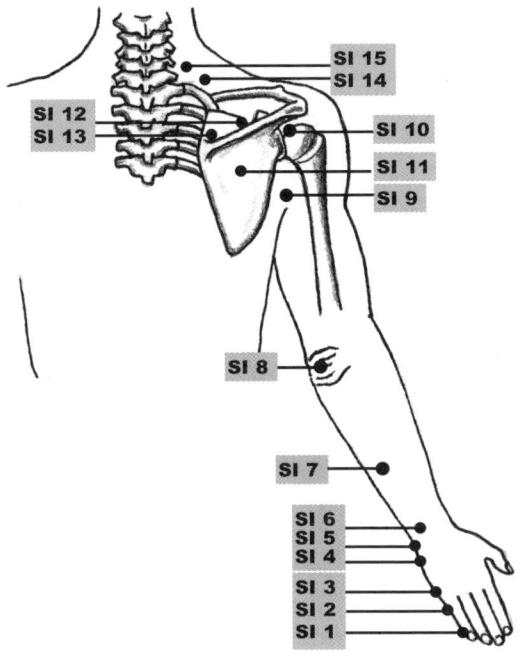
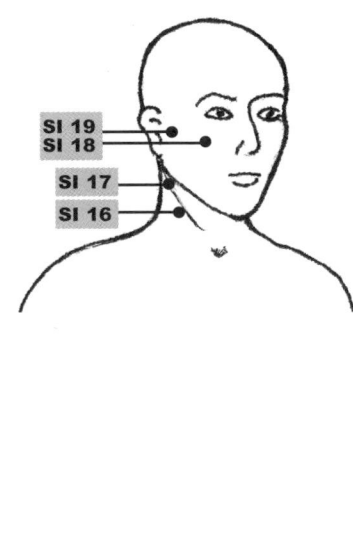

CHANNEL/ORGAN RELATIONSHIPS

• This channel is associated with the Small Intestine & connects with the Heart.

• It is also joined directly with the Stomach.

THERAPEUTIC INDICATIONS

• Diseases of the head, neck, ear, eye, throat; febrile diseases, mental disorders and other diseases of areas this meridian supplies.

PATHOLOGY

Channel: Deafness, yellow sclera, numbness of the mouth and tongue, pain or swelling in the neck or cheek, sore throat, stiff neck, distention and pain in the lower abdomen, and pain along the posterior border of the lateral aspect of the shoulder and arm.

Organ: Pain and distention in the lower abdomen, possibly extending to the waist or the genitals, diarrhea, or dry stool and constipation.

SMALL INTESTINE MERIDIAN OF HAND TAI-YANG

GENERAL PATHWAY	• Originating at the ulnar side of the tip of the little finger, it ascends along the ulnar side of the hand to the wrist, emerging at the styloid process of the ulna. • It then travels directly upward along the posterior aspect of the ulna, passing between the olecranon of the ulna and the medial epicondyle of the humerus at the medial side of the elbow. • It proceeds along the posterior border of the lateral aspect of the upper arm, emerging behind the shoulder joint and circling around the superior & inferior fossa of the scapula. • It meets UB 41, UB 11, & DU 14 in the upper back, then turning downward to the supraclavicular fossa, it connects with the Heart. • From there it descends along the esophagus, passes through the diaphragm & reaches the Stomach. Before reaching its associated organ, the Small Intestine, it intersects the Ren channel internally at Ren 13 & Ren 12. **BRANCHES:** • **BRANCH 1:** A branch travels up from the supraclavicular fossa & crosses the neck and cheek to the outer canthus of the eye, where it meets GB 1. Then it turns back across the temple and enters the ear at SI 19. • **BRANCH 2:** Another branch separates from the former branch at the cheek, ascends to the infraorbital region of the eye & then to the inner canthus, where it meets the Bladder channel at UB 1. It then crosses horizontally to the zygomatic region.
CONNECTING CHANNEL	• After separating from the main channel at SI 7 on the forearm, this channel connects with the Heart channel. • Another branch continues up the arm, crosses the elbow and joins with the shoulder.
DIVERGENT CHANNEL	• After separating from the main channel at the shoulder, this channel enters the axilla, crosses the Heart, and descends to the abdomen where it connects with the Small Intestine.
MUSCULAR REGION	• Beginning on the dorsum of the little finger, it connects at the wrist, and ascends along the forearm to the elbow where it connects with the medial epicondyle of the humerus. • From here, the channel proceeds up the arm and connects below the axilla. **BRANCHES:** • **BRANCH 1:** A branch travels behind the axilla, surrounds the scapula, and follows in front of the Bladder muscle channel on the neck, connecting behind the ear. • **BRANCH 2:** A branch separates behind the auricle and enters the ear itself. After emerging above the auricle, this branch descends across the face and connects beneath the mandible, then ascends to connect at the outer canthus and temple. • **BRANCH 3:** A branch separates at the mandible, ascends around the teeth and in front of the ear, connecting at the outer canthus and the angle of the hairline.

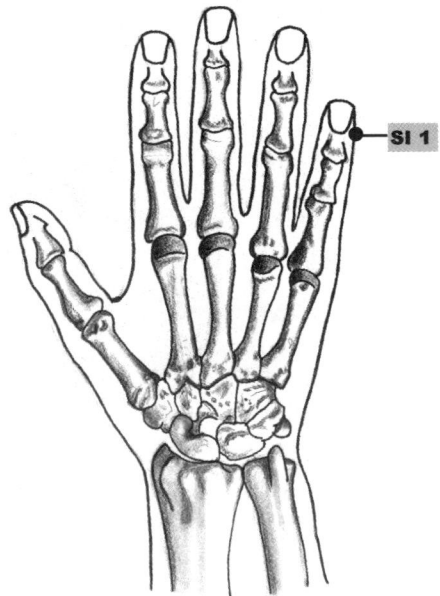

SI 1

LOCATION:
On the ulnar side of the little finger, about 0.1 cun posterior to the corner of the nail.

INDICATIONS:
Headache, febrile diseases, loss of consciousness, insufficient lactation, mastitis, sore throat, redness of the eye, cloudiness of the cornea, pterygium.

METHOD:
Puncture subcutaneously 0.1 cun, or prick with a three-edged needle to cause bleeding.

NOTES:

SI 2
QIANGU

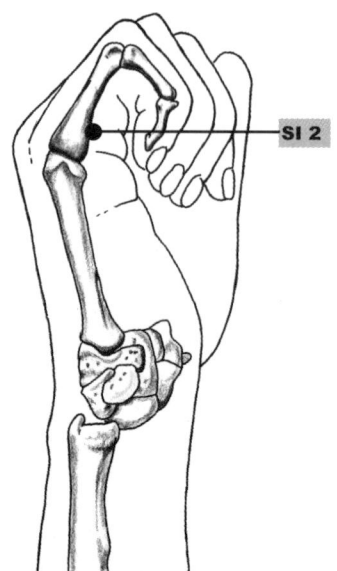

SI 2

LOCATION:
When a loose fist is made, the point is on the ulnar side, distal to the fifth metacarpophalangeal joint, at the junction of the red and white skin.

INDICATIONS:
Numbness of the fingers, febrile diseases, tinnitus, headache, reddish urine, pannus, congested throat, mastitis.

METHOD:
Perpendicularly 0.3-0.5 cun.

NOTES:

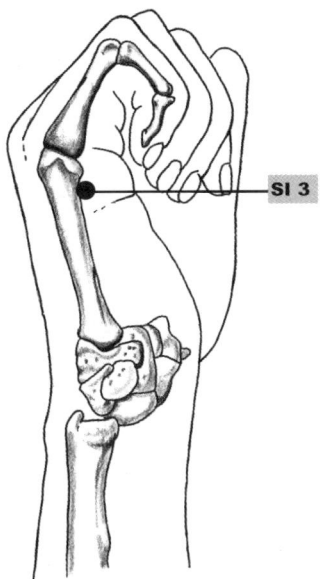

SI 3

LOCATION:

When a loose fist is made, the point is on the ulnar side, proximal to the fifth metacarpophalangeal joint, at the end of the transverse crease and the junction of the red and white skin.

INDICATIONS:

Pain and rigidity of the neck, tinnitus, deafness, sore throat, mania, malaria, seizures, psychosis, hysteria, intercostal neuralgia, acute lumbar sprain, night sweating, febrile diseases, contracture and numbness of the fingers, pain in the shoulder & elbow.

METHOD:

Perpendicularly 0.5-0.7 cun.

NOTES:

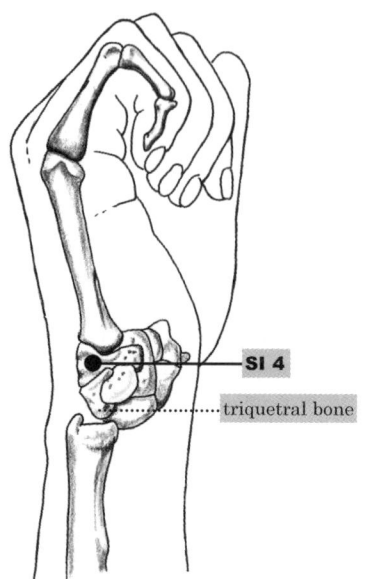

SI 4

triquetral bone

LOCATION:
On the ulnar side of the palm, in the depression between the base of the fifth metacarpal bone and the triquetral bone.

INDICATIONS:
Febrile diseases with anhidrosis, headache, rigidity of the neck, contracture of the fingers, pain and arthritis in the wrist, elbow, and fingers, jaundice, tinnitus, diabetes, gastritis, cholecystitis.

METHOD:
Perpendicularly 0.3-0.5 cun.

NOTES:

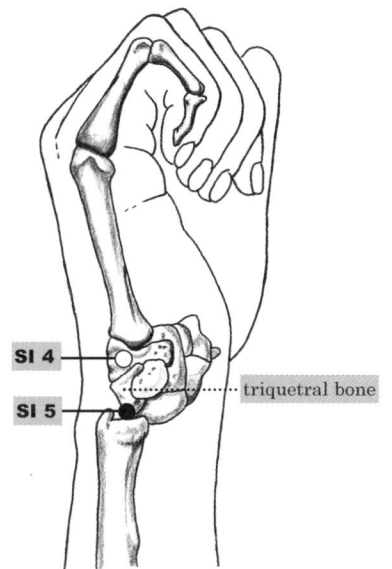

SI 4

SI 5

triquetral bone

LOCATION:
At the ulnar end of the transverse crease on the dorsal aspect of the wrist, in the depression between the styloid process of the ulna and the triquetral bone.

INDICATIONS:
Swelling of the neck and submandibular region, parotitis, pain of the hand and wrist, febrile diseases, insanity, deafness, tinnitus.

METHOD:
Perpendicularly 0.3-0.5 cun.

NOTES:

SI 6
YANGLAO

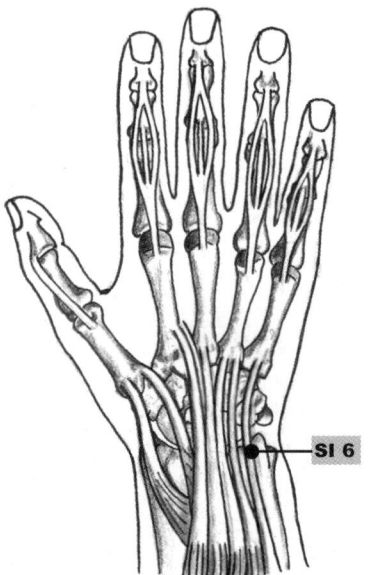

SI 6

LOCATION:
Dorsal to the head of the ulna. When the palm faces the chest, the point is in the bony cleft on the radial side of the styloid process of the ulna.

INDICATIONS:
Blurry vision, pain in the shoulder, elbow, arm and back, arthritis of the upper limb, hemplegia, stiff neck, eye diseases, hernia pain.

METHOD:
Perpendicularly 0.3-0.5 cun.

NOTES:

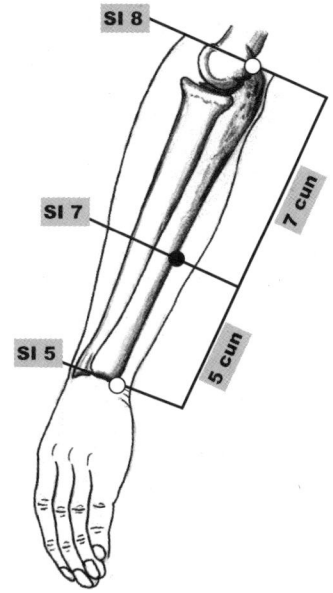

LOCATION:
On the line joining SI 5 and SI 8, 5 cun above SI 5.

INDICATIONS:
Neck rigidity, headache, dizziness, spasmodic pain in the elbow, arm and fingers, febrile diseases, mania, neurasthenia, insanity.

METHOD:
Perpendicularly 0.5-0.8 cun.

NOTES:

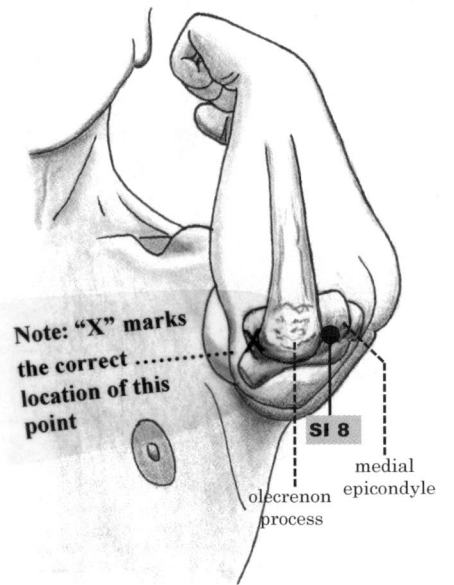

Note: "X" marks the correct location of this point

SI 8

olecrenon process

medial epicondyle

LOCATION:
When the elbow is flexed, the point is located in the depression between the olecrenon of the ulna and the medial epicondyle of the humerus.

INDICATIONS:
Headache, swelling of the cheek, pain in the nape, shoulder, arm and elbow, neuralgia or paralysis of the ulnar nerve, epilepsy, psychosis, chorea.

METHOD:
Perpendicularly 0.3-0.5 cun.

NOTES:

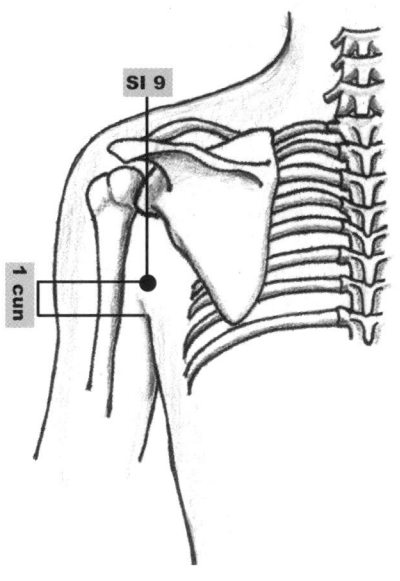

SI 9

1 cun

LOCATION:

Posterior and inferior to the shoulder joint. When the arm is adducted, the point is 1 cun above the posterior end of the axillary fold.

INDICATIONS:

Pain in the scapular region, motor impairment of the hand and arm, diseases of the shoulder and shoulder joint, paralysis of the upper limb, excessive perspiration in the armpits.

METHOD:

Perpendicularly 0.5-1.0 cun.

NOTES:

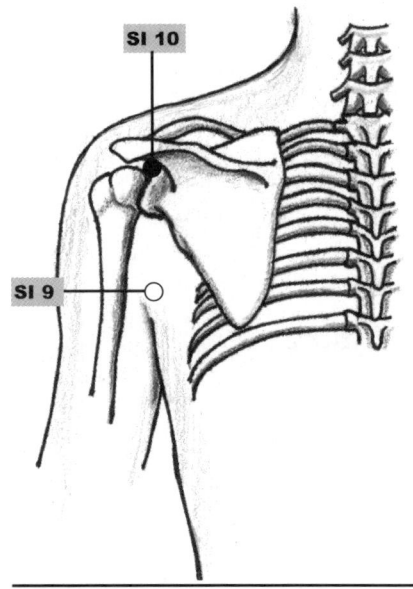

LOCATION:

When the arm is adducted, the point is directly above SI 9, in the depression inferior to the scapular spine.

INDICATIONS:

Swelling of the shoulder, aching and weakness of the shoulder and arm, pain & perifocal inflammation in the shoulder joint, hemiplegia, hypertension, excessive sweating.

METHOD:

Perpendicularly 0.5-1.0 cun.

NOTES:

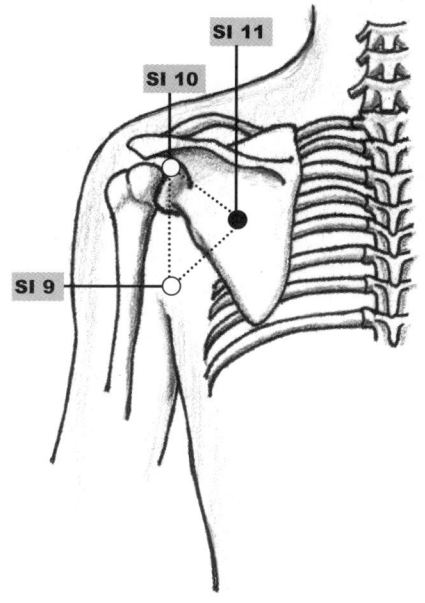

LOCATION:
In the infrascapular fossa, at the junction of the upper and middle third of the distance between the lower border of the scapular spine and the inferior angle of the scapula. (Or draw an equilateral triangle with SI 9 & SI 10, after the patient's shoulder is relaxed.)

INDICATIONS:
Pain in the scapular region and shoulder, pain in the laterosuperior aspect of the elbow and arm, asthma.

METHOD:
Perpendicularly 0.5-1.0 cun.

NOTES:

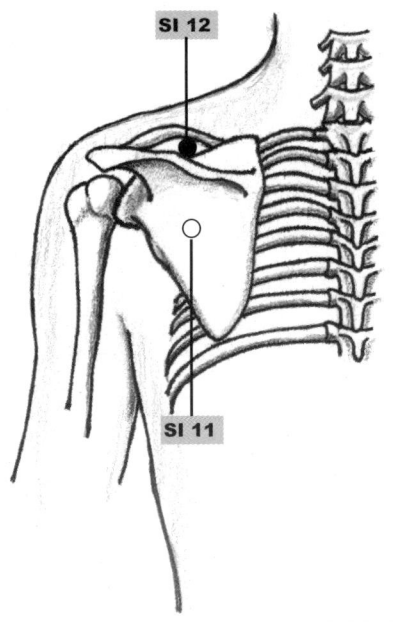

SI 12

LOCATION:
In the center of the suprascapular fossa, directly above SI 11. When the arm is lifted, the point is at the site of the depression.

INDICATIONS:
Pain in the scapular region, numbness and aching of the upper extremities, motor impairment of the shoulder and arm, inflammation of the supraspinatus tendon, soreness & pain of the back of the shoulder.

METHOD:
Perpendicularly 0.5-0.7 cun.

NOTES:

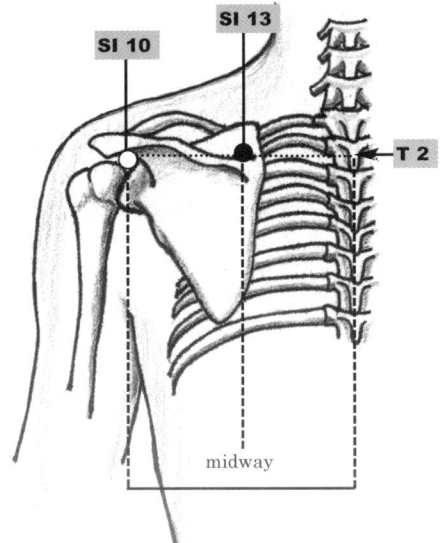

SI 10

SI 13

T 2

midway

LOCATION:
On the medial extremity of the supras-capular fossa, about midway between SI 10 and the spinous process of the 2nd thoracic vertebra.

INDICATIONS:
Pain and stiffness of the scapular region, inflammation of the tendon of the supraspinatus muscle, diseases of the soft tissue of the shoulder joint.

METHOD:
Perpendicularly 0.3-0.5 cun.

NOTES:

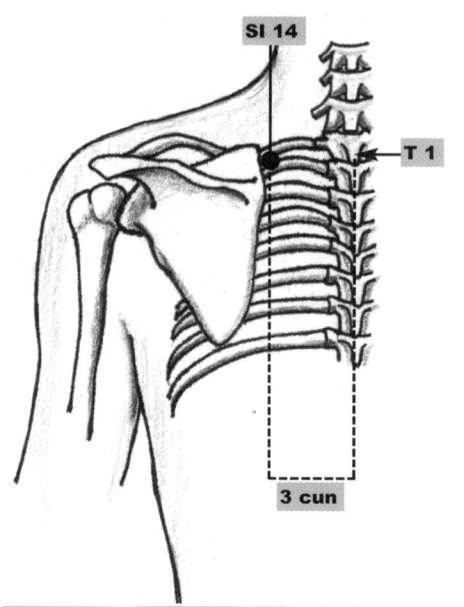

SI 14

JIANWAISHU

LOCATION:
3 cun lateral to the lower border of the 1st thoracic vertebra where DU 13 is located.

INDICATIONS:
Aching of the shoulder and back, pain and rigidity of the neck.

METHOD:
Obliquely 0.3-0.7 cun.

NOTES:

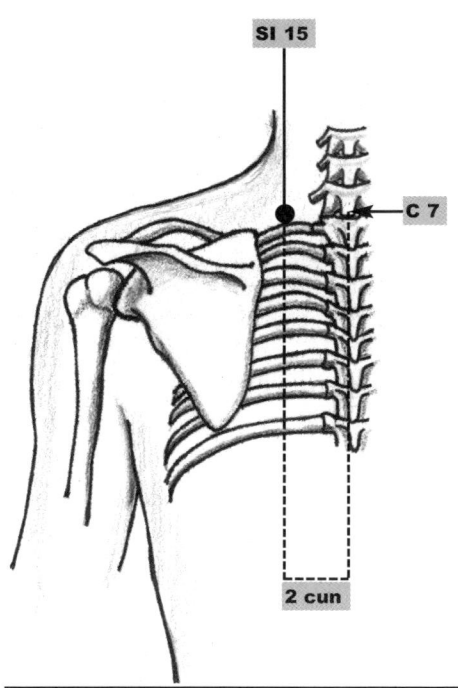

SI 15

JIANZHONGSHU

LOCATION:
2 cun lateral to the lower border of the spinous process of the 7th cervical vertebra (DU 14).

INDICATIONS:
Cough, asthma, bronchitis, bronchiectasis, pain in the shoulder and back, hemoptysis, stiff neck.

METHOD:
Obliquely 0.3-0.6 cun.

NOTES:

149

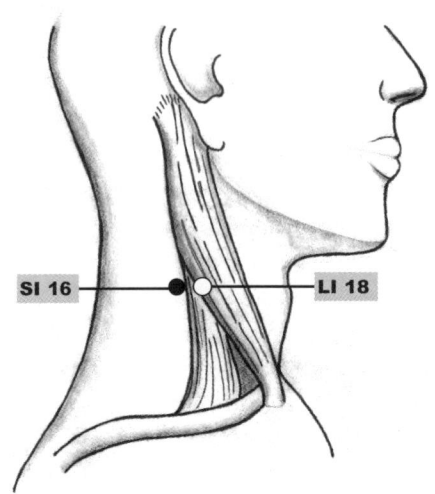

SI 16
TIANCHUANG

LOCATION:
In the lateral aspect of the neck, in the posterior border of m.sternocleidomastoideus, posterior to LI 18.

INDICATIONS:
Sore throat, sudden loss of voice, goiter, deafness, tinnitus, stiffness and pain of the neck.

METHOD:
Perpendicularly 0.3-0.7 cun.

NOTES:

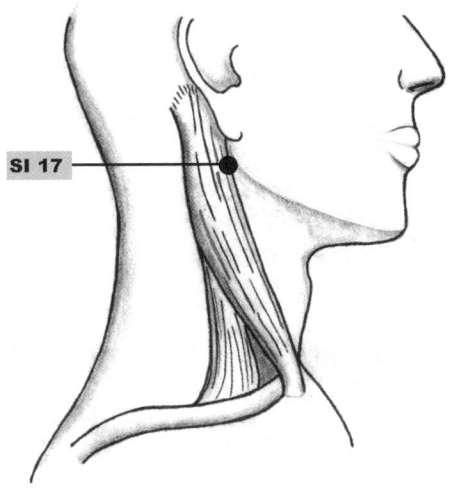

SI 17

LOCATION:
Posterior to the angle of the mandible, in the depression on the anterior border of m.sternocleidomastoideus.

INDICATIONS:
Sore throat, tonsillitis, pharyngitis, sudden loss of voice, deafness, tinnitus, stiffness and pain of the neck, asthma.

METHOD:
Perpendicularly 0.5-0.7 cun.

NOTES:

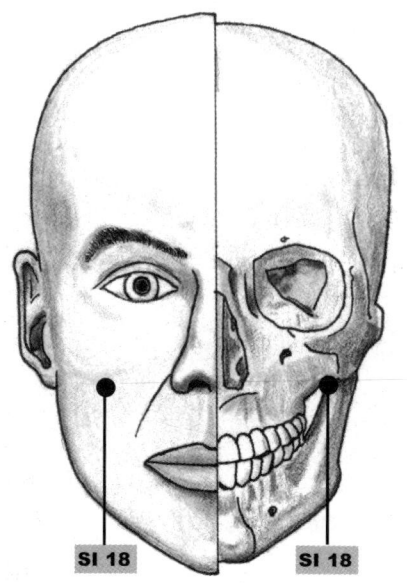

SI 18
QUANLIAO

LOCATION:
Directly below the outer canthus, in the depression on the lower border of the zygoma.

INDICATIONS:
Facial paralysis, trigeminal neuralgia, twitching of the eyelids, pain in the face, toothache, swelling of the cheek, spasm of the facial muscles, yellowish sclera.

METHOD:
Perpendicularly 0.5-0.8 cun.

NOTES:

SI 18   SI 18

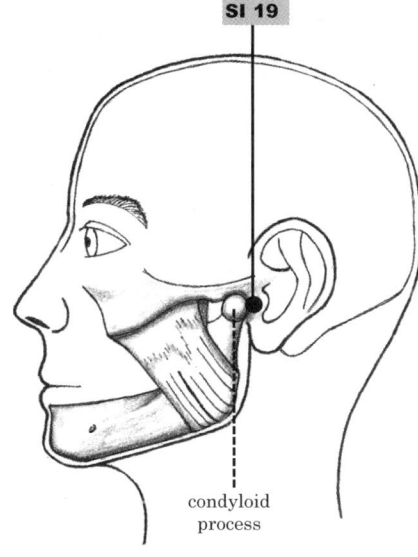

SI 19

condyloid
process

LOCATION:
Anterior to the tragus and posterior to the condyloid process of the mandible, in the depression formed when the mouth is open.

INDICATIONS:
Deafness, deaf-mutism, otitis media, tinnitus, otorrhea, inflammation of the external ear canal, motor impairment of the mandibular joint, toothache.

METHOD:
Perpendicularly 0.5-1.0 cun when the mouth is open.

NOTES:

NOTES

URINARY BLADDER CHANNEL

BLADDER MERIDIAN OF FOOT TAI-YANG

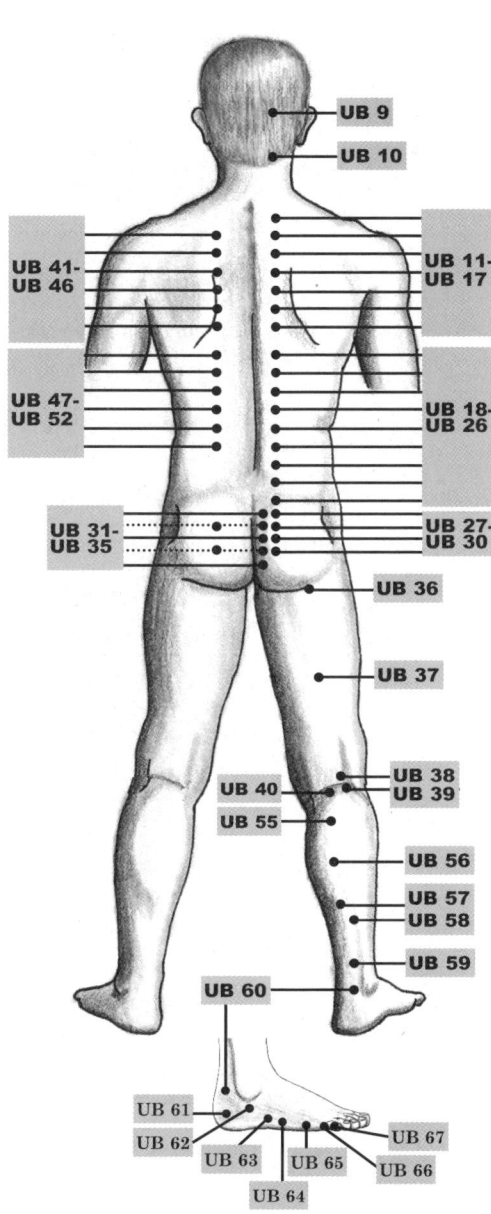

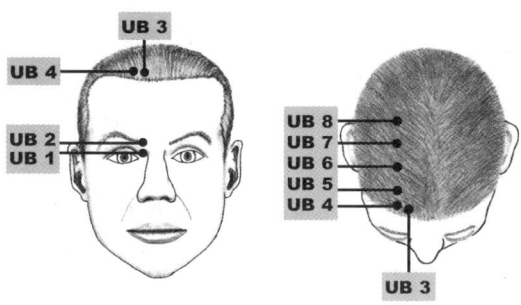

THERAPEUTIC INDICATIONS

●Diseases of the head, neck, eye, back, low back, lower limbs, and mental disorders.

●The Back-Shu points are indicated for diseases of their related zang fu organs and related tissues.

PATHOLOGY

Channel: Alternating chills & fever, malaria, retention of urine, enuresis, manic & depressive mental disorders, eye pain, lacrimation when exposed to wind, headache, stiff neck, nasal congestion, epistaxis, diseases of the eye, pain in nape, back, low back, buttocks, and posterior aspect of the lower limbs.

Organ: Lower abdominal pain, enuresis, retention of urine, painful urination, mental disorders.

CHANNEL/ORGAN RELATIONSHIPS

●This channel is associated with the Bladder & connects with the Kidneys.

●It also joins directly with the brain and Heart.

157

GENERAL PATHWAY	●Begins at the inner canthus at UB 1. ●Ascending to the forehead (intersecting with DU 24 & GB 15), it joins the DU meridian at the vertex at DU 20 where a branch arises, running to the temple. ●The channel then enters & communicates with the brain from the vertex & intersects with DU 17. ●It then emerges & bifurcates to descend along the posterior aspect of the neck. ●Running downward along the medial aspect of the scapula region & parallel to the vertebral column (intersecting with DU 13 & DU 14), it reaches the lumbar region, where it enters the body cavity via the paravertebral muscle to connect with the Kidney and join its pertaining organ, the Bladder. BRANCHES: ●**BRANCH 1:** From the vertex a branch descends to the area above the ear, joining the GB channel at GB 7, GB 8, & GB 12. ●**BRANCH 2:** The branch of the lumbar region descends through the gluteal region & ends in the popliteal fossa. ●**BRANCH 3:** A branch separates from the main channel at the back of the neck & descends, parallel to the spine, from the medial side of the scapula to the gluteal region. It crosses the buttock to connect with GB 30 & then descends across the lateral posterior aspect of the thigh to join with the other branch of the UB channel at the popliteal fossa. Going downward through the gastrocnemius muscle, the channel emerges behind the external malleolus, then follows the 5th metatarsal bone, crossing its tuberosity to the lateral tip of the little toe at UB 67.
CONNECTING CHANNEL	●This channel separates from the main channel at UB 58 on the lateral aspect of the lower leg, then connects with the Kidney channel.
DIVERGENT CHANNEL	●After diverging from the main channel in the popliteal fossa, this channel travels to a point 5 cun below the sacrum. ●It then detours to the anal region, connects with the Bladder and disperses in the Kidneys. ●From here it follows the spine and disperses in the cardiac region before emerging at the neck where it rejoins the Bladder main channel.
MUSCULAR REGION	●This channel originates at the little toe, proceeds upward to the external malleolus and then to the knee. BRANCHES: ●**BRANCH 1:** A lower branch extends below the external malleolus to the heel, then ascends to the lateral margin of the popliteal fossa. ●**BRANCH 2:** Another branch separates at the convergence of the medial & lateral heads of the gastrocnemius muscle and ascends to the medial margin of the popliteal fossa. ●These two branches join in the gluteal region and continue upward along the side of the spine to the nape of the neck, where a branch reaches inward to the root of the tongue. ●Above the neck, the channel joins with the occipital bone & proceeds over the head to the bridge of the nose. ●**BRANCH 3:** A branch spreads around the eye & knots at the side of the nose below. ●**BRANCH 4:** A branch extends from the lateral side of the posterior axillary fold to LI 15 on the shoulder. ●**BRANCH 5:** A branch crosses below the axilla and over the chest, emerging at the supraclavicular fossa and ascends to GB 12 . ●**BRANCH 6:** Another branch, after emerging from the supraclavicular fossa, traverses the face to emerge beside the nose.

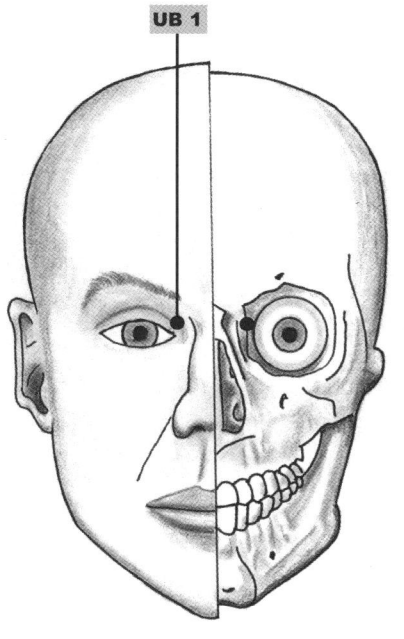

UB 1

LOCATION:
0.1 cun superior to the inner canthus.

INDICATIONS:
Redness, swelling and pain of the eye, itching of the canthus, lacrimation, acute & chronic conjunctivitis, night blindness, color blindness, blurring of vision, myopia, hypermetropia, astigmatism, atrophy of the optic nerve, optic neuritis, inflammation of the ora serrata, glaucoma, early stages of cataract, keratoleukoma, pterygium.

METHOD:
Ask the patient to close his eyes when pushing gently the eyeball to the lateral side. Puncture slowly & perpendicularly 0.3-0.7 cun along the orbital wall. It is not advisable to twist or lift and thrust the needle vigorously. To avoid bleeding, press the puncturing site for a few seconds after withdrawal of the needle. Moxibustion is forbidden.

NOTES:

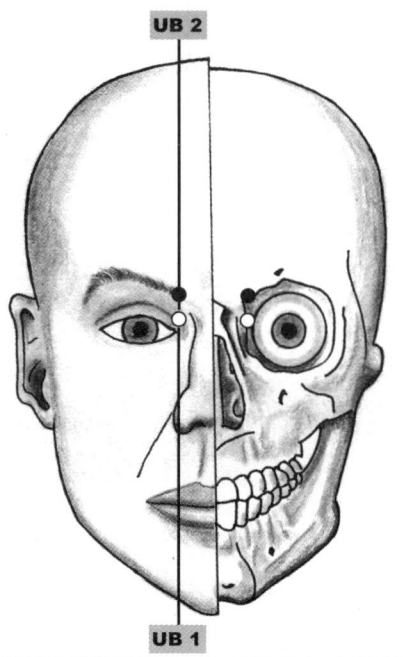

UB 2

UB 1

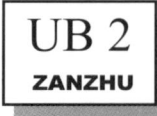

LOCATION:
On the medial extremity of the eyebrow, or on the supraorbital notch.

INDICATIONS:
Headache, blurring and failing vision, pain in the supraorbital region, excessive lacrimation, redness, swelling and pain of the eye, twitching of the eyelids, glaucoma, myopia, acute conjunctivitis, keratoleukoma, facial paralysis.

METHOD:
Puncture subcutaneously 0.3-0.5 cun, or prick with three-edged needle to cause bleeding.

NOTES:

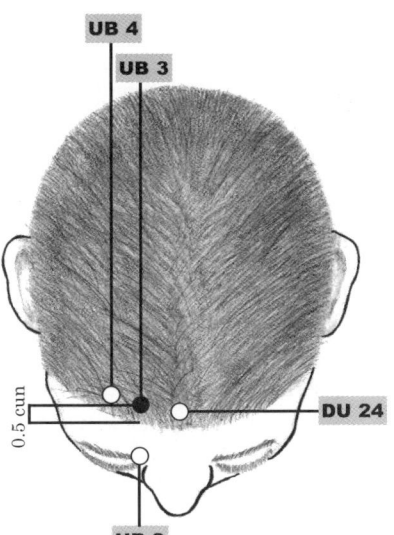

UB 4

UB 3

0.5 cun

DU 24

UB 2

LOCATION:
Directly above the medial end of the eyebrow, 0.5 cun within the anterior hairline, between DU 24 and UB 4.

INDICATIONS:
Headache, giddiness, epilepsy, nasal obstruction, vertigo.

METHOD:
Puncture subcutaneously 0.3-0.5 cun.

NOTES:

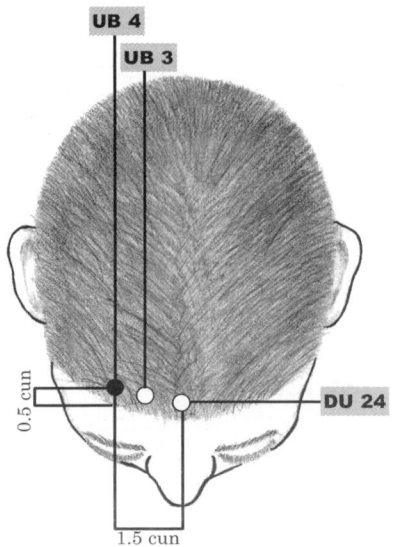

UB 4 ... UB 3 ... DU 24 ... 0.5 cun ... 1.5 cun

LOCATION:
1.5 cun lateral to DU 24 at the junction of the medial third and lateral two-thirds of the distance from DU 24 to ST 8.

INDICATIONS:
Headache, nasal obstruction, epistaxis, blurring and failing vision, eye diseases.

METHOD:
Puncture subcutaneously 0.3-0.5 cun.

NOTES:

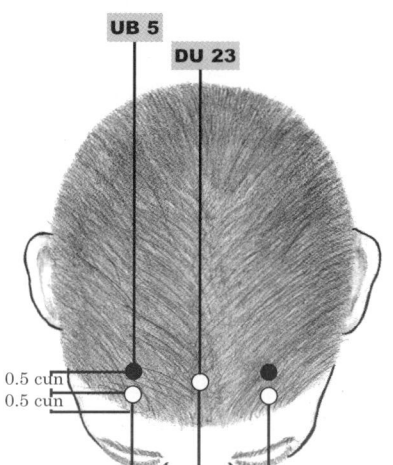

UB 5
DU 23
0.5 cun
0.5 cun
1.5 cun
UB 4

LOCATION:
1.5 cun lateral to DU 23, or 0.5 cun directly above UB 4.

INDICATIONS:
Headache, vertigo, rhinitis, blurry vision, epilepsy, convulsion.

METHOD:
Puncture subcutaneously 0.3-0.5 cun.

NOTES:

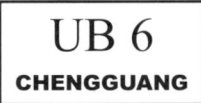

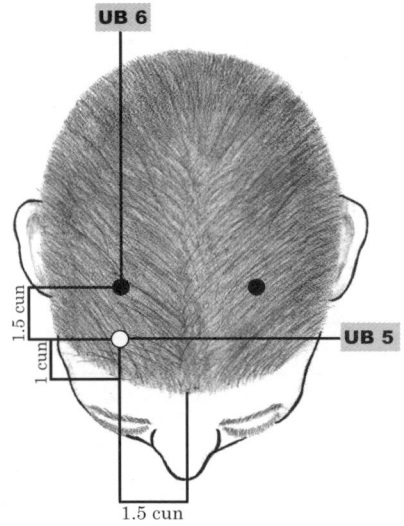

UB 6

1.5 cun

1 cun

UB 5

1.5 cun

LOCATION:
1.5 cun posterior to UB 5, 1.5 cun lateral to the DU meridian.

INDICATIONS:
Headache, common cold, pannus, rhinitis, vertigo, blurring of vision, nasal obstruction.

METHOD:
Puncture subcutaneously 0.3-0.5 cun.

NOTES:

164

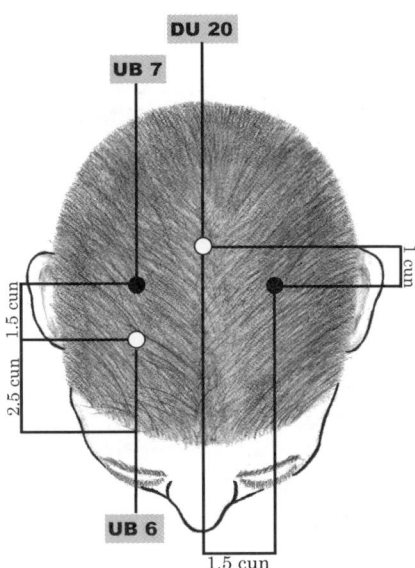

LOCATION:
1.5 cun posterior to UB 6, 1.5 cun lateral to the DU meridian.

INDICATIONS:
Headache, giddiness, nasal obstruction, epistaxis, rhinorrhea, rhinitis.

METHOD:
Puncture subcutaneously 0.3-0.5 cun.

NOTES:

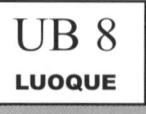

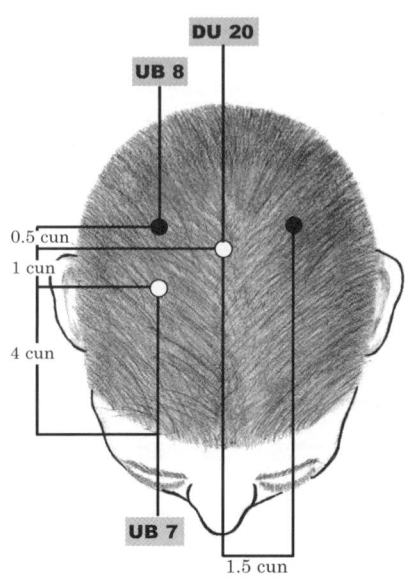

LOCATION:
1.5 cun posterior to UB 7, 1.5 cun lateral to the DU meridian.

INDICATIONS:
Headache, vertigo, facial paralysis, giddiness, nasal obstruction, rhinitis, epistaxis, rhinorrhea, goiter, vomiting.

METHOD:
Puncture subcutaneously 0.3-0.5 cun.

NOTES:

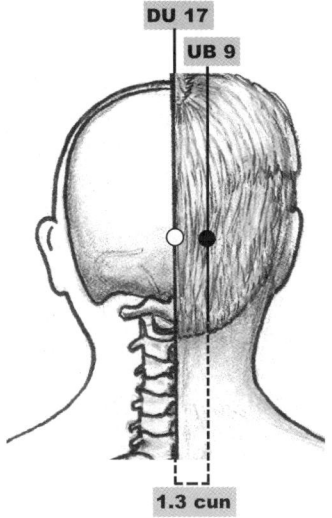

DU 17

UB 9

1.3 cun

LOCATION:
1.3 cun lateral to DU 17, on the lateral side of the superior border of the external occipital protuberance.

INDICATIONS:
Headache and neck pain, dizziness, vertigo, opthalmalgia, myopia, nasal obstruction.

METHOD:
Puncture subcutaneously 0.3-0.5 cun.

NOTES:

167

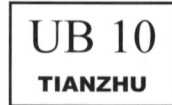

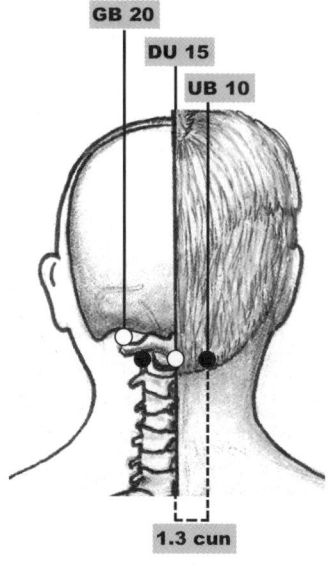

GB 20

DU 15

UB 10

1.3 cun

LOCATION:
1.3 cun lateral to DU 15, in the depression on the lateral aspect of m.trapezius.

INDICATIONS:
Occipital headache, nasal obstruction, sore throat, neck rigidity, pain in the shoulder and back, hysteria, neurasthenia.

METHOD:
Perpendicularly 0.5-0.8 cun.

NOTES:

168

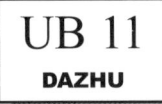
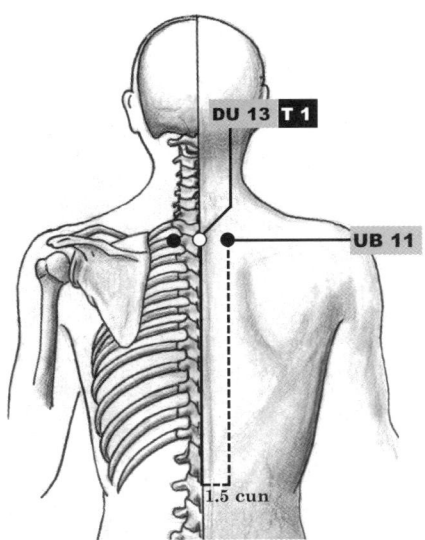

LOCATION:
1.5 cun lateral to DU 13, at the level of the spinous process of the 1st thoracic vertebra.

INDICATIONS:
Headache, pain in the neck and back, pain and soreness in the scapular region, numbness in the limbs, fever, cough, common cold, bronchitis, pneumonia, pleurisy, tuberculosis of the bones, arthritis, neck rigidity.

METHOD:
Obliquely 0.5-0.7 cun.

NOTES:

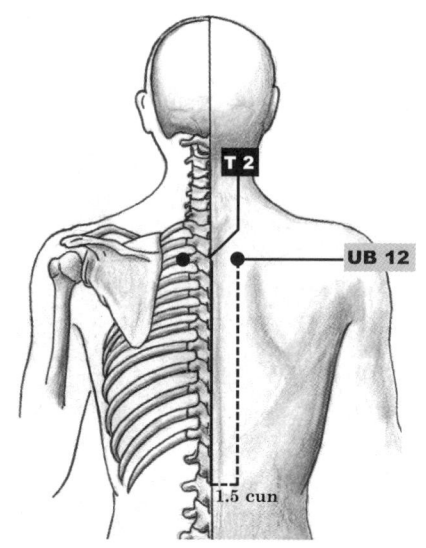

LOCATION:
1.5 cun lateral to the DU meridian, at the level of the lower border of the spinous process of the 2nd thoracic vertebra.

INDICATIONS:
Common cold, cough, bronchitis, pneumonia, pleurisy, asthma, urticaria, fever and headache, neck rigidity, backache, shoulder sprain.

METHOD:
Obliquely 0.5-0.7 cun.

NOTES:

BACK-SHU POINT OF THE LUNG

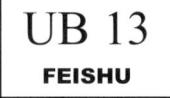

UB 13
FEISHU

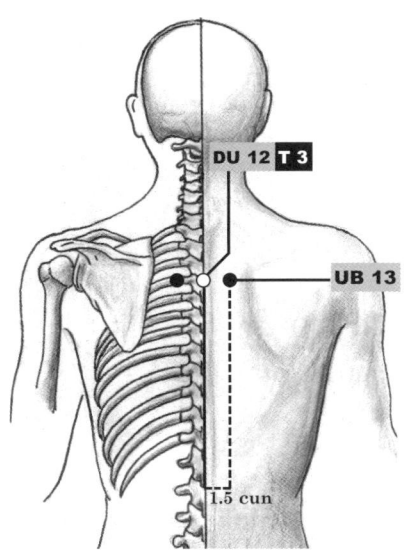

LOCATION:
1.5 cun lateral to DU 12, at the level of the lower border of the spinous process of the 3rd thoracic vertebra.

INDICATIONS:
Cough, bronchitis, pneumonia, asthma, chest pain, spitting of blood, pulmonary tuberculosis, pleurisy, afternoon fever,spontaneous sweating, night sweating.

METHOD:
Obliquely 0.5-0.7 cun.

NOTES:

UB 14
JUEYINSHU

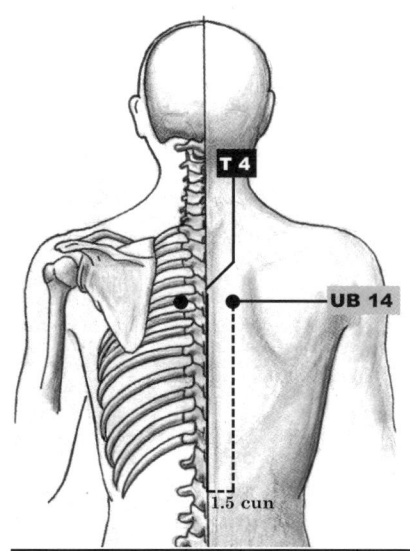

T 4

UB 14

1.5 cun

LOCATION:
1.5 cun lateral to the DU meridian, at the level of the lower border of the spinous process of the 4th thoracic vertebra.

INDICATIONS:
Cough, cardiac pain, rheumatic heart disease, neurasthenia, intercostal neuralgia, palpitation, stuffy chest, vomiting.

METHOD:
Obliquely 0.5-0.7 cun.

NOTES:

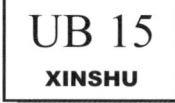

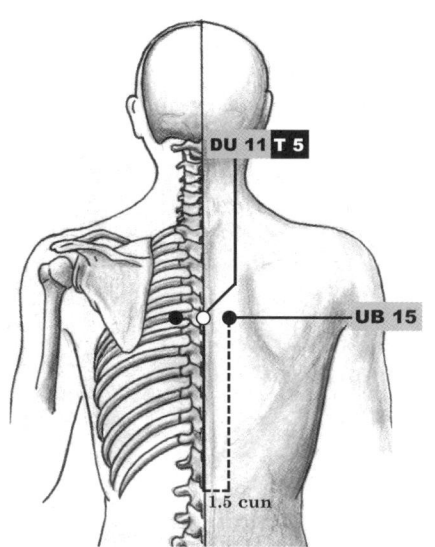

DU 11 T 5

UB 15

1.5 cun

LOCATION:
1.5 cun lateral to DU 11, at the level of the lower border of the spinous process of the 5th thoracic vertebra.

INDICATIONS:
Cardiac pain, rheumatic heart disease, atrial fibrillation, tachycardia, intercostal neuralgia, panic, hysteria, psychosis, loss of memory, palpitation, cough, spitting of blood, nocturnal emission, night sweating, mania, neurasthenia, epilepsy.

METHOD:
Obliquely 0.5-0.7 cun.

NOTES:

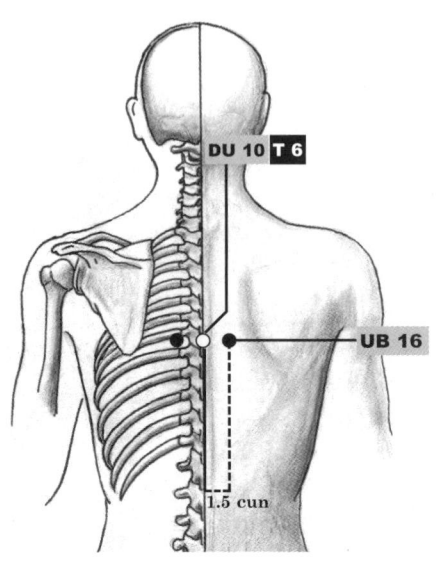

LOCATION:
1.5 cun lateral to DU 10, at the level of the lower border of the spinous process of the 6th thoracic vertebra.

INDICATIONS:
Abdominal pain, chest pain, endocarditis, pericarditis, borborygmus, rebellious Qi, spasms of the diaphragm, mastitis, alopecia, pruritis, psoriasis.

METHOD:
Obliquely 0.5-0.7 cun.

NOTES:

174

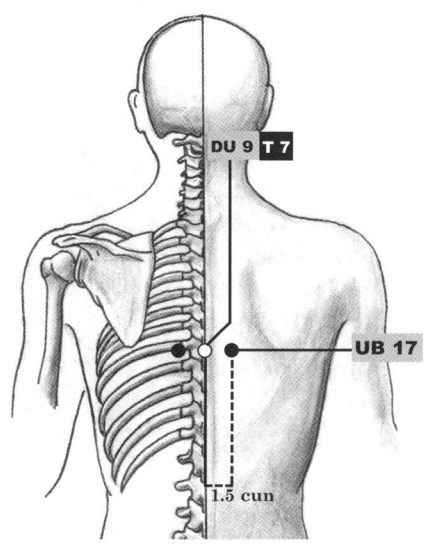

LOCATION:
1.5 cun lateral to DU 9, at the level of the lower border of the spinous process of the 7th thoracic vertebra.

INDICATIONS:
Vomiting, hiccup, belching, difficulty in swallowing, asthma, cough, spitting of blood, afternoon fever, night sweating, measles, anemia, chronic hemorrhagic disorders, spasms of the diaphragm, nervous vomiting, urticaria, tuberculosis of the lymph glands, stomach cancer, constriction of the esophagus.

METHOD:
Obliquely 0.5-0.7 cun.

NOTES:

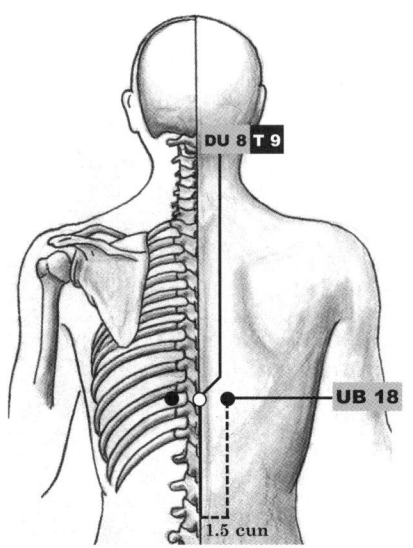

LOCATION:
1.5 cun lateral to DU 8, at the level of the lower border of the spinous process of the 9th thoracic vertebra.

INDICATIONS:
Jaundice, chronic & acute hepatitis, cholecystitis, stomach diseases, pain in the hypochondriac region, intercostal neuralgia, redness of the eye, blurring of vision, night blindness, eye diseases, mental disorders, epilepsy, backache, spitting of blood, epistaxis, neurasthenia, irregular menstruation.

METHOD:
Obliquely 0.5-0.7 cun.

NOTES:

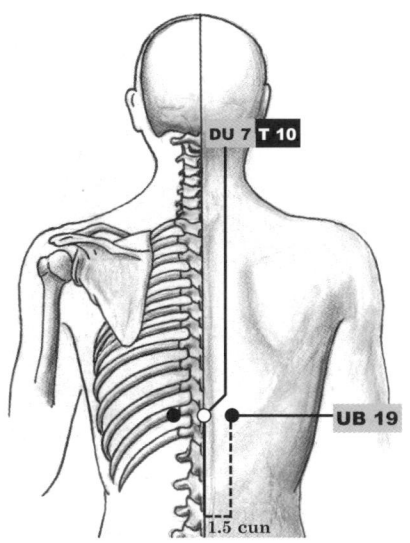

LOCATION:

1.5 cun lateral to DU 7, at the level of the lower border of the spinous process of the 10th thoracic vertebra.

INDICATIONS:

Jaundice, hepatitis, cholecystitis, gastritis,abdominal distention, roundworm in the bile duct, bitter taste in the mouth, pain in the chest and hypochondriac region, sciatica, pulmonary tuberculosis, tuberculosis of the lymph nodes, afternoon fever.

METHOD:

Obliquely 0.5-0.8 cun.

NOTES:

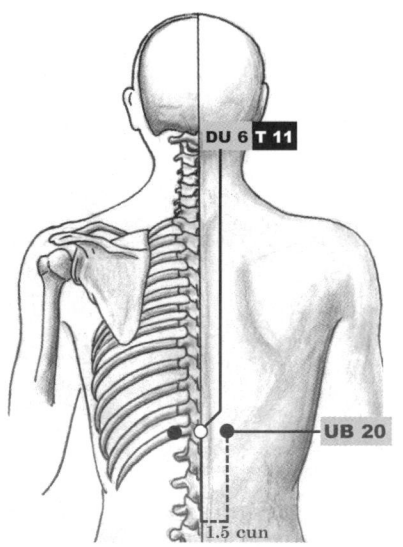

DU 6 T 11

UB 20

1.5 cun

LOCATION:
1.5 cun lateral to DU 6, at the level of the lower border of the spinous process of the 11th thoracic vertebra.

INDICATIONS:
Epigastric pain, gastritis, ulcers, prolapsed stomach, abdominal distention, indigestion, hepatitis, enteritis, jaundice, vomiting, diarrhea, enlargement of the liver and spleen, dysentery, bloody stools, profuse menstruation, prolapsed uterus, chronic hemorrhagic diseases, edema, anorexia, anemia, backache, urticaria, weakness in the limbs.

METHOD:
Obliquely 0.5-0.7 cun.

NOTES:

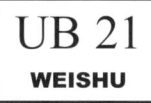
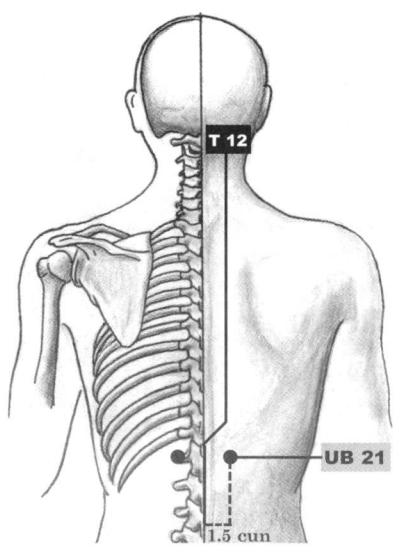

LOCATION:
1.5 cun lateral to the DU meridian, at the level of the lower border of the spinous process of the 12th thoracic vertebra.

INDICATIONS:
Pain in the chest, hypochondriac, and epigastric regions, pain along the spine, anorexia, abdominal distention, stomach ache, gastritis, enteritis, gastric distention, prolapsed stomach, ulcer, pancreatitis, hepatitis, borborygmus, diarrhea, nausea, vomiting, insomnia.

METHOD:
Obliquely 0.5-0.8 cun.

NOTES:

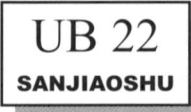

UB 22
SANJIAOSHU

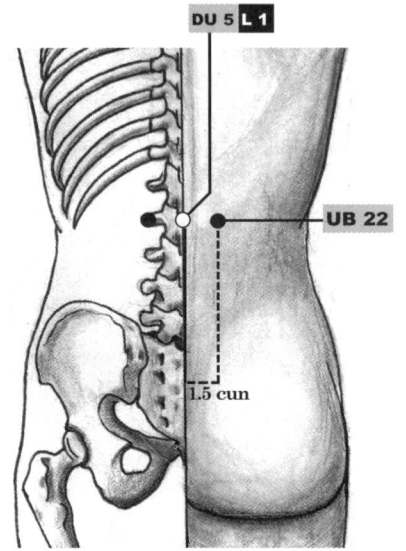

DU 5 L 1

UB 22

1.5 cun

LOCATION:
1.5 cun lateral to DU 5, at the level of the lower border of the spinous process of the 1st lumbar vertebra.

INDICATIONS:
Borborygmus, abdominal distention, indigestion, gastritis, enteritis, vomiting, diarrhea, dysentery, edema, nephritis, ascites, urinary retention, enuresis, neurasthenia, pain and stiffness of the lower back.

METHOD:
Perpendicularly 0.5-1.0 cun.

NOTES:

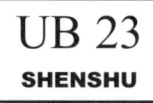
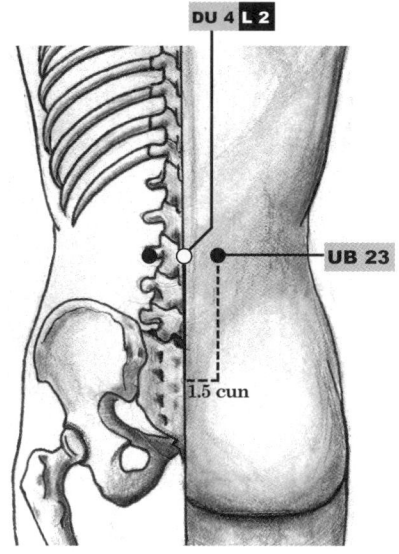

DU 4 L 2

UB 23

1.5 cun

LOCATION:
1.5 cun lateral to DU 4, at the level of the lower border of the spinous process of the 2nd lumbar vertebra.

INDICATIONS:
Nocturnal emission, impotence, spermatorrhea, enuresis, nephritis, nephroptosis, renal colic, irregular menstruation, leukorrhea, low back pain, injury to soft tissues of the lower back, weakness of the knee, sequelae of infantile paralysis, blurry vision, dizziness, tinnitus, deafness, edema, bronchial asthma, diarrhea, alopecia, anemia.

METHOD:
Perpendicularly 1.0-1.2 cun.

NOTES:

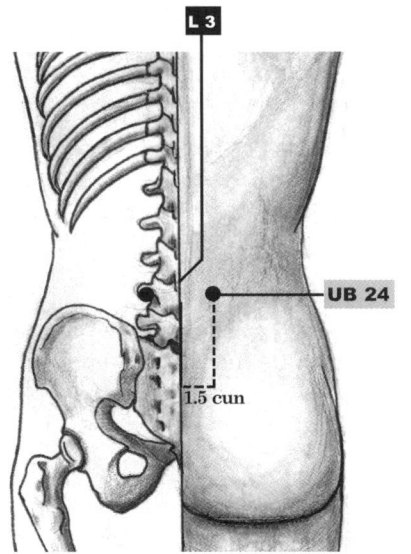

LOCATION:
1.5 cun lateral to the DU meridian, at the level of the lower border of the spinous process of the 3rd lumbar vertebra.

INDICATIONS:
Low back pain, paralysis of the lower limbs, irregular menstruation, dysmennoreah, functional uterine bleeding, asthma, hemorrhoids.

METHOD:
Perpendicularly 0.8-1.2 cun.

NOTES:

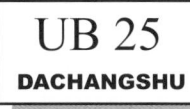

UB 25
DACHANGSHU

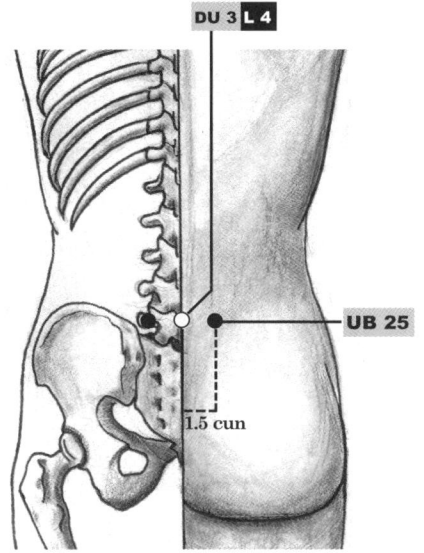

DU 3 L 4

UB 25

1.5 cun

LOCATION:

1.5 cun lateral to DU 3, at the level of the lower border of the spinous process of the 4th lumbar vertebra.

INDICATIONS:

Low back pain or sprain, pain in the sacroiliac joint, borborygmus, abdominal distention, diarrhea, constipation, enteritis, dysentery, muscular atrophy, pain, numbness, and motor impairment of the lower extremities, sciatica.

METHOD:

Perpendicularly 0.8-1.2 cun.

NOTES:

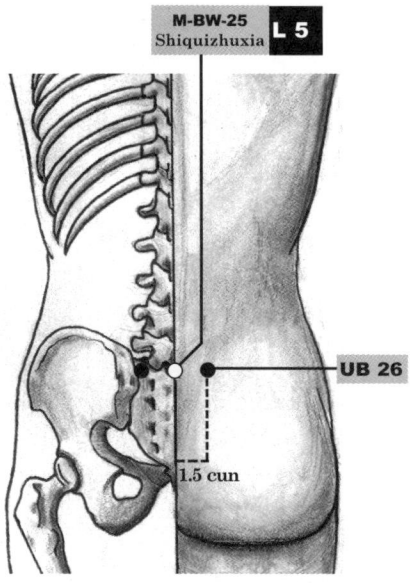

M-BW-25
Shiquizhuxia **L 5**

UB 26

1.5 cun

LOCATION:
1.5 cun lateral to the DU meridian, at the level of the lower border of the spinous process of the 5th lumbar vertebra.

INDICATIONS:
Low back pain, abdominal distention, chronic peritonitis, chronic enteritis, diabetes, anemia, diarrhea, enuresis, sciatica, frequent urination, cystitis.

METHOD:
Perpendicularly 0.8-1.2 cun.

NOTES:

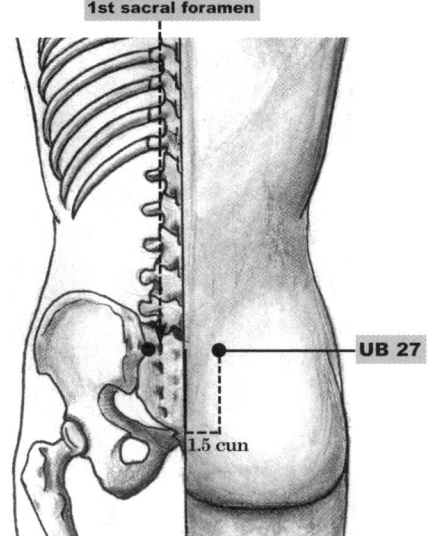

1st sacral foramen

UB 27

1.5 cun

LOCATION:
1.5 cun lateral to the DU meridian, at the level of the 1st posterior sacral foramen.

INDICATIONS:
Lower abdominal pain and distention, dysentery, enteritis, constipation, peritonitis, nocturnal emission, spermatorrhea, hematuria, enuresis, morbid leukorrhea, lower back pain, pain in the sacroiliac and diseases of the sacroiliac joint, sciatica.

METHOD:
Perpendicularly 0.8-1.2 cun.

NOTES:

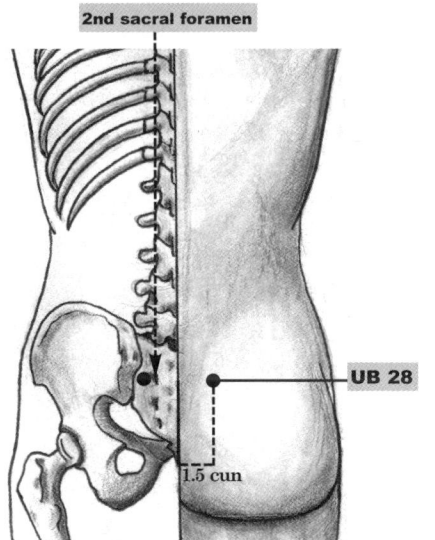

2nd sacral foramen

UB 28

1.5 cun

LOCATION:
1.5 cun lateral to the DU meridian, at the level of the 2nd posterior sacral foramen.

INDICATIONS:
Retention of urine, enuresis, frequent urination, diseases of the urogenital system, diabetes, diarrhea, constipation, stiffness and pain of the lower back and sacral areas, sciatica.

METHOD:
Perpendicularly 0.8-1.2 cun.

NOTES:

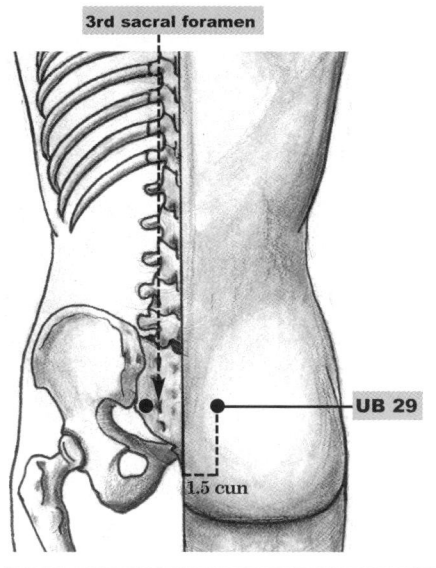

3rd sacral foramen

UB 29

1.5 cun

LOCATION:
1.5 cun lateral to the DU meridian, at the level of the 3rd posterior sacral foramen.

INDICATIONS:
Diarrhea, enteritis, hernia, rigidity and pain of the lower back and sacrum, sciatica.

METHOD:
Perpendicularly 0.8-1.2 cun.

NOTES:

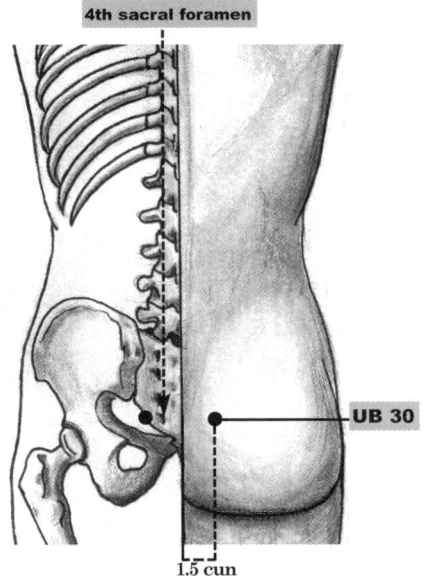

4th sacral foramen

UB 30

1.5 cun

LOCATION:
1.5 cun lateral to the DU meridian, at the level of the 4th posterior sacral foramen.

INDICATIONS:
Enuresis, pain due to hernia, morbid leukorrhea, irregular menstruation, endometritis, cold sensation and pain of the lower back, pain in the lumbo-sacral region, sciatica, dysuria, constipation, tenesmus, prolapse of the rectum, anal diseases, sequelae of infantile paralysis.

METHOD:
Perpendicularly 0.8-1.2 cun.

NOTES:

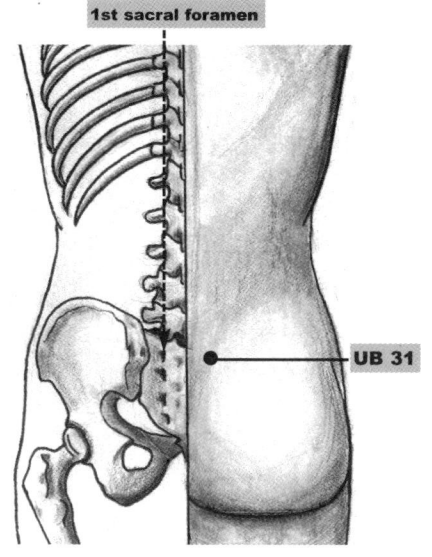

1st sacral foramen

UB 31

LOCATION:
In the 1st posterior sacral foramen.

INDICATIONS:
Low back pain, diseases of the lumbosacral joint, sciatica, dysuria, constipation, irregular menstruation, inducing labor, morbid leukorrhea, peritonitis, orchitis, paralysis of lower limbs, sequelae of infantile paralysis.

METHOD:
Perpendicularly 0.8-1.2 cun.

NOTES:

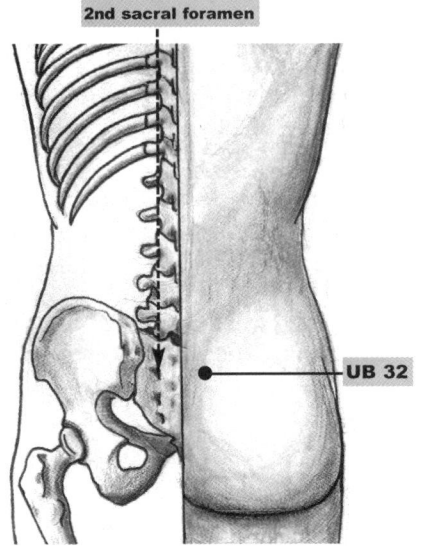

2nd sacral foramen

UB 32

LOCATION:
In the 2nd posterior sacral foramen.

INDICATIONS:
Low back pain, diseases of the lumbarsacral joint, sciatica, hernia, irregular menstruation, leukorrhea, dysmenorrhea, nocturnal emission, impotence, enuresis, dysuria, muscular atrophy, pain, numbness and motor impairment of the lower extremities, inducing labor, peritonitis, orchitis, sequelae of infantile paralysis.

METHOD:
Perpendicularly 0.8-1.2 cun.

NOTES:

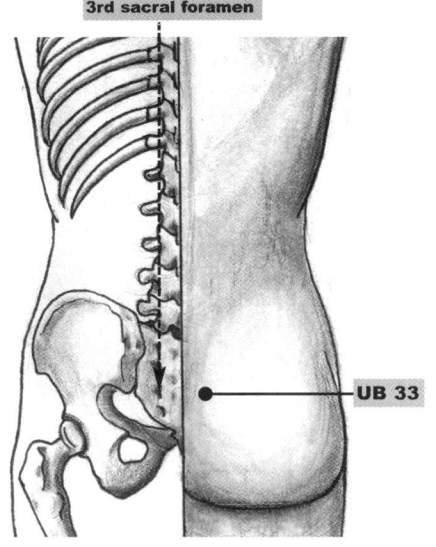

3rd sacral foramen

UB 33

LOCATION:
In the 3rd posterior sacral foramen.

INDICATIONS:
Low back pain, diseases of the lumbosacral joint, sciatica, constipation, diarrhea, peritonitis, dysuria, irregular menstruation, morbid leukorrhea, inducing labor, orchitis, paralysis of the lower limbs, sequelae of infantile paralysis.

METHOD:
Perpendicularly 0.8-1.2 cun.

NOTES:

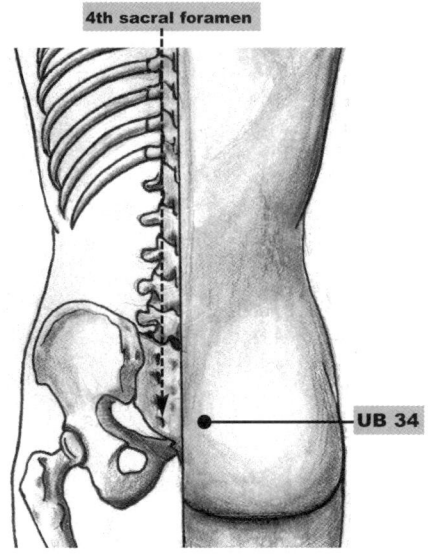

4th sacral foramen

UB 34

LOCATION:
In the 4th posterior sacral foramen.

INDICATIONS:
Low back pain, diseases of the lumbosacral joint, sciatica, irregular menstruation, inducing labor, lower abdominal pain, dysuria, constipation, peritonitis, orchitis, morbid leukorrhea, paralysis of the lower limbs, sequelae of infantile paralysis.

METHOD:
Perpendicularly 0.8-1.2 cun.

NOTES:

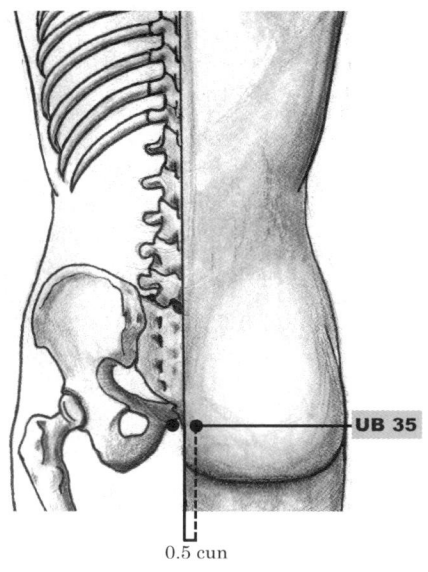

0.5 cun

LOCATION:
On either side of the tip of the coccyx, 0.5 cun lateral to the DU meridian.

INDICATIONS:
Dysentery, bloody stools, diarrhea, hemorrhoids, impotence, morbid leukorrhea, pain in the lower back during menstruation.

METHOD:
Perpendicularly 0.5-1.0 cun.

NOTES:

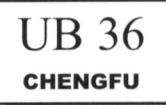

UB 36
CHENGFU

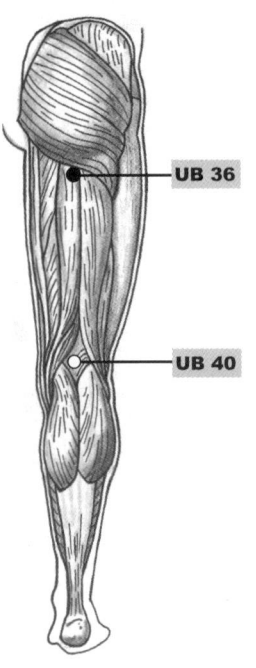

UB 36

UB 40

LOCATION:
In the middle of the transverse gluteal fold. Locate the point in the prone position.

INDICATIONS:
Pain in the lower back and gluteal region, constipation, hemorrhoids, retention of urine, muscular atrophy, pain, numbness and motor impairment of the lower extremities, sciatica.

METHOD:
Perpendicularly 1.0-1.5 cun.

NOTES:

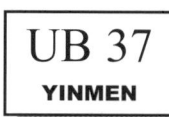

UB 37
YINMEN

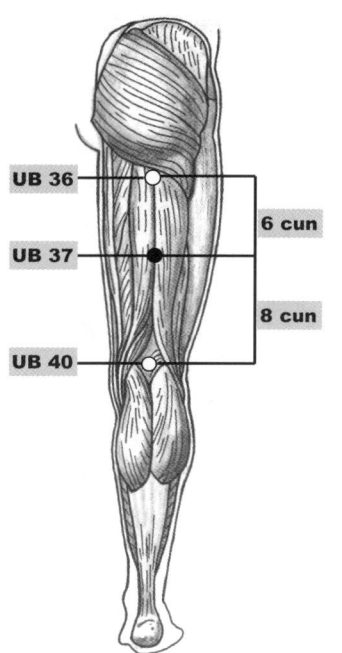

UB 36

6 cun

UB 37

8 cun

UB 40

LOCATION:
6 cun below UB 36, on the line joining UB 36 and UB 40.

INDICATIONS:
Pain in the lower back and thigh, herniated disc, sciatica, occipital headache, muscular atrophy, pain, numbness and motor impairment of the lower extremities, hemiplegia, paralysis.

METHOD:
Perpendicularly 1.0-2.0 cun.

NOTES:

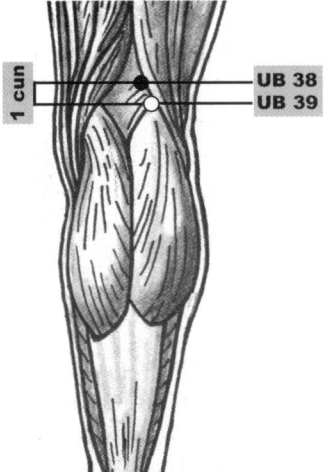

1 cun

UB 38
UB 39

LOCATION:

1 cun above UB 39 on the medial side of the tendon of m.biceps femoris. The point is located with the knee slightly flexed.

INDICATIONS:

Numbness of the gluteal and femoral regions, contracture of the tendons of the popliteal fossa, paralysis along the lateral aspect of lower extremities, acute gastroenteritis, cystitis, constipation.

METHOD:

Perpendicularly 0.5-1.0 cun.

NOTES:

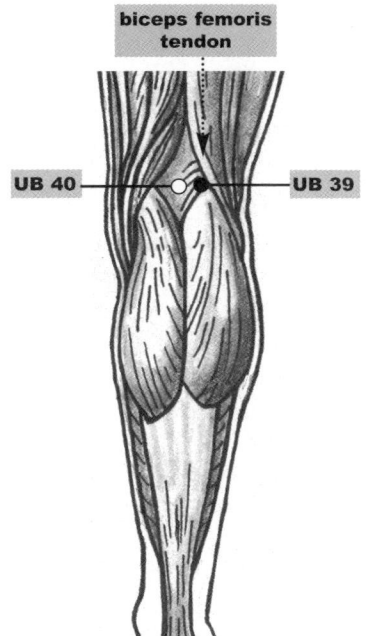

biceps femoris
tendon

UB 40

UB 39

LOCATION:
Lateral to UB 40, on the medial border of the tendon of m. biceps femoris.

INDICATIONS:
Stiffness and pain of the lower back, distention and fullness of the lower abdomen, edema, dysuria, nephritis, cystitis, chyluria, cramping of the leg and foot, spasm of gastrocnemius muscle.

METHOD:
Perpendicularly 0.5-1.0 cun.

NOTES:

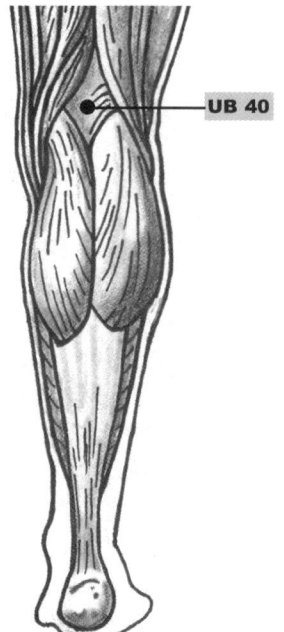

UB 40

LOCATION:
Midpoint of the transverse crease of the popliteal fossa, between the tendons of m.biceps femoris and m.semitendinosus.

INDICATIONS:
Numbness of the gluteal and femoral regions, contracture of the tendons of the popliteal fossa, arthritis of the knee, paralysis of the lower limbs, spasm of the gastrocnemius muscle, low back pain, sciatica, heat exhaustion, acute gastroenteritis.

METHOD:
Perpendicularly 0.5-1.0 cun.

NOTES:

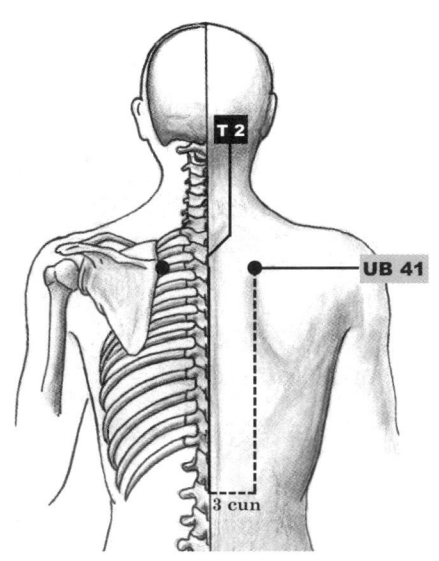

T 2

UB 41

3 cun

LOCATION:
3 cun lateral to the DU meridian, at the level of the lower border of the spinous process of the 2nd thoracic vertebra, on the spinal border of the scapula.

INDICATIONS:
Stiffness and pain of the shoulder, back and neck, numbness of the elbow and arm.

METHOD:
Perpendicularly 0.3-0.5 cun.

NOTES:

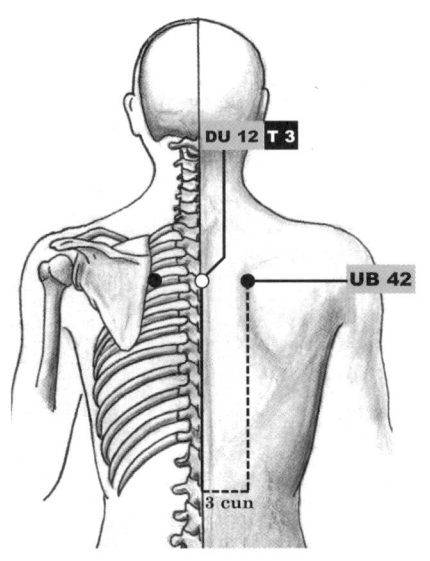

LOCATION:
3 cun lateral to the DU meridian, at the level of the lower border of the spinous process of the 3rd thoracic vertebra, on the spinal border of the scapula.

INDICATIONS:
Pulmonary tuberculosis, hemoptysis, cough, bronchitis, atelectasis, asthma, neck rigidity, pain in the shoulder and back.

METHOD:
Obliquely 0.3-0.5 cun.

NOTES:

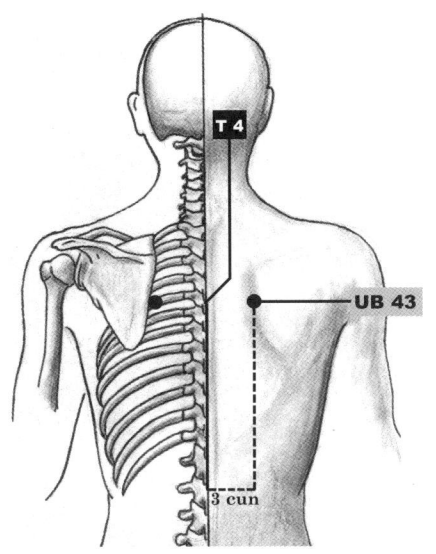

LOCATION:
3 cun lateral to the DU meridian, at the level of the lower border of the spinous process of the 4th thoracic vertebra, on the spinal border of the scapula.

INDICATIONS:
Pulmonary tuberculosis, cough, bronchitis, pleurisy, asthma, spitting of blood, night sweating, poor memory, nocturnal emission, neurasthenia, general weakness caused by prolonged illness.

METHOD:
Perpendicularly 0.3-0.5 cun.

NOTES:

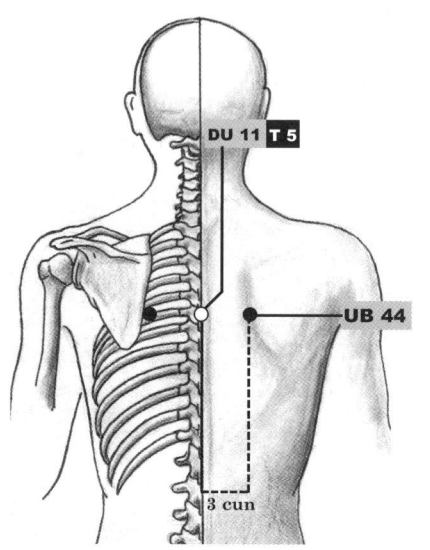

DU 11 T 5

UB 44

3 cun

LOCATION:
3 cun lateral to DU 11, at the level of the lower border of the spinous process of the 5th thoracic vertebra, on the spinal border of the scapula.

INDICATIONS:
Asthma, cardiac pain, heart disease, palpitation, stuffy chest, cough, bronchitis, intercostal neuralgia, stiffness and pain of the back.

METHOD:
Obliquely 0.3-0.5 cun.

NOTES:

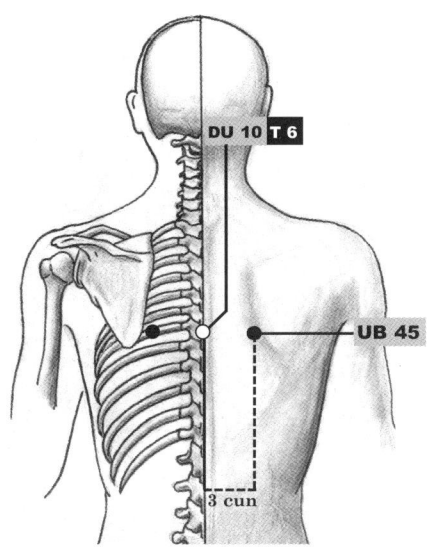

LOCATION:
3 cun lateral to DU 10, at the level of the lower border of the spinous process of the 6th thoracic vertebra, on the spinal border of the scapula.

INDICATIONS:
Cough, asthma, pericarditis, pain of the shoulder and back, malaria, intercostal neuralgia, hiccups.

METHOD:
Puncture obliquely downward 0.3-0.5 cun.

NOTES:

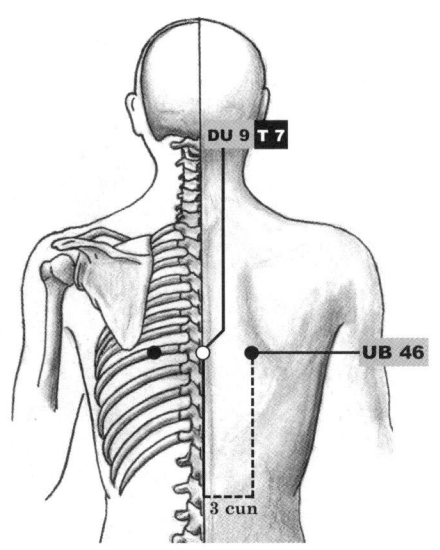

LOCATION:
3 cun lateral to DU 9, at the level of the lower border of the spinous process of the 7th thoracic vertebra, approximately at the level of the inferior angle of the scapula.

INDICATIONS:
Dysphagia, hiccup, spasms of esophagus, gastric hemorrhage, vomiting, belching, pain and stiffness of the back, intercostal neuralgia.

METHOD:
Obliquely 0.3-0.5 cun.

NOTES:

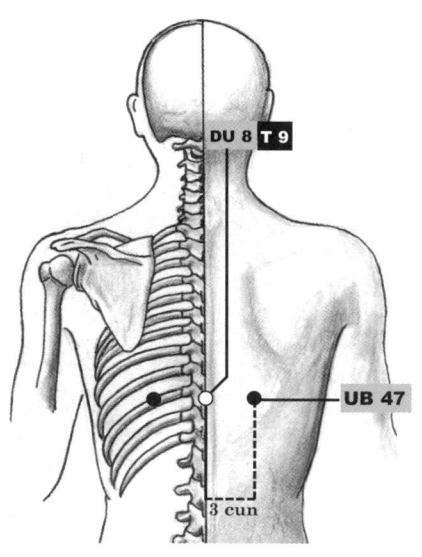

LOCATION:
3 cun lateral to DU 8, at the level of the lower border of the spinous process of the 9th thoracic vertebra.

INDICATIONS:
Pain in the chest and hypochondriac region, pleurisy, diseases of the liver & gallbladder, back pain, vomiting, diarrhea, stomach ache, neurasthenia.

METHOD:
Obliquely 0.3-0.5 cun.

NOTES:

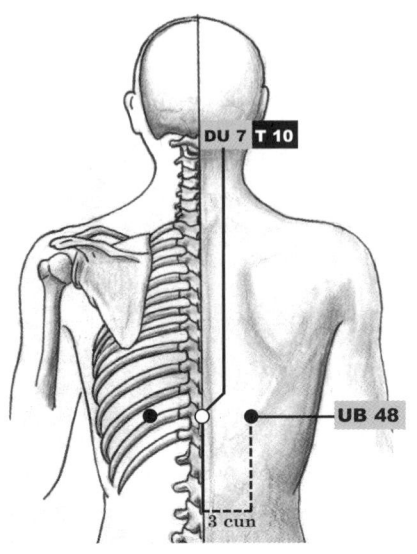

LOCATION:
3 cun lateral to DU 7, at the level of the lower border of the spinous process of the 10th thoracic vertebra.

INDICATIONS:
Borborygmus, abdominal pain, gastritis, diarrhea, pain in the hypochondriac region, jaundice, hepatitis, cholecystitis.

METHOD:
Obliquely 0.3-0.5 cun.

NOTES:

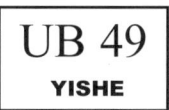

UB 49
YISHE

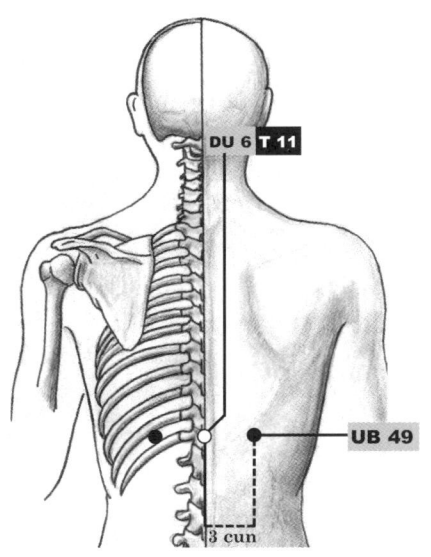

LOCATION:
3 cun lateral to DU 6, at the level of the lower border of the spinous process of the 11th thoracic vertebra.

INDICATIONS:
Abdominal distention, gastritis, borborygmus, vomiting, diarrhea, difficulty in swallowing, hepatitis, cholecystitis.

METHOD:
Obliquely 0.3-0.5 cun.

NOTES:

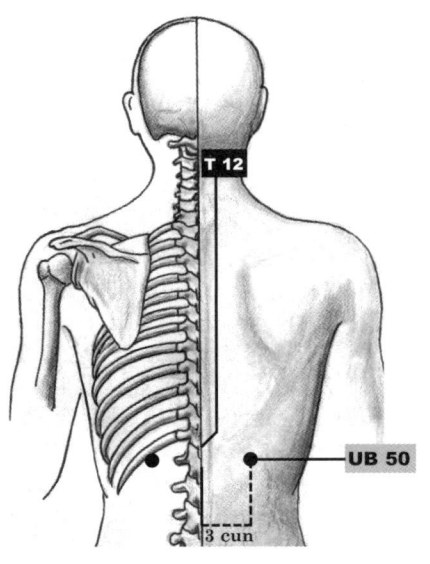

LOCATION:
3 cun lateral to the DU meridian, at the level of the lower border of the 12th thoracic vertebra.

INDICATIONS:
Abdominal distention & pain, pain in the epigastric region and back, stomach ache, gastritis, infantile indigestion.

METHOD:
Obliquely 0.3-0.5 cun.

NOTES:

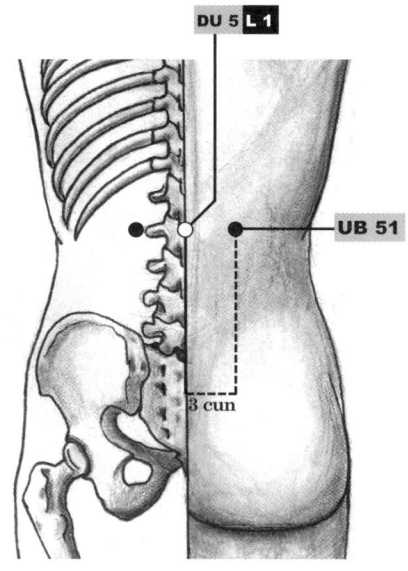

DU 5 L 1

UB 51

3 cun

LOCATION:
3 cun lateral to DU 5, at the level of the lower border of the spinous process of the 1st lumbar vertebra.

INDICATIONS:
Abdominal pain, pain in the upper abdomen, constipation, abdominal mass, mastitis, low back pain, paralysis of the lower limbs.

METHOD:
Obliquely 0.3-0.5 cun.

NOTES:

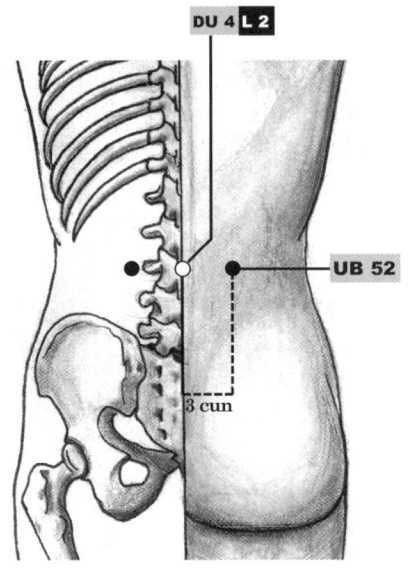

DU 4 L 2

UB 52

3 cun

LOCATION:
3 cun lateral to DU 4, at the level of the lower border of the spinous process of the 2nd lumbar vertebra.

INDICATIONS:
Nocturnal emission, spermatorrhea, impotence, prostatitis, eczema of the scrotum, enuresis, frequency of urination, dysuria, painful urination, nephritis, irregular menstruation, pain in the back and knee, low back pain, edema, paralysis of the lower limbs.

METHOD:
Perpendicularly 0.5-1.0 cun.

NOTES:

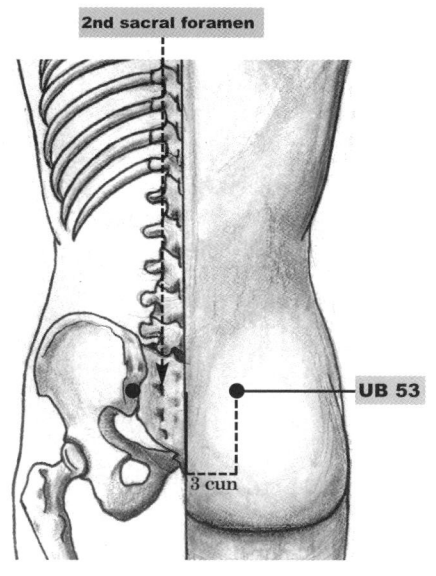

2nd sacral foramen

UB 53

3 cun

LOCATION:
3 cun lateral to the DU meridian, at the level of the 2nd sacral posterior foramen.

INDICATIONS:
Borborygmus, abdominal distention or pain, pain in the lower back, anuria, sciatica.

METHOD:
Perpendicularly 0.8-1.2 cun.

NOTES:

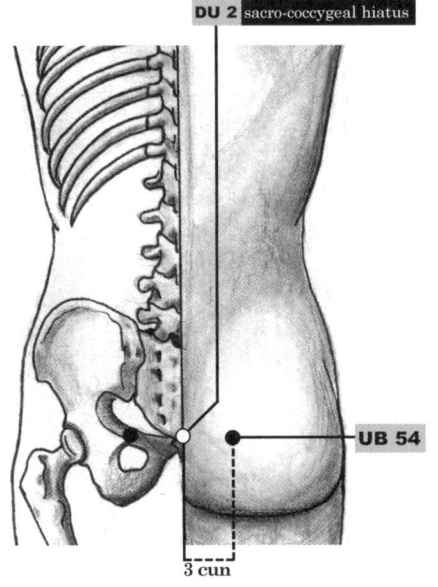

DU 2 sacro-coccygeal hiatus

UB 54

3 cun

LOCATION:
Lateral to the hiatus of the sacrum, 3 cun lateral to DU 2.

INDICATIONS:
Pain in the lumbosacral region, sciatica, muscular atrophy, motor impairment or paralysis of the lower extremities, strained muscles of the buttocks, dysuria, swelling around external genitalia, hemorrhoids, constipation, diseases of the reproductive organs and anus.

METHOD:
Perpendicularly 1.5-2.0 cun.

NOTES:

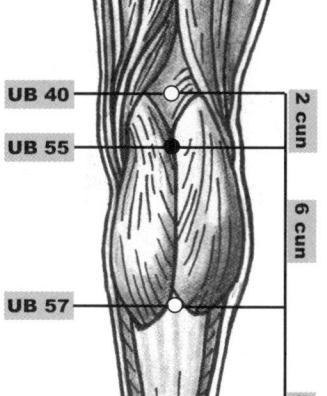

UB 40
UB 55
UB 57

2 cun
6 cun
8 cun

UB 55
HEYANG

LOCATION:
2 cun directly below UB 40, between the medial and lateral heads of m.gastrocnemius, on the line joining UB 40 and UB 57.

INDICATIONS:
Lower back pain, soreness from lower back to knee, pain and paralysis of the lower extremities, abnormal uterine bleeding.

METHOD:
Perpendicularly 0.7-1.0 cun.

NOTES:

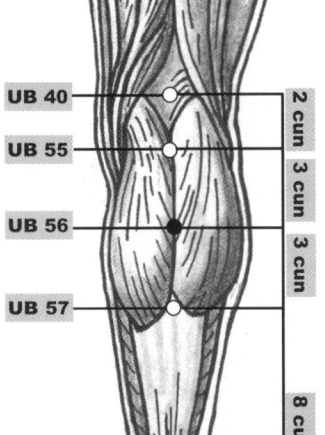

LOCATION:
Midway between UB 55 and UB 57, in the center of the belly of m.gastrocnemius.

INDICATIONS:
Spasm of the gastrocnemius, pain in the calf, paralysis of lower limbs, hemorrhoids, acute lower back pain, headache.

METHOD:
Perpendicularly 0.8-1.2 cun.

NOTES:

214

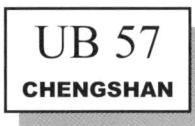

UB 57
CHENGSHAN

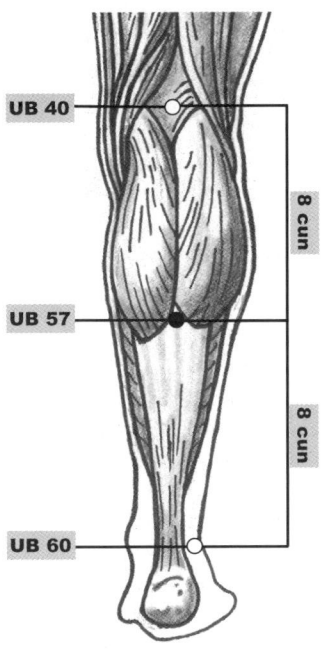

UB 40

8 cun

UB 57

8 cun

UB 60

LOCATION:
Directly below the belly of m.gastrocne-mius, on the line joining UB 40 and tendo calcaneus, about 8 cun below UB 40. (about midway between UB 40 and UB 60.)

INDICATIONS:
Low back pain, leg pain, spasm of the gastrocnemius, sciatica, paralysis of the lower limb, prolapsed anus, hemorrhoids, constipation, beriberi.

METHOD:
Perpendicularly 0.8-1.2 cun.

NOTES:

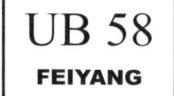
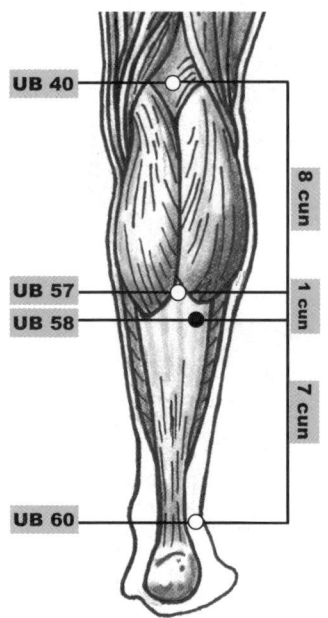

UB 40

8 cun

UB 57

1 cun

UB 58

7 cun

UB 60

LOCATION:

7 cun directly above UB 60, on the posterior border of the fibula, about 1 cun inferior and lateral to UB 57.

INDICATIONS:

Headache, blurry vision, nasal obstruction, epistaxis, low back pain, leg pain, hemorrhoids, weakness of the leg, rheumatoid arthritis, nephritis, cystitis, beri beri, seizures.

METHOD:

Perpendicularly 0.7-1.0 cun.

NOTES:

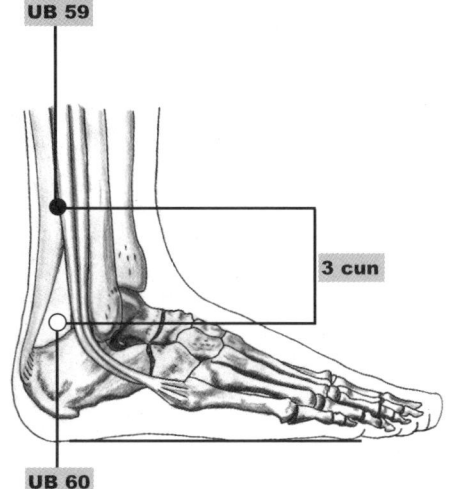

UB 59

3 cun

UB 60

LOCATION:
3 cun directly above UB 60.

INDICATIONS:
Heavy sensation of the head, headache, low back pain, redness and swelling of the external malleolus, inflammation of the ankle joint, paralysis of the lower extremities.

METHOD:
Perpendicularly 0.5-1.0 cun.

NOTES:

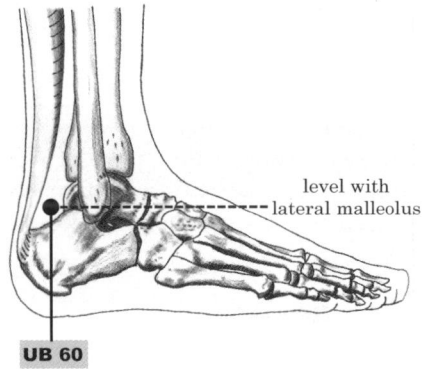

level with
lateral malleolus

UB 60

LOCATION:
In the depression between the external malleolus and tendo calcaneus.

INDICATIONS:
Headache, blurry vision, neck rigidity, goiter, epistaxis, pain in the shoulder, back, and arm, low back pain, sciatica, paralysis of the lower limb, swelling and pain of the heel, diseases of the ankle joint & surrounding soft tissues, difficult labor, epilepsy.

METHOD:
Perpendicularly 0.5-1.0 cun. Contraindicated during pregancy.

NOTES:

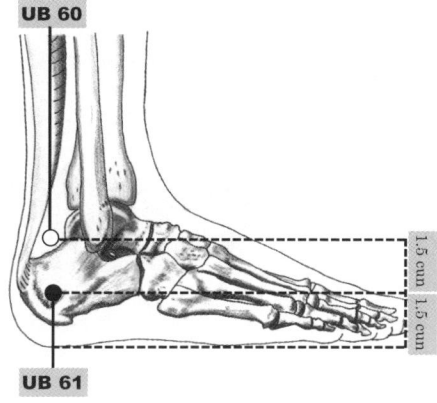

UB 60

UB 61

1.5 cun | 1.5 cun

LOCATION:
Posterior and inferior to the external malle-olus, directly below UB 60, in the depression of calcaneum at the junction of the red and white skin.

INDICATIONS:
Muscular atrophy, weakness, or paralysis of the lower extremities, low back pain, pain in the heel, ankle & foot, beri beri.

METHOD:
Perpendicularly 0.3-0.5 cun.

NOTES:

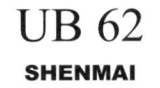

UB 62
SHENMAI

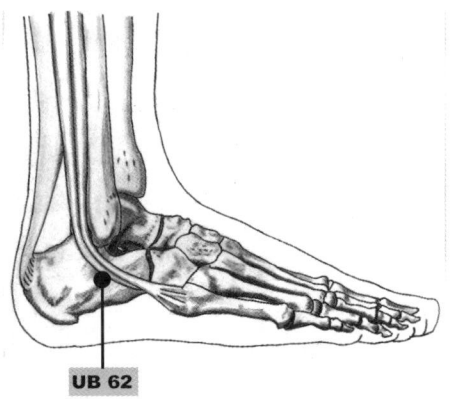

UB 62

LOCATION:
In the depression directly below the external malleolus.

INDICATIONS:
Epilepsy, mania, headache, meningitis, Meniere's disease, seizures, psychosis, dizziness, insomnia, backache, aching of the leg, arthritis in the ankle, pain of the lower back & leg.

METHOD:
Perpendicularly 0.3-0.5 cun.

NOTES:

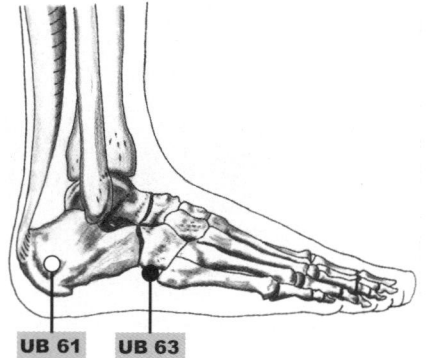

UB 61   UB 63

LOCATION:
Anterior and inferior to UB 62, in the depression lateral to the cuboid bone, posterior to the tuberosity of the fifth metarsal bone.

INDICATIONS:
Mania, epilepsy, infantile convulsion, seizures, backache, pain in the external malleolus, motor impairment and pain of the lower extremities, pain in the bottom of the foot.

METHOD:
Perpendicularly 0.3-0.5 cun.

NOTES:

221

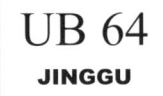
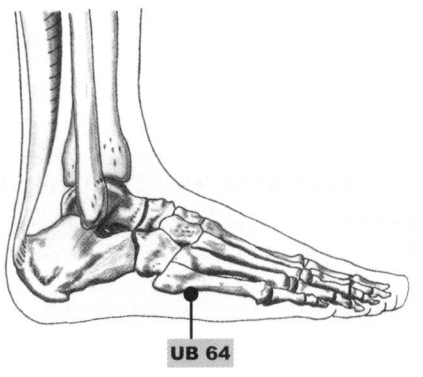

UB 64

LOCATION:
Below the tuberosity of the 5th metatarsal bone, at the junction of the red and white skin.

INDICATIONS:
Headache, neck rigidity, myocarditis, meningitis, pain in the lower back and leg, seizures, epilepsy.

METHOD:
Perpendicularly 0.3-0.5 cun.

NOTES:

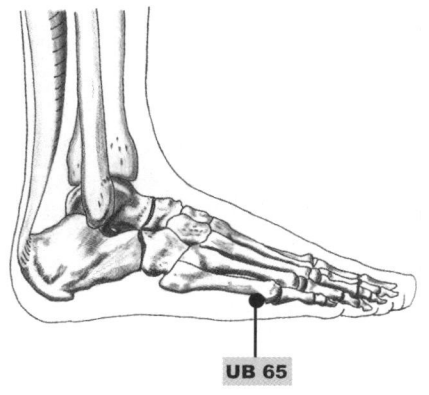

UB 65

LOCATION:
Posterior to the head of the 5th metatarsal bone, at the junction of the red and white skin.

INDICATIONS:
Mania, mental illness, headache, neck rigidity, blurry vision, backache, pain in the lower extremities, malaria, panus, seizures.

METHOD:
Perpendicularly 0.3-0.5 cun.

NOTES:

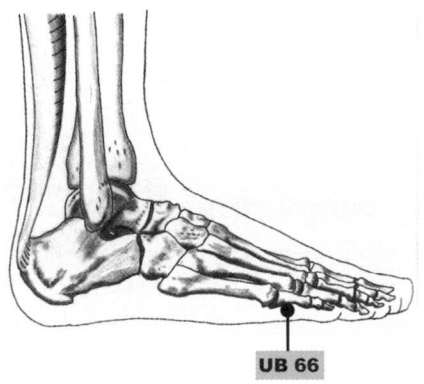

UB 66

LOCATION:
In the depression anterior to the 5th metarsophalangeal joint.

INDICATIONS:
Headache, vertigo, asthma, neck rigidity, blurry vision, epistaxis, mania, mental illness.

METHOD:
Perpendicularly 0.2-0.3 cun.

NOTES:

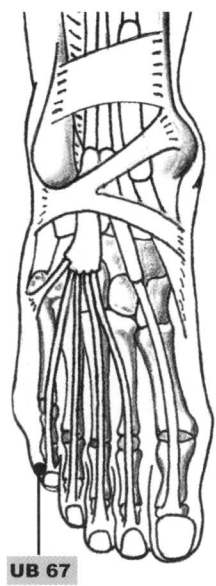

UB 67

INDICATIONS:
Headache, nasal obstruction, epistaxis, ophthalmalgia, malposition of fetus, difficult fetus, difficult labor, detention of afterbirth, feverish sensation in the sole, stroke.

LOCATION:
On the lateral side of the small toe, about 0.1 cun posterior to the corner of the nail.

METHOD:
Puncture superficially 0.1 cun. Contraindicated during pregnancy.

NOTES:

NOTES

226

NOTES

KIDNEY
CHANNEL

KIDNEY MERIDIAN OF FOOT SHAO-YIN

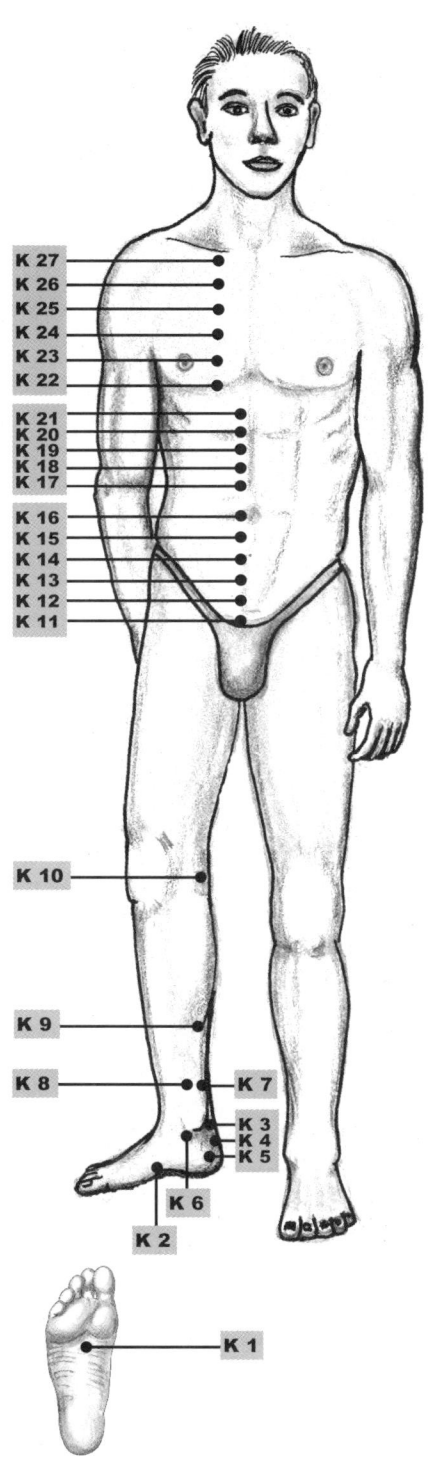

K 27
K 26
K 25
K 24
K 23
K 22
K 21
K 20
K 19
K 18
K 17
K 16
K 15
K 14
K 13
K 12
K 11

K 10

K 9

K 8
K 7
K 3
K 4
K 5
K 6
K 2

K 1

PATHOLOGY

Channel: Enuresis, frequent urination, nocturnal emission, impotence, irregular menstruation, edema, asthma, hemoptysis, dryness of the mouth or tongue, congested or sore throat, pain in the lumbar region and in the posteriomedial aspect of the thigh, weakness of the lower limbs, coldness in the feet, motor impairment or muscular atrophy of the foot, pain in the sole of the foot, and heat sensation in the soles.

Organ: Chronic diarrhea or constipation, loose stool, abdominal distention, impotence, vomiting, vertigo, blurry vision, shortness of breath, irritability, drowsiness, facial edema, ashen complexion.

THERAPEUTIC INDICATIONS

• Diseases of gynecology, external genitalia, kidney, lung and throat, and other diseases of areas it supplies.

CHANNEL/ORGAN RELATIONSHIPS

• This channel is associated with the Kidneys and connects with the Bladder.
• It also joins directly with the Liver, Lungs, and Heart.

KIDNEY MERIDIAN OF FOOT SHAO-YIN

GENERAL PATHWAY	• Begins beneath the little toe, crosses the sole of the foot, & emerges at K 2 on the inferior aspect of the navicular tuberosity at the instep. • It then travels posterior to the medial malleolus, enters the heel, and proceeds upward along the medial aspect of the lower leg where it intersects the Spleen channel at SP 6. • It continues up the leg within the gastrocnemius muscle to the medial side of the popliteal fossa at K10 and along the postero-medial aspect of the thigh to the tip of the coccyx where it intersects the DU channel at DU 1. • Here, it goes beneath the spine to enter its associated organ, the Kidney, and to communicate with the Bladder. • It intersects the Ren channel at Ren 3 and Ren 4. **BRANCHES:** • **BRANCH 1:** A branch ascends directly from the Kidney, crosses the Liver & diaphragm, enters the Lung, and follows the throat to the root of the tongue. • **BRANCH 2:** A branch separates in the Lung, connects with the Heart, and disperses in the chest.
CONNECTING CHANNEL	• This channel separates from the main channel at UB 58 on the lateral aspect of the lower leg, then connects with the Kidney channel.
DIVERGENT CHANNEL	• After separating from the main channel in the popliteal fossa, it intersects the Divergent channel of the Bladder on the thigh. • It proceeds upward, connecting first with the Kidney before crossing the Dai channel at about T7. • Here the channel ascends to the base of the tongue & continues upward, emerging at the nape of the neck to converge with the Bladder main channel.
MUSCULAR REGION	• Originating beneath the little toe, together with the Spleen channel, it crosses below the internal malleolus & connects at the heel where it converges with the Bladder muscle channel. • It then proceeds up the leg & connects at the lower, medial aspect of the knee. • Next, it joins with the Spleen channel and proceeds upward along the medial aspect of the thigh to the genital region. **BRANCH:** • A branch ascends along the side of the spine to the nape of the neck, where it connects with the occipital bone & converges with the Bladder muscle channel.

JING-WELL & WOOD POINT

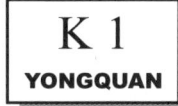

K 1
YONGQUAN

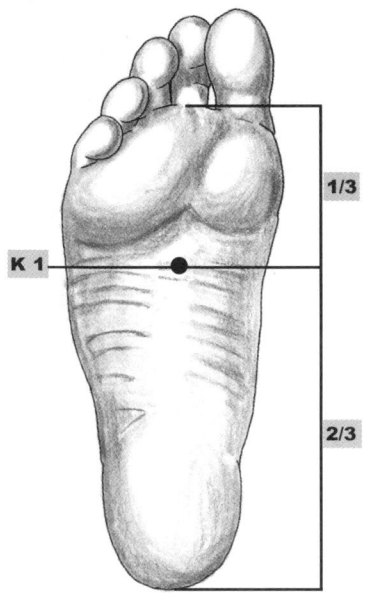

1/3

K 1

2/3

LOCATION:

On the sole, in the depression when the foot is in plantar flexion, approximately at the junction of the anterior third and posterior two thirds of the sole.

INDICATIONS:

Vertex headache, blurry vision, dizziness, sore throat, dryness of the tongue, loss of voice, dysuria, infantile convulsion, seizures, feverish sensation in the sole, loss of consciousness, psychosis, mental illness, shock, heat exhaustion, insomnia, stroke, hypertension, paralysis of the lower limbs.

METHOD:

Perpendicularly 0.3-0.5 cun.

NOTES:

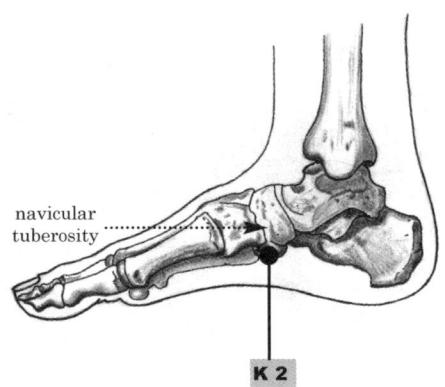

navicular
tuberosity

K 2

LOCATION:
Anterior and inferior to the medial malleolus, in the depression on the lower border of the tuberosity of the navicular bone.

INDICATIONS:
Pruritus vulvae, prolapse of uterus, irregular menstruation, nocturnal emission, hemoptysis, thirst, pharyngitis, cystitis, diabetes, tetanus, diarrhea, swelling and pain of the dorsum of the foot.

METHOD:
Perpendicularly 0.3-0.5 cun.

NOTES:

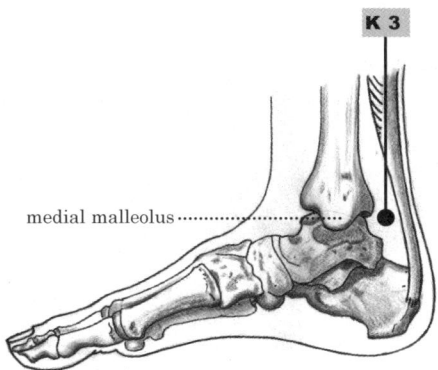

K 3

medial malleolus ·······

LOCATION:
In the depression between the medial malleolus and tendo calcaneus, at the level with the tip of the medial malleolus.

INDICATIONS:
Sore throat, chronic laryngitis, toothache, deafness, tinnitus, dizziness, spitting of blood, asthma, emphysema, thirst, irregular menstruation, insomnia, nocturnal emission, spermattorhea, impotence, frequency of micturition, nephritis, cystitis, enuresis, pain in the lower back, paralysis of lower limbs (upturned foot), pain in the sole of the foot, alopecia, neurasthenia.

METHOD:
Perpendicularly 0.3-0.5 cun.

NOTES:

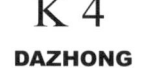
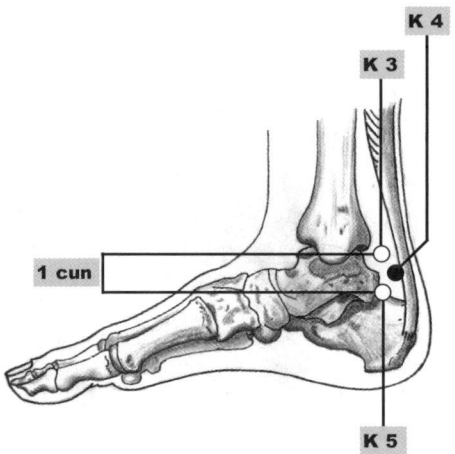

K 4

K 3

1 cun

K 5

LOCATION:
Posterior and inferior to the medial malleolus, in the depression medial to the attachment of tendo calcaneus. Approximately 0.5 cun posterior to the midpoint of the line drawn between K3 and K 5.

INDICATIONS:
Spitting of blood, soreness in the pharynx, asthma, stiffness and pain of the lower back, dysuria, retention of urine, constipation, pain in the heel, dementia, malaria, neurasthenia, hysteria.

METHOD:
Perpendicularly 0.3-0.5 cun.

NOTES:

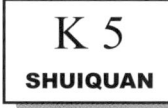

K 5
SHUIQUAN

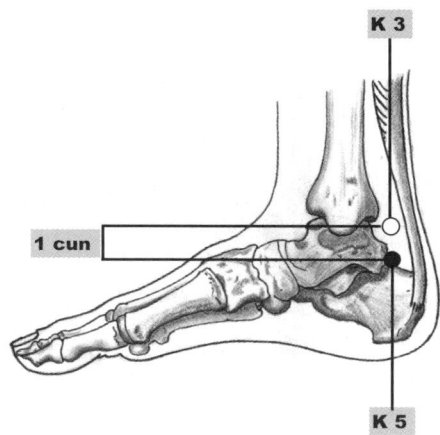

K 3

1 cun

K 5

LOCATION:
1 cun directly below K 3, in the depression anterior and superior to the medial side of the tuberosity of the calcaneum.

INDICATIONS:
Amenorrhea, irregular menstruation, dysmenorrhea, prolapse of the uterus, dysuria, blurring of vision, myopia.

METHOD:
Perpendicularly 0.3-0.5 cun.

NOTES:

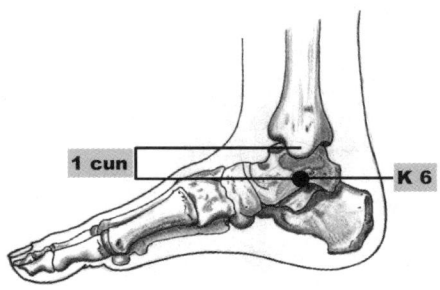

LOCATION:
In the depression of the lower border of the medial malleolus, or 1 cun below the medial malleolus.

INDICATIONS:
Irregular menstruation, morbid leukorrhea, prolapsed uterus, pruritus vulvae, frequency of micturition, retention of urine, constipation, epilepsy, seizures, insomnia, sore throat, pharyngitis, tonsillitis, asthma, neurasthenia, psychosis.

METHOD:
Perpendicularly 0.3-0.5 cun.

NOTES:

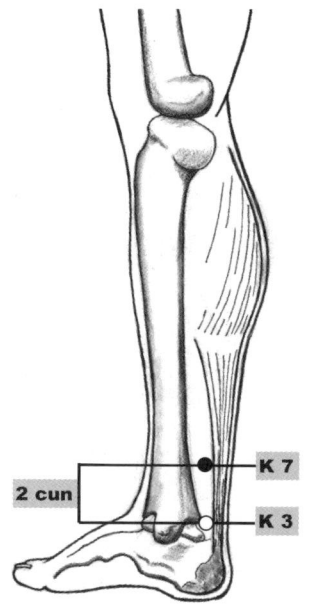

2 cun — K 7
— K 3

LOCATION:
2 cun directly above K 3, on the anterior border of tendo calcaneus.

INDICATIONS:
Edema, nephritis, urinary tract infection, leukorrhea, orchitis, functional uterine bleeding, abdominal distention, diarrhea, borborygmus, muscular atrophy of the leg, low back pain, night sweating, spontaneous sweating, febrile diseases without sweating.

METHOD:
Perpendicularly 0.5-0.7 cun.

NOTES:

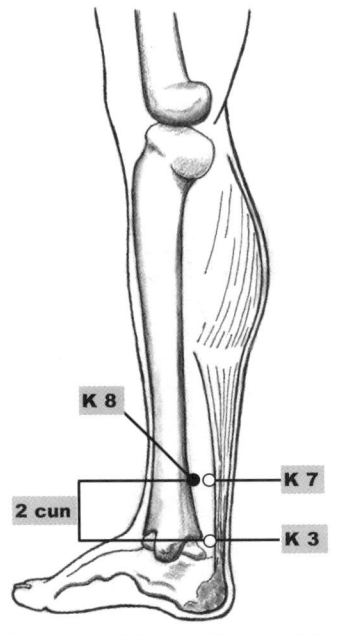

K 8

2 cun

K 7

K 3

LOCATION:
0.5 cun anterior to K 7, 2 cun above K 3 posterior to the medial border of the tibia.

INDICATIONS:
Irregular menstruation, dysmenorrhea, uterine bleeding, retention of urine, prolapse of the uterus, diarrhea, constipation, pain and swelling of the testis, pain in medial aspect of lower limb.

METHOD:
Perpendicularly 0.5-0.7 cun.

NOTES:

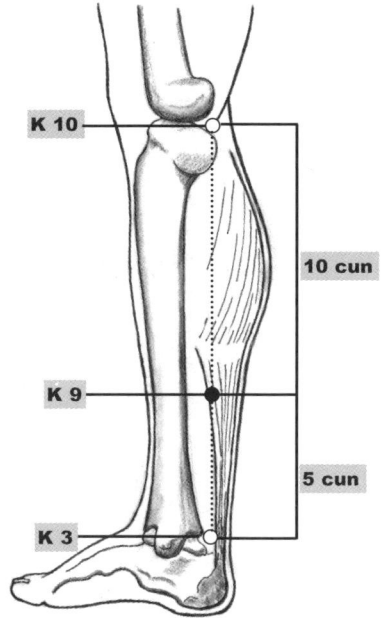

K 10

10 cun

K 9

5 cun

K 3

LOCATION:
5 cun directly above K 3 at the lower end of the belly of m.gastrocnemius, on the line drawn from K 3 to K 10.

INDICATIONS:
Mental disorders, pain in the foot and lower leg, spasm of gastrocnemius muscle, hernia, nephritis, cystitis, orchitis, pelvic inflammatory disease, seizures, psychosis.

METHOD:
Perpendicularly 0.5-0.7 cun.

NOTES:

m. semitendinosus
m. semimembranosus

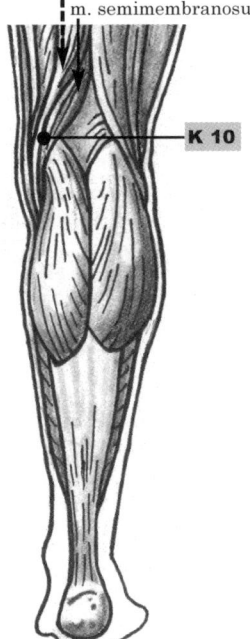

K 10

LOCATION:
When the knee is flexed, the point is on the medial side of the popliteal fossa, between the tendons of m.semitendinosus and semimembranosus, at the level with UB 40.

INDICATIONS:
Impotence, hernia, uterine bleeding, dysuria, diseases of the urogenital system, pain in the knee and popliteal fossa, arthritis of the knee, mental disorders.

METHOD:
Perpendicularly 0.8-1.0 cun.

NOTES:

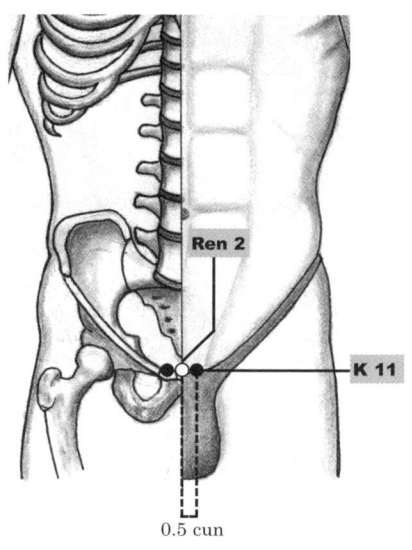

Ren 2

K 11

0.5 cun

LOCATION:
5 cun below the umbilicus, on the superior border of symphysis pubis, 0.5 cun lateral to Ren 2.

INDICATIONS:
Fullness and pain of the lower abdomen, hernia, urethritis, dysuria, enuresis, incontinence of urine, spermatorrhea, nocturnal emission, impotence, pain of the genitalia.

METHOD:
Perpendicularly 0.5-1.0 cun.

NOTES:

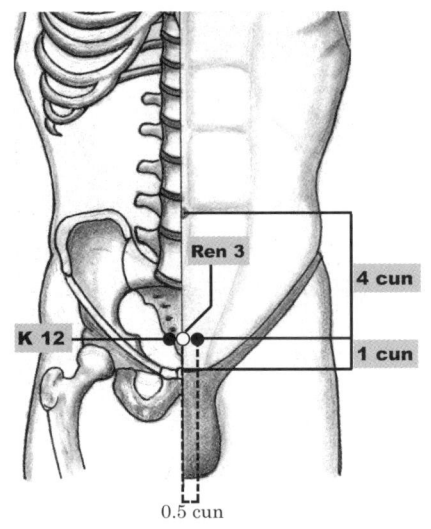

Ren 3

4 cun

K 12

1 cun

0.5 cun

LOCATION:
4 cun below the umbilicus, 0.5 cun lateral to Ren 3.

INDICATIONS:
Nocturnal emission, impotence, spermatorrhea, neuralgia of the spermatic cord, morbid leukorrhea, pain in the external genitalia, prolapse of the uterus.

METHOD:
Perpendicularly 0.5-1.0 cun.

NOTES:

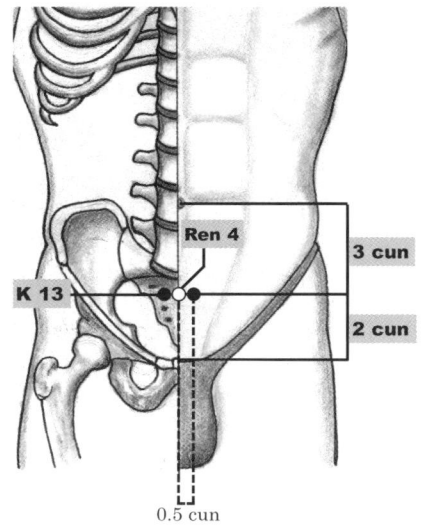

Ren 4

K 13

3 cun

2 cun

0.5 cun

LOCATION:
3 cun below the umbilicus, 0.5 cun lateral to Ren 4.

INDICATIONS:
Irregular menstruation, dysmennorrhea, dysuria, urinary tract infection, leukorrhea, sterility, abdominal pain, diarrhea.

METHOD:
Perpendicularly 0.5-1.0 cun.

NOTES:

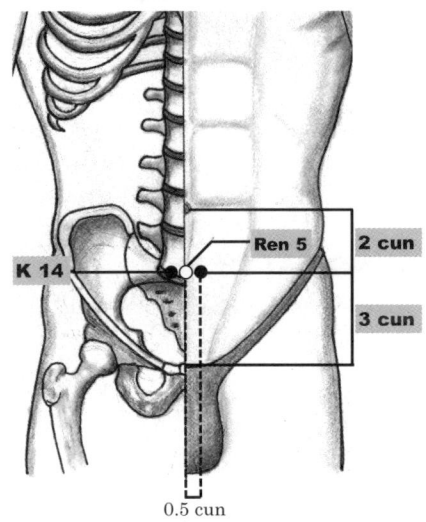

LOCATION:
2 cun below the umbilicus, 0.5 cun lateral to Ren 5.

INDICATIONS:
Abdominal pain and distention, diarrhea, nocturnal emission, irregular menstruation, dysmenorrhea, leukorrhea, sterility, urinary tract infection, post-partum abdominal pain.

METHOD:
Perpendicularly 0.5-1.0 cun.

NOTES:

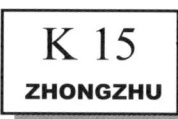

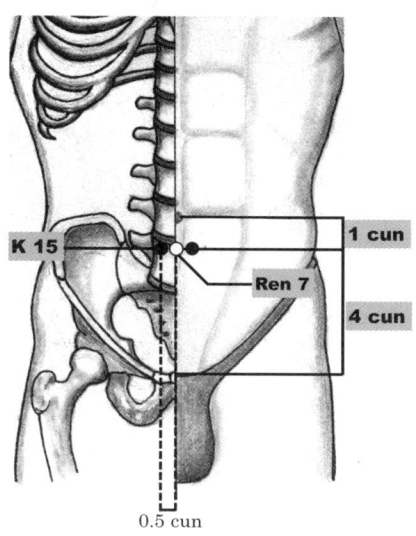

K 15

Ren 7

1 cun

4 cun

0.5 cun

LOCATION:
1 cun below the umbilicus, 0.5 cun lateral to Ren 7.

INDICATIONS:
Irregular menstruation, abdominal pain, constipation, low back pain.

METHOD:
Perpendicularly 0.5-1.0 cun.

NOTES:

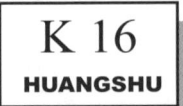

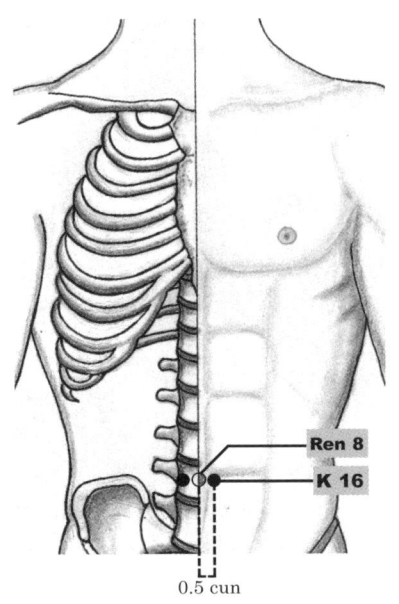

Ren 8

K 16

0.5 cun

LOCATION:
0.5 cun lateral to the umbilicus, level with Ren 8.

INDICATIONS:
Abdominal pain and distention, stomach spasms, vomiting, constipation, diarrhea, enteritis, hiccups, hernial pain.

METHOD:
Perpendicularly 0.5-1.0 cun.

NOTES:

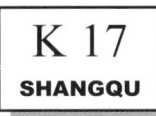

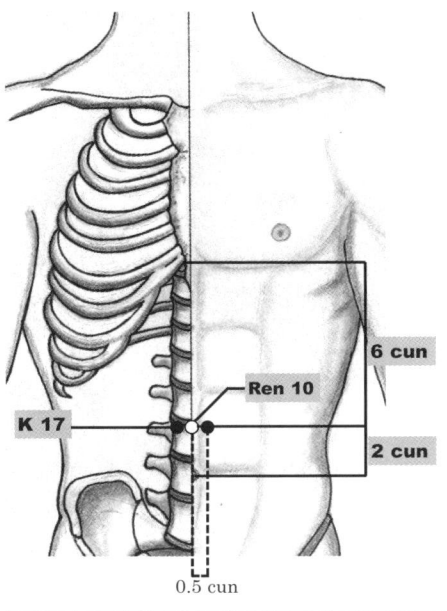

6 cun

Ren 10

K 17

2 cun

0.5 cun

LOCATION:
2 cun above the umbilicus, 0.5 cun lateral to Ren 10.

INDICATIONS:
Abdominal pain, stomach ache, colic, peritonitis, diarrhea, constipation.

METHOD:
Perpendicularly 0.5-1.0 cun.

NOTES:

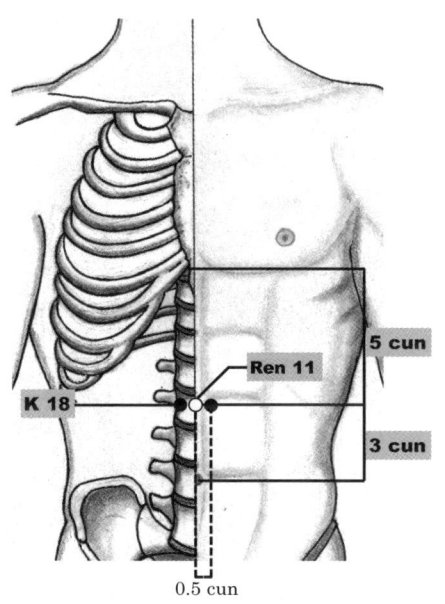

LOCATION:

3 cun above the umbilicus, 0.5 cun lateral to Ren 11.

INDICATIONS:

Vomiting, spasms of esophagus, abdominal pain, stomach ache, hiccups, constipation, postpartum abdominal pain, sterility.

METHOD:

Perpendicularly 0.5-1.0 cun.

NOTES:

248

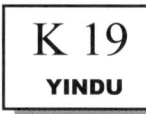

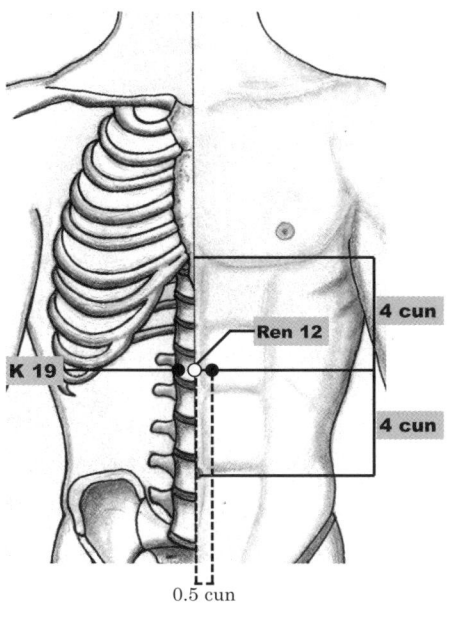

Ren 12

4 cun

K 19

4 cun

0.5 cun

LOCATION:
4 cun above the umbilicus, 0.5 cun lateral to Ren 12.

INDICATIONS:
Borborygmus, abdominal distention or pain, epigastric pain, constipation, vomiting, emphysema, pleurisy, malaria.

METHOD:
Perpendicularly 0.5-1.0 cun.

NOTES:

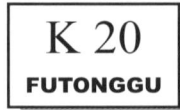
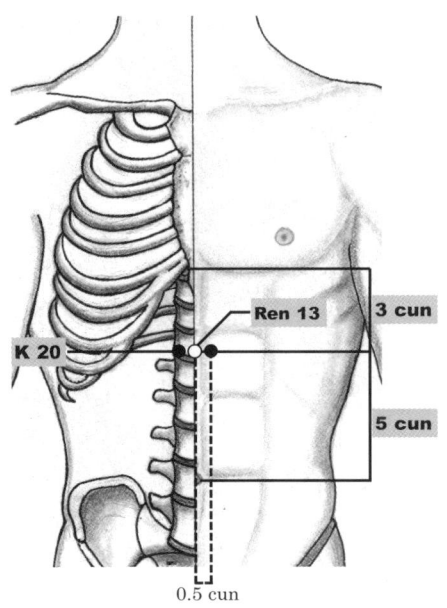

Ren 13

3 cun

K 20

5 cun

0.5 cun

LOCATION:
5 cun above the umbilicus, 0.5 cun lateral to Ren 13.

INDICATIONS:
Abdominal pain and distention, vomiting, indigestion, diarrhea, stiff neck, seizures, palpitations, intercostal neuralgia.

METHOD:
Perpendicularly 0.5-1.0 cun.

NOTES:

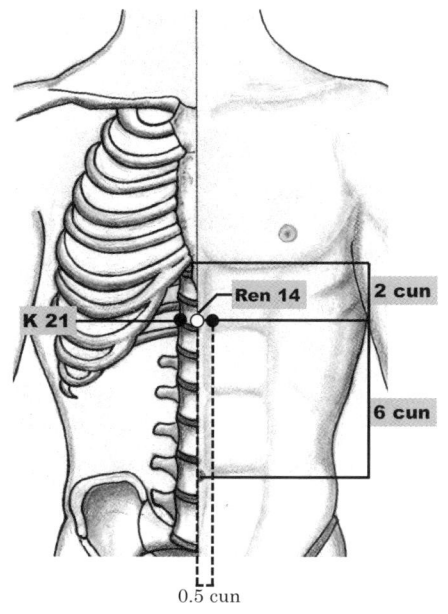

LOCATION:
6 cun above the umbilicus, 0.5 cun lateral to Ren 14.

INDICATIONS:
Abdominal pain and distention, distended stomach, stomach spasms, chronic gastritis, indigestion, vomiting, diarrhea, nausea, morning sickness, intercostal neuralgia.

METHOD:
Perpendicularly 0.3-0.7 cun. To avoid injuring the liver, deep insertion is not advisable.

NOTES:

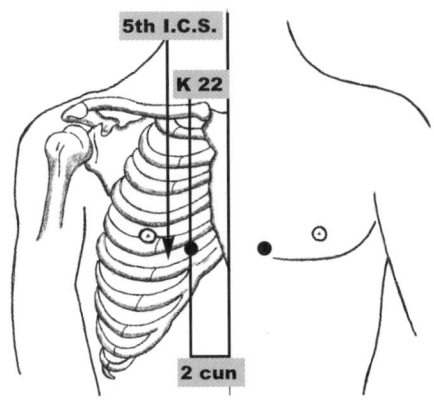

LOCATION:
In the fifth intercostal space, 2 cun lateral to the Ren meridian.

INDICATIONS:
Cough, bronchitis, pleurisy, asthma, rhinitis, distention and fullness in the chest and hypochondriac region, intercostal neuralgia, vomiting, gastritis, anorexia.

METHOD:
Obliquely 0.3-0.5 cun. To avoid injuring the heart, deep insertion is not advisable.

NOTES:

252

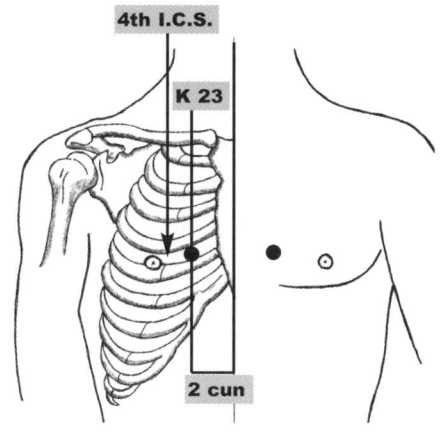

LOCATION:
In the fourth intercostal space, 2 cun lateral to the Ren meridian.

INDICATIONS:
Cough, bronchitis, pleurisy, asthma, fullness in the chest and hypochondriac region, intercostal neuralgia, mastitis.

METHOD:
Puncture obliquely 0.3-0.5 cun.

NOTES:

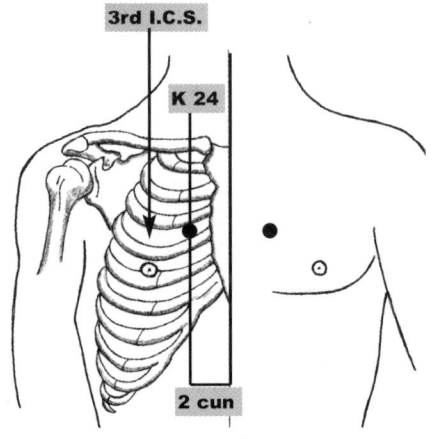

LOCATION:
In the third intercostal space, 2 cun lateral to the Ren meridian.

INDICATIONS:
Cough, bronchitis, asthma, vomiting, fullness in the chest and hypochondriac region, intercostal neuralgia, mastitis.

METHOD:
Puncture obliquely 0.3-0.5 cun.

NOTES:

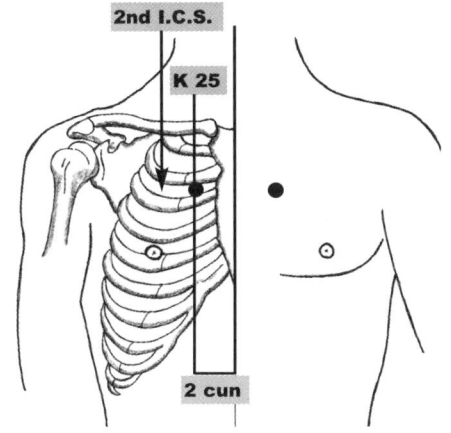

LOCATION:
In the second intercostal space, 2 cun lateral to the Ren meridian.

INDICATIONS:
Cough, bronchitis, asthma, chest pain, intercostal neuralgia, vomiting.

METHOD:
Puncture obliquely 0.3-0.5 cun.

NOTES:

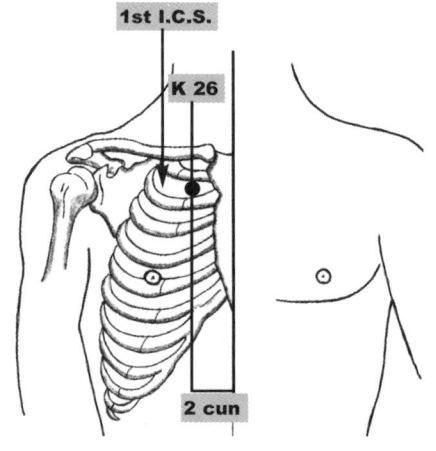

LOCATION:
In the first intercostal space, 2 cun lateral to the Ren meridian.

INDICATIONS:
Cough, asthma, bronchitis, accumulation of phlegm, fullness in the chest and hypochondriac region, intercostal neuralgia, vomiting.

METHOD:
Puncture obliquely 0.3-0.5 cun.

NOTES:

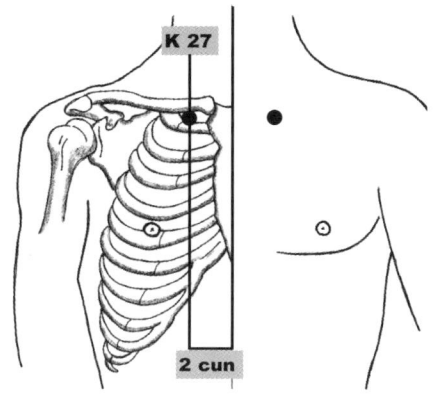

K 27

2 cun

LOCATION:
In the depression on the lower border of the clavicle, 2 cun lateral to the Ren meridian.

INDICATIONS:
Cough, asthma, bronchitis, chest pain, vomiting, abdominal distention.

METHOD:
Puncture obliquely 0.3-0.5 cun.

NOTES:

NOTES

NOTES

PERICARDIUM CHANNEL

PERICARDIUM MERIDIAN OF HAND JUE-YIN

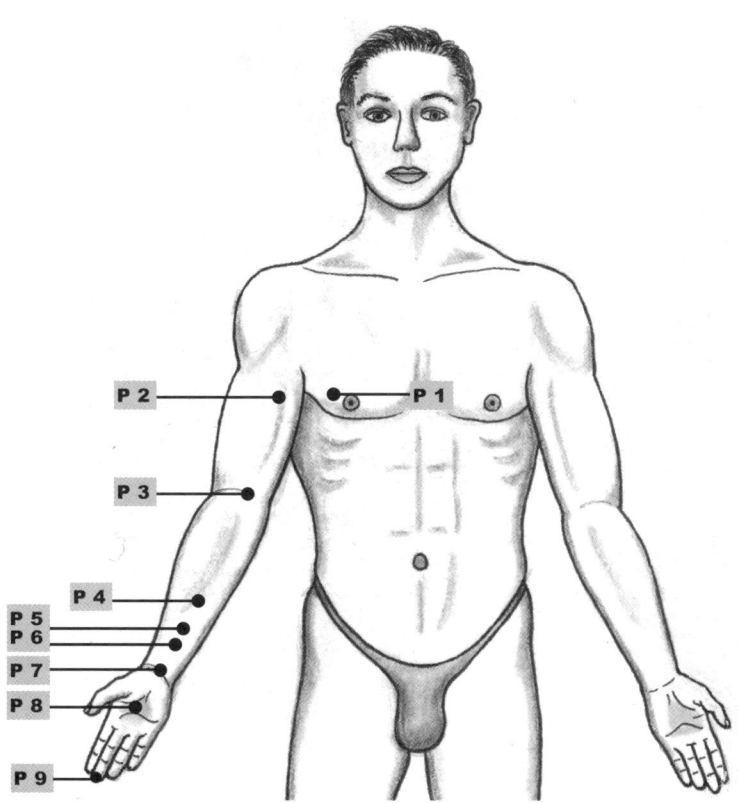

P 2
P 1
P 3
P 4
P 5
P 6
P 7
P 8
P 9

CHANNEL/ORGAN RELATIONSHIPS

•This channel is associated with the Pericardium and is connected with the Triple Burner.

THERAPEUTIC INDICATIONS

•Diseases of the heart, chest, and stomach, mental disorders, and other diseases of areas this meridian supplies.

PATHOLOGY

Channel: Cardiac pain, palpitations, mental restlessness, chest distention, depressive & manic mental disorders, stiff neck, spasms in the arm or leg, flushed face, eye pain, subaxillary swelling, spasms and contracture of the upper limbs, restricted movement, hot palms.

Organ: Impaired speech, motor impairment of the tongue, fainting, irritability, chest fullness or pain, palpitations, mental disorders.

261

GENERAL PATHWAY	•This channel begins in the chest, where it joins with its associated organ, the Pericardium. •It then descends across the diaphragm and into the abdomen, where it connects successively with the upper, middle, and lower jiaos of the San Jiao. •Following the medial aspect of the upper arm, it runs downward between the Lung and Heart meridians to the cubital fossa, & then downward to the forearm between the two tendons of m.palmaris longus and m.flexor carpi radialis. •Entering the palm, it follows the ulnar aspect of the middle finger until it reaches the finger tip. **BRANCHES:** •**BRANCH 1:** A branch arising from the chest moves inside the chest emerging superficially in the costal region at a point 3 cun below the anterior axillary fold & then ascends to the inferior aspect of the axilla. •**BRANCH 2:** A branch arises from the palm at P 8, runs along the ring finger to its tip (SJ 1), and links with the San Jiao meridian.
CONNECTING CHANNEL	•After separating from the main channel at P 6 on the wrist, this channel spreads out between the two tendons and follows the Pericardium channel upward to the Pericardium, after which it connects with the Heart.
DIVERGENT CHANNEL	•After separating from the main channel at a point 3 cun below the axilla, this channel enters the chest and communicates with the San Jiao. •**BRANCH:** A branch ascends across the throat, emerging behind the ear where it converges with the San Jiao channel.
MUSCULAR REGION	•This channel begins on the palmar aspect of the middle finger and follows the Muscle Channel of the Lung upward, connecting first at the medial aspect of the elbow, and again below the axilla. •From here, the channel descends, spreading over the front and back sides of the ribs. •**BRANCH:** A branch enters the chest below the axilla and spreads over the chest, connecting at the diaphragm.

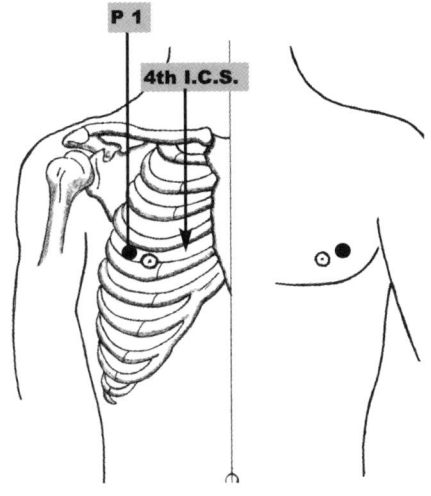

P 1

4th I.C.S.

LOCATION:
In the fourth intercostal space, 1 cun lateral to the nipple.

INDICATIONS:
Suffocating sensation in the chest, pain in the hypochondriac region, intercostal neuralgia, angina pectoris, swelling and pain of the axillary region.

METHOD:
Puncture obliquely 0.2-0.4 cun. Deep puncture is not advisable.

NOTES:

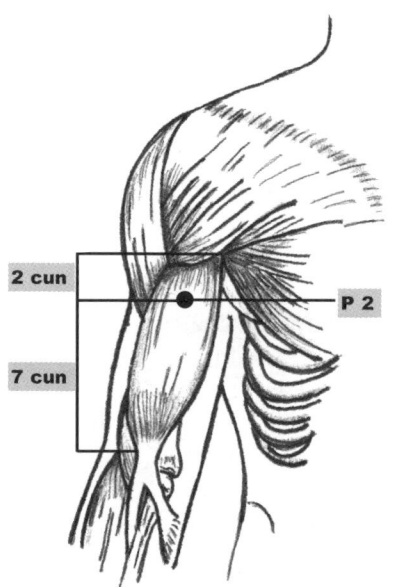

2 cun

P 2

7 cun

LOCATION:
2 cun below the level of the anterior axillary fold, between the two heads of m.biceps brachii.

INDICATIONS:
Cardiac pain, angina, palpitation, distention of the hypochondriac region, cough, pain in the chest, back, flank, and the medial aspect of the arm.

METHOD:
Puncture perpendicularly 0.5-0.7 cun.

NOTES:

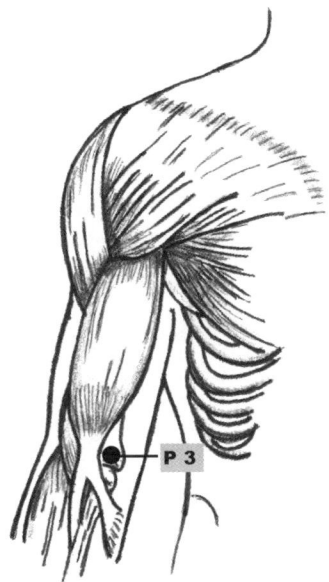

P 3

LOCATION:
On the transverse cubital crease, at the ulnar side of the tendon of m. biceps brachii.

INDICATIONS:
Cardiac pain, rheumatic heart disease, myocarditis, bronchitis, palpitation, febrile diseases, irritability, stomachache, acute gastroenteritis, enteritis, vomiting, pain in the elbow and arm, tremor of the hand and arm, heat exhaustion.

METHOD:
Puncture perpendicularly 0.5-0.7 cun, or prick with a three-edged needle to cause bleeding.

NOTES:

XI-CLEFT POINT

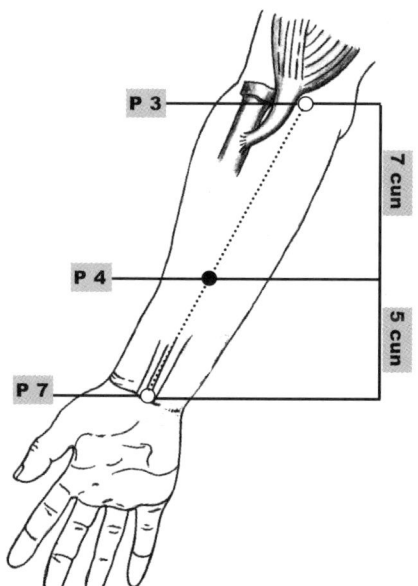

LOCATION:
5 cun above the transverse crease of the wrist, on the line connecting P 3 and P 7, between the tendons of m. palmaris longus and m. flexor carpi radialis.

INDICATIONS:
Cardiac pain, angina pectoris, rheumatic heart disease, myocarditis, palpitation, epistaxis, hematemesis, hemoptysis, chest pain, pleurisy, furuncle, mastitis, epilepsy, spasms of the diaphragm, hysteria.

METHOD:
Puncture perpendicularly 0.5-1.0 cun.

NOTES:

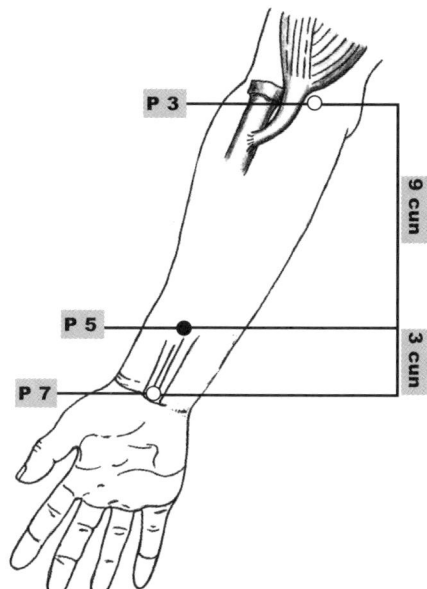

P 3

9 cun

P 5

3 cun

P 7

LOCATION:
3 cun above the transverse crease of the wrist, between the tendons of m.palmaris longus and m.flexor carpi radialis.

INDICATIONS:
Cardiac pain, rheumatic heart disease, palpitation, stomach ache, vomiting, febrile diseases, irritability, malaria, mental disorders, hysteria, psychosis, epilepsy, seizures, swelling of the axilla, contracture of the elbow and arm.

METHOD:
Puncture perpendicularly 0.5-1.0 cun.

NOTES:

267

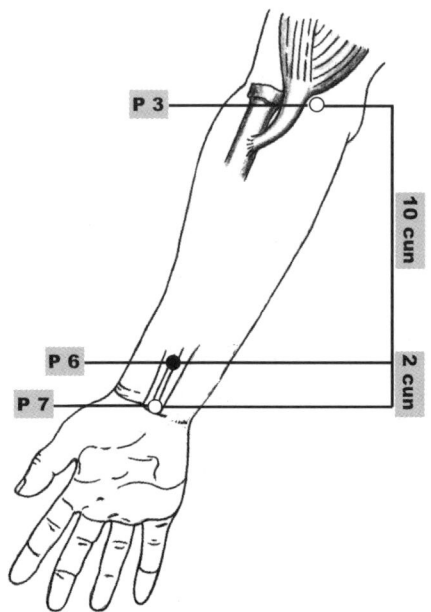

P 3

10 cun

P 6

2 cun

P 7

LOCATION:
2 cun above the transverse crease of the wrist, between the tendons of m.palmaris longus and m.flexor carpi radialis.

INDICATIONS:
Cardiac pain, angina pectoris, rheumatic heart disease, palpitation, stuffy chest, chest pain, asthma, pain in the hypochondriac region, spasms of the diaphragm, stomach ache, abdominal pain, nausea, vomiting, hiccup, mental disorders, epilepsy, seizures, insomnia, febrile diseases, irritability, hysteria, malaria, contracture and pain of the elbow and arm, shock, migraine headache, hyperthyroidism, swollen & painful throat, pain associated with surgery.

METHOD:
Puncture perpendicularly 0.5-0.8 cun.

NOTES:

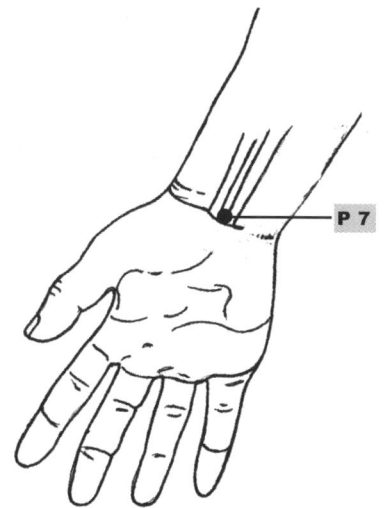

LOCATION:

In the middle of the transverse crease of the wrist, between the tendons of m.palmaris longus and m.flexor carpi radialis.

INDICATIONS:

Cardiac pain, myocarditis, palpitation, stomachache, vomiting, gastritis, mental disorders, epilepsy, stuffy chest, pain in the hypochondriac region, intercostal neuralgia, convulsion, insomnia, irritability, foul breath, tonsillitis, diseases and pain of the wrist joint.

METHOD:

Puncture perpendicularly 0.3-0.5 cun.

NOTES:

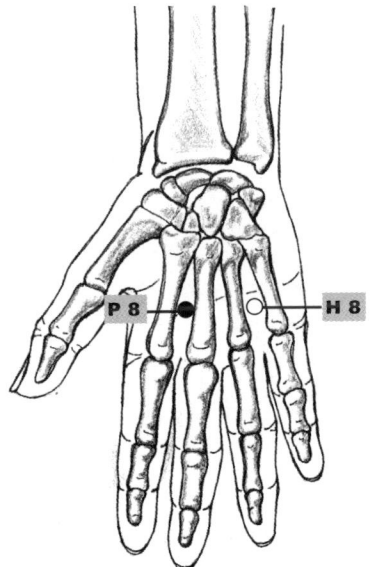

LOCATION:
On the transverse crease of the palm, between the second and third metacarpal bones. When the fist is clenched, the point is just below the tip of the middle finger.

INDICATIONS:
Cardiac pain, angina pectoris, mental disorder, epilepsy, gastritis, foul breath, stomatitis, fungus infection of the hand and foot, excessive sweating of the palms, numb fingers, vomiting, nausea, coma from stroke, heat exhaustion, frightened fainting among infants, hysteria.

METHOD:
Puncture perpendicularly 0.3-0.5 cun.

NOTES:

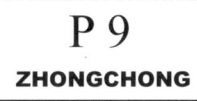
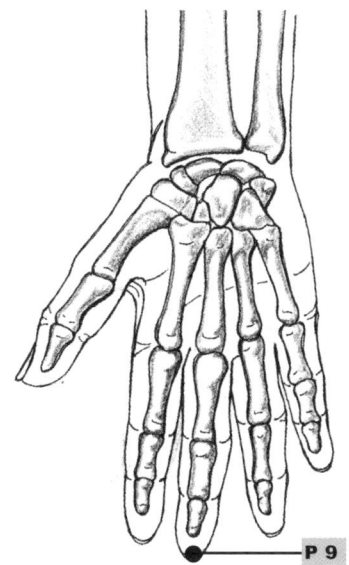

P 9

LOCATION:
In the center of the tip of the middle finger.

INDICATIONS:
Cardiac pain, angina pectoris, palpitation, loss of consciousness, shock, apoplectic coma, aphasia with stiffness and swelling of the tongue, febrile diseases, heat stroke, convulsion, high fever, feverish sensation in the palm.

METHOD:
Puncture superficially 0.1 cun or prick with a three-edged needle to cause bleeding.

NOTES:

NOTES

NOTES

SAN JIAO
CHANNEL

SAN JIAO MERIDIAN OF HAND SHAO-YANG

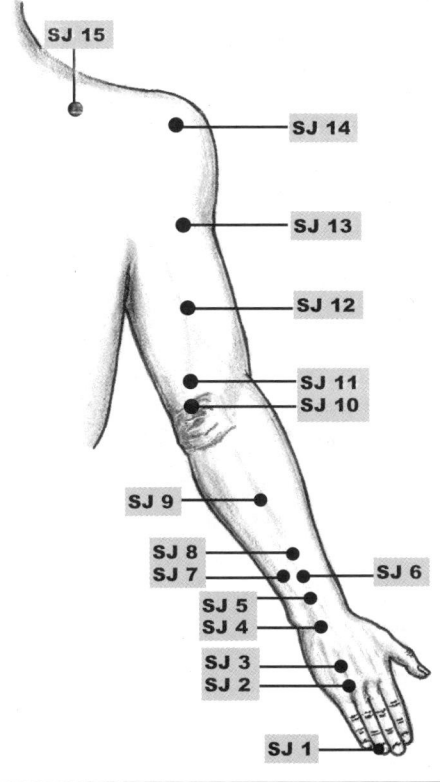

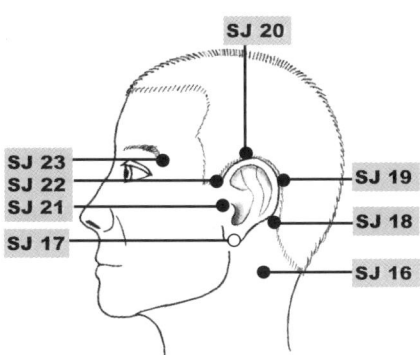

CHANNEL/ORGAN RELATIONSHIPS

• This channel is associated with the San Jiao channel and is connected with the Pericardium.

THERAPEUTIC INDICATIONS

• Diseases of the lateral aspect of the head, of the ear, eye, chest, hypochondrium and throat; febrile diseases and other diseases of areas this meridian supplies.

PATHOLOGY

Channel: Swelling and pain in the throat, pain or swelling in the cheek and jaw, abdominal distention, edema, enuresis, dysuria, redness in the eyes, deafness, tinnitus, pain in the retroauricular region or along the lateral aspect of the shoulder, upper arm, and elbow, and pain in the outer canthus.

Organ: Abdominal distention & hardness, enuresis, frequent urination, edema, dysuria.

SAN JIAO MERIDIAN OF HAND SHAO-YANG

GENERAL PATHWAY	● Originating on the ulnar aspect of the 4th ringer tip, it ascends between the 4th & 5th metacarpal bones on the dorsum of the wrist. ● It then traverses the forearm between the ulna and radius & continues upward across the olecrenon and the lateral aspect of the upper arm to the shoulder. ● Here it intersects the Small Intestine channel at SI 12 and meets the DU channel at DU 14 before crossing back over the shoulder. ● It then intersects the Gall Bladder channel at GB 21, from which it enters the supraclavicular fossa & travels to the mid-chest region at Ren 17. ● From here, the channel joins with the pericardium & descends across the diaphragm to the abdomen, linking successively with the upper, middle, & lower jiaos of the San Jiao. **BRANCHES:** ● **BRANCH 1:** A branch of the main channel separates in the chest at Ren 17 and ascends to emerge superficially at the neck. Here, it proceeds upward behind the ear, intersecting the Gall Bladder channel at GB 6 and GB 4 on the forehead before winding downward across the cheek to below the eye. It intersects the Small Intestine channel at SI 18. ● **BRANCH 2:** A branch separates behind the auricle & enters the ear. It then emerges in front of the ear where it intersects with the Small Intestine channel at SI 19, crosses in front of the Gall Bladder channel at GB 3, and traverses the cheek to terminate at the outer canthus at SJ 23.
CONNECTING CHANNEL	● After separating from the main channel at SJ 5 on the wrist, this channel proceeds up the posterior aspect of the arm and over the shoulder, converging with the Pericardium channel in the chest.
DIVERGENT CHANNEL	● After separating from the main channel at the vertex, this channel descends into the supraclavicular fossa and across the San Jiao, dispersing in the chest.
MUSCULAR REGION	● This channel arises at the tip of the 4th finger and connects at the dorsum of the wrist. ● From here, the channel proceeds upward along the forearm and connects with the olecrenon of the elbow before continuing upward along the lateral aspect of the upper arm. ● It then passes over the shoulder to the neck, where it joins with the Small Intestine muscle channel. **BRANCHES:** ● **BRANCH 1:** A branch separates at the angle of the mandible and connects with the base of the tongue. ● **BRANCH 2:** Another branch travels from the mandible upward in front of the ear to the outer canthus, then across the temple where it connects at the side of the forehead.

SJ 1
GUANCHONG

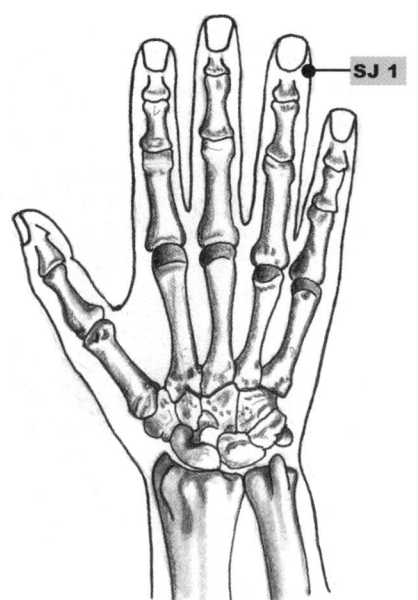

SJ 1

LOCATION:
On the lateral side of the ring finger, about 0.1 cun posterior to the corner of the nail.

INDICATIONS:
Headache, redness of the eyes, conjunctivitis, sore throat, stiffness of the tongue, laryngitis, febrile diseases, irritability.

METHOD:
Puncture superficially 0.1 cun, or prick with a three-edged needle to cause bleeding.

NOTES:

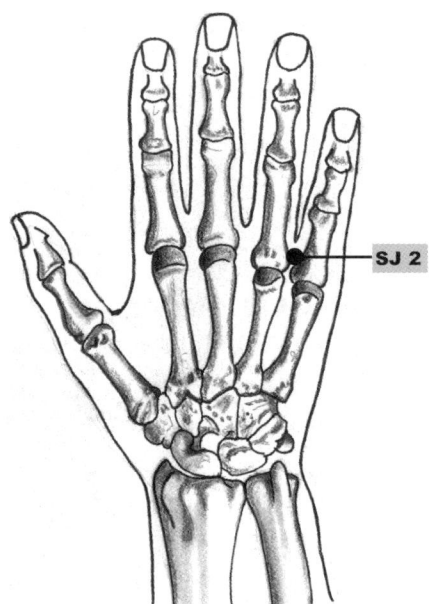

SJ 2

LOCATION:
When the fist is clenched, the point is located in the depression proximal to the margin of the web between the ring and small fingers.

INDICATIONS:
Headache, redness of the eyes, sudden deafness, sore throat, laryngopharyngitis, malaria, pain in the hand & arm, pain & swelling of the fingers.

METHOD:
Puncture obliquely 0.3-0.5 cun towards the interspace of the metacarpal bones.

NOTES:

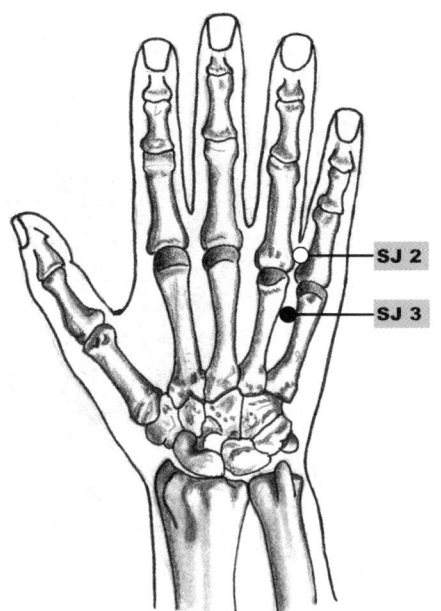

SJ 2

SJ 3

LOCATION:
When the fist is clenched, the point is on the dorsum of the hand between the fourth and fifth metacarpal bones, in the depression proximal to the metacarpophalangeal joint.

INDICATIONS:
Headache, redness of the eyes, deafness, deaf-mutism, tinnitus, sore throat, febrile diseases, pain in the shoulder, back, elbow and arm, motor impairment of the fingers, intercostal neuralgia.

METHOD:
Puncture perpendicularly 0.3-0.5 cun.

NOTES:

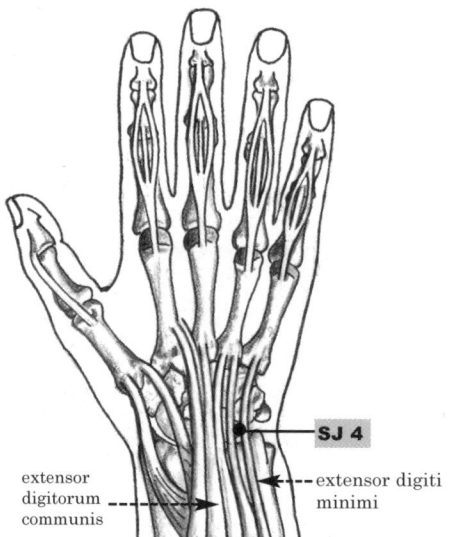

SJ 4

extensor
digitorum - - - -
communis

- - extensor digiti
minimi

LOCATION:
On the transverse crease of the dorsum of the wrist, in the depression lateral to the tendon of m.extensor digitorum communis.

INDICATIONS:
Pain in the arm, shoulder and wrist, pain & diseases of the soft tissue of the wrist, common cold, tonsillitis, malaria, deafness, thirst.

METHOD:
Puncture perpendicularly 0.3-0.5 cun.

NOTES:

LUO-CONNECTING POINT
CONFLUENT POINT OF THE YANG WEI

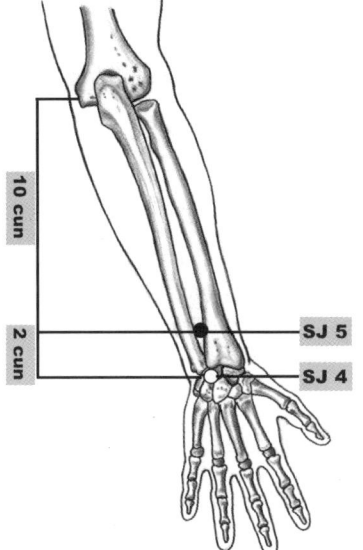

LOCATION:
2 cun above SJ 4, between the radius and the ulna.

INDICATIONS:
Febrile diseases, common cold, high fever, pneumonia, perotitis, migraine headache, headache, stiff neck, pain in the cheek, strained neck, deafness, tinnitus, enuresis, pain in the hypochondriac region, motor impairment of the elbow and arm, pain of the fingers, pain in the joints of the upper limb & hand, tremor, hemiplegia, paralysis.

METHOD:
Puncture perpendicularly 0.5-1.0 cun.

NOTES:

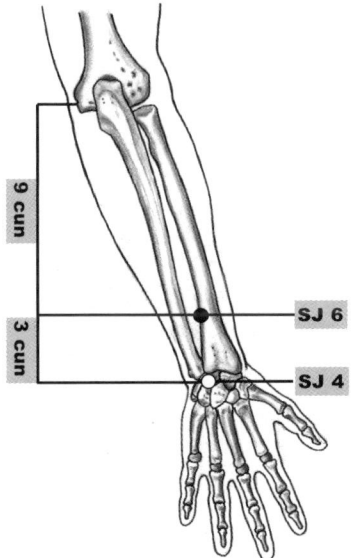

9 cun

3 cun

SJ 6

SJ 4

LOCATION:
3 cun above SJ 4, between the radius and the ulna, on the radial side of m.extensor digitorum.

INDICATIONS:
Tinnitus, deafness, pain in the hypochondriac region, angina pectoris, intercostal neuralgia, pleurisy, insufficient lactation, vomiting, constipation, febrile diseases, aching and heavy sensation of the shoulder and back, pain in the shoulder & arm, sudden hoarseness of voice.

METHOD:
Puncture perpendicularly 0.8-1.2 cun.

NOTES:

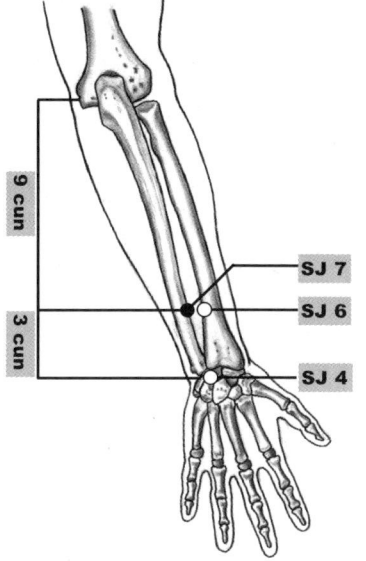

9 cun

3 cun

SJ 7

SJ 6

SJ 4

LOCATION:
At the level with SJ 6, about one finger-breadth lateral to SJ 6, on the radial side of the ulna.

INDICATIONS:
Deafness, pain in the ear, epilepsy, seizures, pain of the arm.

METHOD:
Puncture perpendicularly 0.5-1.0 cun.

NOTES:

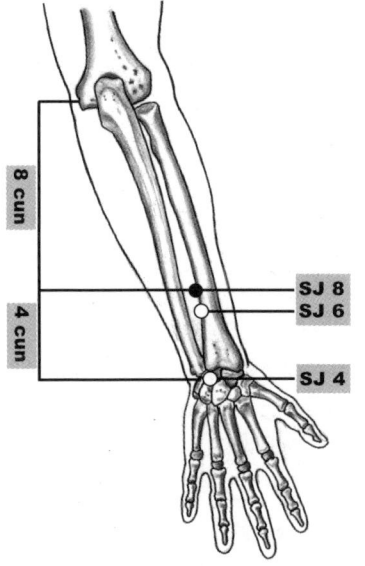

LOCATION:
4 cun above SJ 4, between the radius and the ulna.

INDICATIONS:
Deafness, aphasia, sudden hoarseness of the voice, pain in the chest and hypochondriac region, pain in the hand and arm, toothache, post-operative pain associated with pneumonectomy.

METHOD:
Puncture perpendicularly 0.5-1.0 cun.

NOTES:

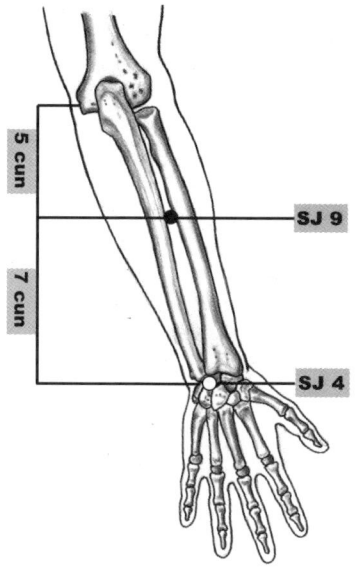

5 cun

7 cun

SJ 9

SJ 4

LOCATION:
On the lateral side of the forearm, 5 cun below the olecrenon, between the radius and the ulna.

INDICATIONS:
Deafness, toothache, migraine, headache, vertigo, sudden hoarseness of voice, pain in the forearm, paralysis of the upper limb, neurasthenia, nephritis.

METHOD:
Puncture perpendicularly 0.5-1.0 cun.

NOTES:

285

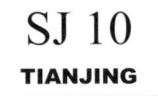
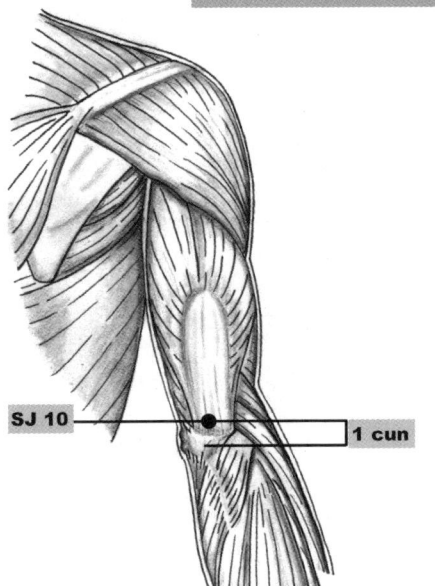

SJ 10 ——— | 1 cun

LOCATION:
When the elbow is flexed, the point is in the depression about 1 cun superior to the olecrenon.

INDICATIONS:
Migraine, pain in the neck, shoulder, and arm, diseases of the soft tissue of the elbow, epilepsy, scrofula (use moxibustion), goiter, tonsillitis, urticaria.

METHOD:
Puncture perpendicularly 0.3-0.5 cun.

NOTES:

286

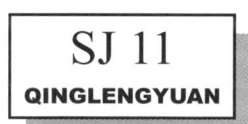

SJ 11
QINGLENGYUAN

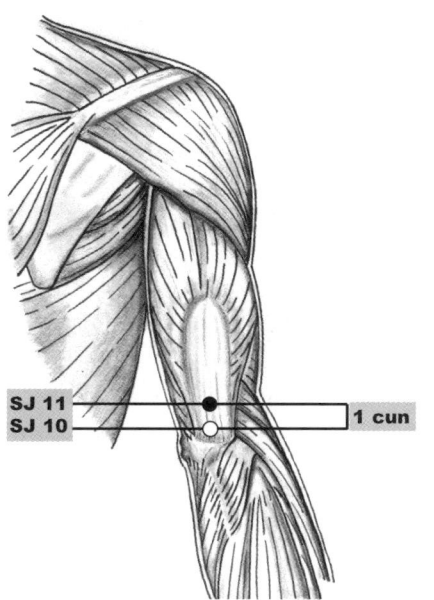

SJ 11
SJ 10
1 cun

LOCATION:
1 cun above SJ 10 when the elbow is flexed.

INDICATIONS:
Motor impairment and pain of the shoulder and arm, migraine, headache, pain in the eyes.

METHOD:
Puncture perpendicularly 0.3-0.5 cun.

NOTES:

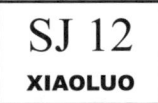

SJ 12
XIAOLUO

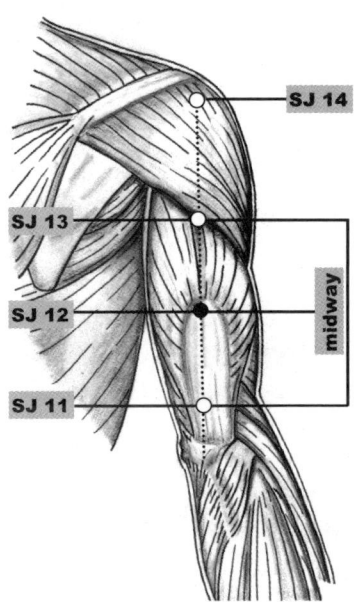

SJ 14

SJ 13

midway

SJ 12

SJ 11

LOCATION:
On the line joining the olecrenon and SJ 14, midway between SJ 11 and SJ 13.

INDICATIONS:
Headache, neck rigidity, toothache, motor impairment and pain of the arm, seizures.

METHOD:
Puncture perpendicularly 0.5-0.7 cun.

NOTES:

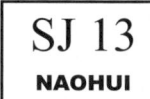
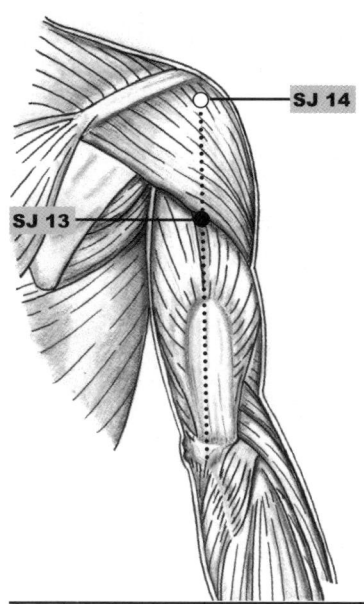

SJ 14

SJ 13

LOCATION:
On the line joining SJ 14 and the olecrenon, on the posterior border of m.deltoideus.

INDICATIONS:
Goiter, pain in the shoulder and arm.

METHOD:
Puncture perpendicularly 0.5-0.8 cun.

NOTES:

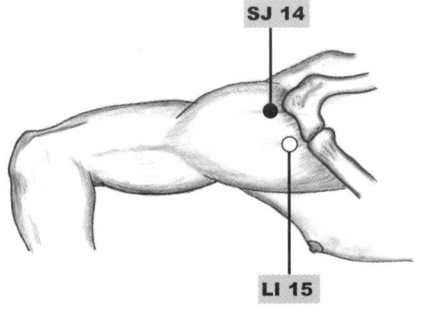

SJ 14

LI 15

LOCATION:

Posterior and inferior to the acromion, in the depression about 1 cun posterior to LI 15 when the arm is abducted.

INDICATIONS:

Pain and motor impairment of the shoulder and upper arm, pain in the shoulder joint, perifocal inflammation of the shoulder joint, hemiplegia, hypertension, excessive sweating.

METHOD:

Puncture perpendicularly 0.7-1.0 cun.

NOTES:

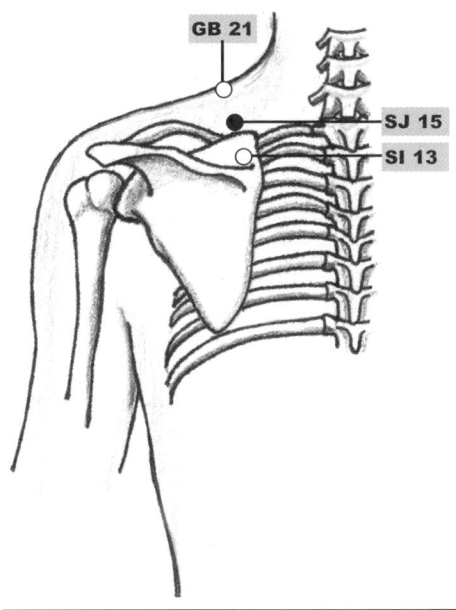

LOCATION:

Midway between GB 21 and SI 13, on the superior angle of the scapula.

INDICATIONS:

Pain in the shoulder and elbow, stiffness of the neck, pain or soreness in the region of the scapula and back of the neck, inflammation of the supraspinatus tendon, fever.

METHOD:

Puncture perpendicularly 0.3-0.5 cun.

NOTES:

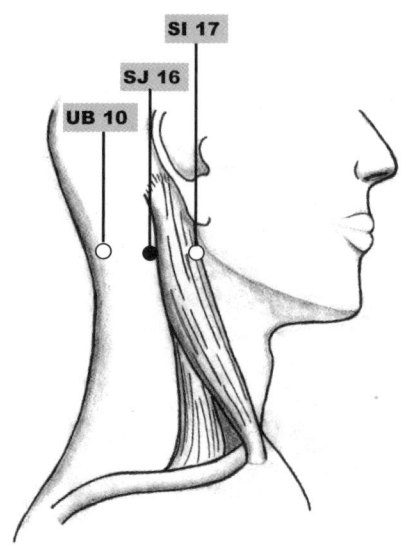

SI 17
SJ 16
UB 10

LOCATION:
Posterior and inferior to the mastoid process, on the posterior border of m.sternocleidomastoideus, almost level with SI 17 and UB 10.

INDICATIONS:
Headache, neck rigidity, facial swelling, blurry vision, tinnitus, sore throat, sudden deafness.

METHOD:
Puncture perpendicularly 0.3-0.5 cun.

NOTES:

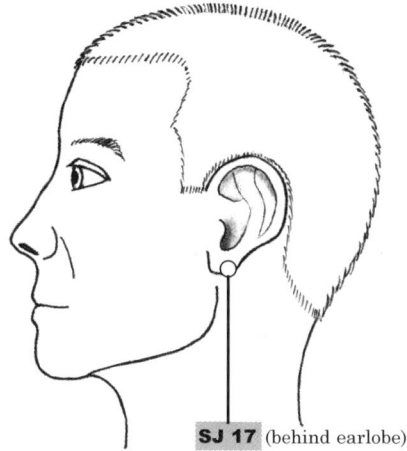

SJ 17 (behind earlobe)

LOCATION:
Posterior to the lobule of the ear, in the depression between the mandible and the mastoid process.

INDICATIONS:
Tinnitus, deafness, deaf-mutism, parotitis, otorrhea, facial paralysis, toothache, swelling of the cheek, sore eyes, scrofula, trismus, temporomandibular arthritis.

METHOD:
Puncture perpendicularly 0.5-1.0 cun.

NOTES:

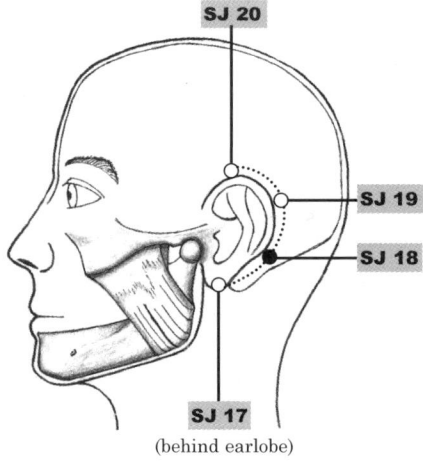

SJ 20

SJ 19

SJ 18

SJ 17
(behind earlobe)

LOCATION:

In the center of the mastoid process, at the junction of the middle and lower third of the curve formed by SJ 17 and SJ 20 posterior to the helix.

INDICATIONS:

Headache, tinnitus, deafness, infantile convulsion.

METHOD:

Puncture subcutaneously 0.3-0.5 cun or prick with a three-edged needle to cause bleeding.

NOTES:

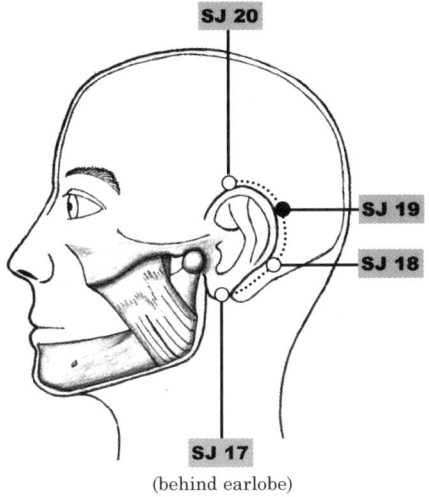

SJ 20

SJ 19

SJ 18

SJ 17
(behind earlobe)

LOCATION:
Posterior to the ear, at the junction of the upper and middle third of the curve formed by SJ 17 and SJ 20 behind the helix.

INDICATIONS:
Headache, tinnitus, deafness, ear ache, pain in the ear, otitis media, infantile convulsion, vomiting.

METHOD:
Puncture obliquely 0.3-0.5 cun.

NOTES:

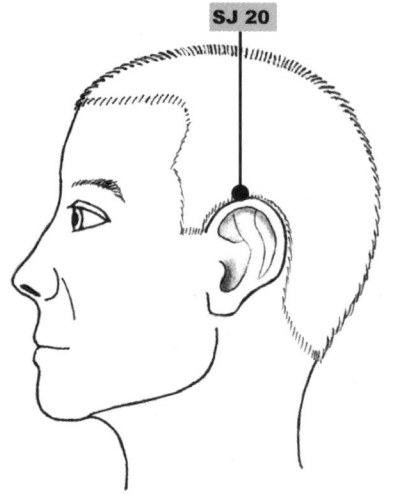

SJ 20

SJ 20
JIAOSUN

LOCATION:
Directly above the ear apex, when the ear is folded forwards, within the hair line.

INDICATIONS:
Tinnitus, redness, pain and swelling of the eye, swelling of the gum, toothache, parotitis, panus, red & swollen ear lobe.

METHOD:
Puncture subcutaneously 0.3-0.5 cun.

NOTES:

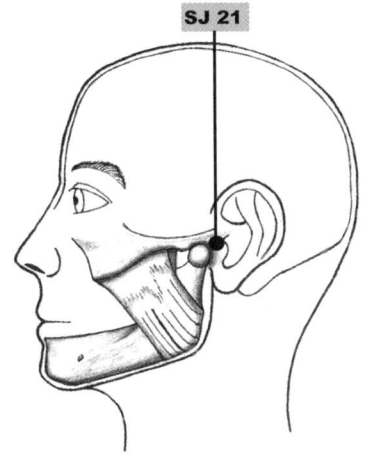

SJ 21

LOCATION:

In the depression anterior to the supratragic notch and slightly superior to the condyloid process of the mandible. The point is located with the mouth open.

INDICATIONS:

Tinnitus, deafness, deaf-mutism, otorrhea, toothache, stiffness of the lip, temporomandibular arthritis.

METHOD:

Puncture perpendicularly 0.3-0.5 cun.

NOTES:

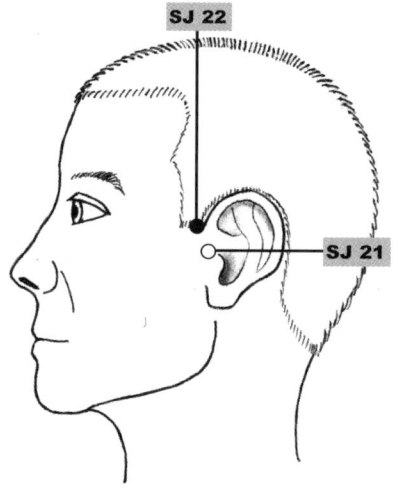

LOCATION:
Anterior and superior to SJ 21, at the level with the root of the auricle, on the posterior border of the hairline of the temple where the superficial temporal artery passes.

INDICATIONS:
Migraine, headache, tinnitus, lockjaw, facial paralysis.

METHOD:
Puncture obliquely 0.1-0.3 cun. Avoid puncturing the artery.

NOTES:

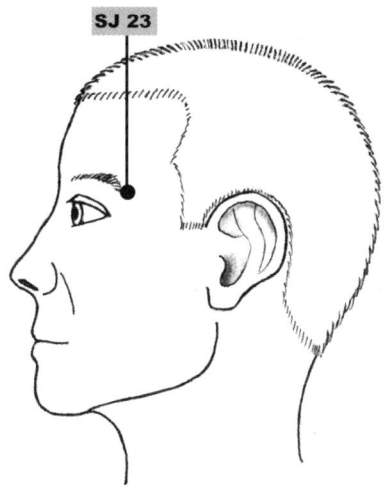

SJ 23

LOCATION:
In the depression at the lateral end of the eyebrow.

INDICATIONS:
Headache, redness & pain of the eye, blurry vision, eye diseases, twitching of the eyelid, toothache, facial paralysis.

METHOD:
Puncture subcutaneously 0.3-0.5 cun.

NOTES:

NOTES

NOTES

GALLBLADDER CHANNEL

GALLBLADDER MERIDIAN OF FOOT SHAO-YANG

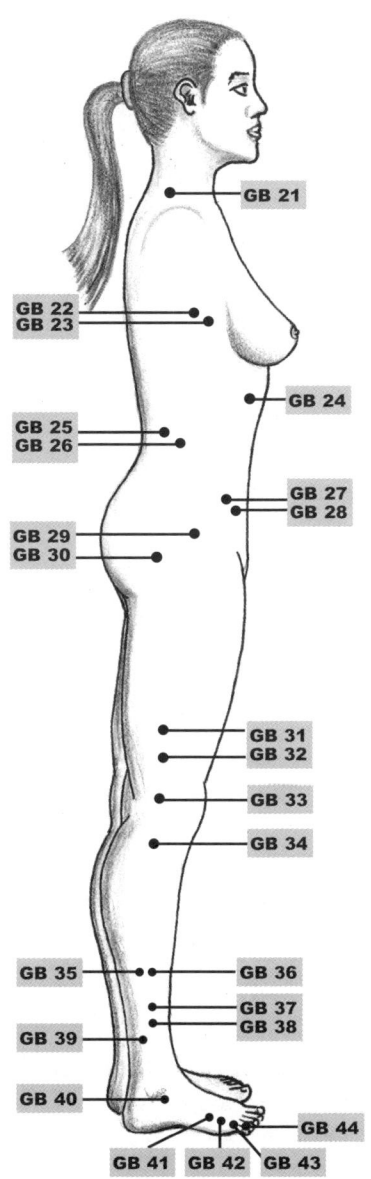

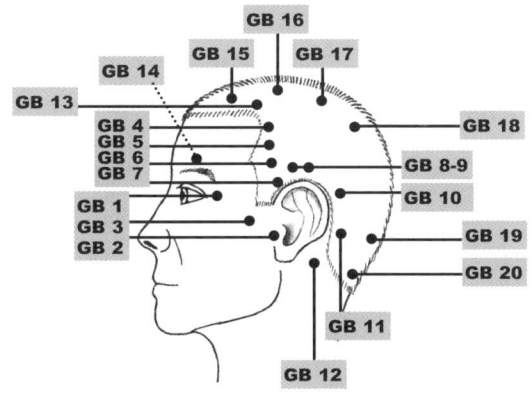

GB 16
GB 15 GB 17
GB 14
GB 13
GB 4
GB 5
GB 6
GB 7
GB 18
GB 8-9
GB 1
GB 3
GB 2
GB 10
GB 19
GB 20
GB 11
GB 12

GB 21

GB 22
GB 23

GB 24

GB 25
GB 26

GB 27
GB 28

GB 29
GB 30

GB 31
GB 32

GB 33

GB 34

GB 35
GB 36

GB 37
GB 38
GB 39

GB 40

GB 44

GB 41 GB 42 GB 43

PATHOLOGY

Channel: Headache, alternating fever & chills, ashen complexion, pain in the outer canthus, eye or jaw, blurry vision, bitter taste in the mouth, scrofula, deafness, swelling or pain in the sub-axillary region or supraclavicular fossa, pain along the lateral aspect of the chest, hypochondrium, thigh and lower limbs.

Organ: Pain in the costal region or chest, vomiting, bitter taste in the mouth.

CHANNEL/ORGAN RELATIONSHIPS

● This channel is associated with the Gallbladder & connects with the Liver.

● It is also joined directly with the Heart.

THERAPEUTIC INDICATIONS

● Diseases of the lateral head, eye, ear, and throat; mental disorders, febrile diseases, and other diseases of areas the meridian supplies.

GENERAL PATHWAY	• This channel begins at the outer canthus of the eye and traverses the temple to SJ 22. It then ascends to the corner of the forehead where it intersects ST 8 before descending behind the ear. • From here, it proceeds along the neck in front of the San Jiao channel & crosses the Small Intestine channel at SI 17. • Next, at the top of the shoulder it turns back and runs behind the San Jiao channel to intersect the DU channel at DU 14 on the spine. • The channel then turns downward into the supraclavicular fossa. • Next, the channel runs downward from the supraclavicular fossa, passes in front of the axilla along the lateral aspect of the chest and through the free ends of the floating ribs to the hip region where it meets Branch #2. • Then it descends along the lateral aspect of the thigh to the lateral side of the knee. • Going further downward along the anterior aspect of the fibula extending to its lower end, it reaches the anterior aspect of the external malleolus. • It then follows the dorsum of the foot to the lateral side of the tip of the 4th toe. **BRANCHES:** • **BRANCH 1:** One branch of the main channel emerges behind the auricle and enters the ear at SJ 17. Emerging in front of the ear, this branch intersects the Small Intestine channel at SI 19, and the Stomach channel at ST 7 before terminating behind the outer canthus. • **BRANCH 2:** A branch separates at the outer canthus and proceeds downward to ST 5 on the jaw. Then, crossing the San Jiao channel, it returns upward to the infraorbital region before descending again to the neck, where it joins the main channel in the supraclavicular fossa. It then descends further into the chest, crossing the diaphragm & connecting with the Liver before joining with its associated organ, the Gall Bladder. Moving along the inside of the ribs, it emerges in the inguinal region of the lower abdomen & winds around the genitals, submerging again in the hip at GB 30. • **BRANCH 3:** The branch of the dorsum of the foot leaves from GB 41, runs between the 1st & 2nd metatarsal bones to the medial tip of the big toe, then crosses under the toenail to join with the Liver channel at LIV 1.
CONNECTING CHANNEL	• After separating from the main channel at GB 37 on the lateral aspect of the lower leg, this channel connects with the Liver channel, proceeds downward and disperses over the dorsum of the foot.

304

DIVERGENT CHANNEL	• After diverging from the main channel on the thigh, this channel crosses over & enters the lower abdomen in the pelvic region where it converges with the Divergent channel of the Liver. • From here it crosses between the lower ribs, connects with the Gall Bladder and spreads through the Liver before proceeding upward across the Heart & esophagus, dispersing in the face. • Here it connects with the eye and rejoins the Gall Bladder main channel at the outer canthus.
MUSCULAR REGION	• Beginning at the 4th toe, it joins with the external malleolus, then proceeds up the lateral side of the leg where it connects with the knee. • It then proceeds upward across the ribs & anterior to the axilla, connecting with the breast and then above the collar bone (ST 12). • Another part of the main channel extends from the axilla upward across the clavicle, emerging in front of the Spleen channel, then continues upward behind the ear to the temple. • From here, it continues to the vertex, where it joins its bilateral counterpart. **BRANCHES:** • **BRANCH 1:** A branch starts at the upper fibula and ascends along the thigh. **SUB-BRANCH 1:** A sub-branch of Branch #1 travels anteriorly, joining the thigh above point ST 32. **SUB-BRANCH 2:** Another sub-branch of Branch #1 travels posteriorly, & joins with the sacrum. • **BRANCH 2:** A branch descends from the temple across the cheek before joining with the bridge of the nose. **SUB-BRANCH:** A sub-branch of Branch #2 connects with the outer canthus.

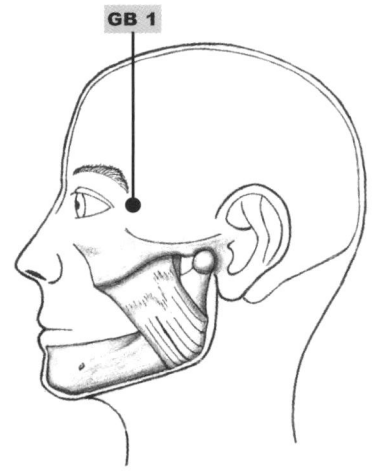

GB 1

LOCATION:
0.5 cun lateral to the outer canthus, in the depression on the lateral side of the orbit.

INDICATIONS:
Headache, keratitis, ametropia, night blindness, atrophy of the optic nerve, redness and pain of the eyes, failing vision, lacrimation, deviation of the eye and mouth.

METHOD:
Puncture subcutaneously 0.3-0.5 cun.

NOTES:

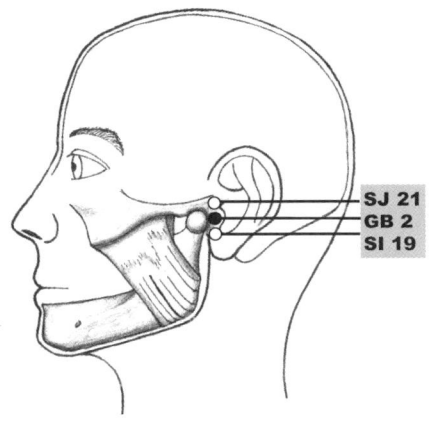

LOCATION:

Anterior to the intertragic notch, at the posterior border of the condyloid process of the mandible. The point is located with the mouth open.

INDICATIONS:

Deafness, deaf-mutism, tinnitus, otitis media, toothache, motor impairment of the temporomandibular joint, mumps, deviation of the eye and mouth, facial paralysis.

METHOD:

Puncture perpendicularly 0.5-0.7 cun, with the mouth open.

NOTES:

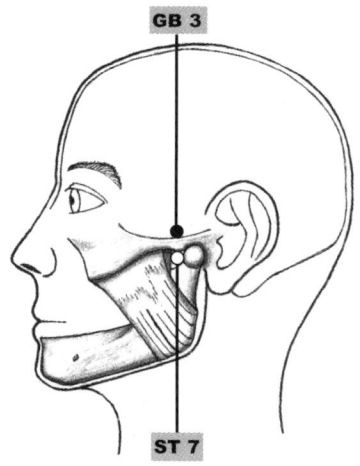

LOCATION:
In the front of the ear, on the upper border of the zygomatic arch, in the depression directly above ST 7.

INDICATIONS:
Headache, deafness, tinnitus, otitis media, diplacusis, deviation of the eye and mouth, toothache, "lockjaw", facial paralysis.

METHOD:
Puncture perpendicularly 0.3-0.5 cun. Deep puncture is not advisable.

NOTES:

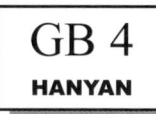

GB 4
HANYAN

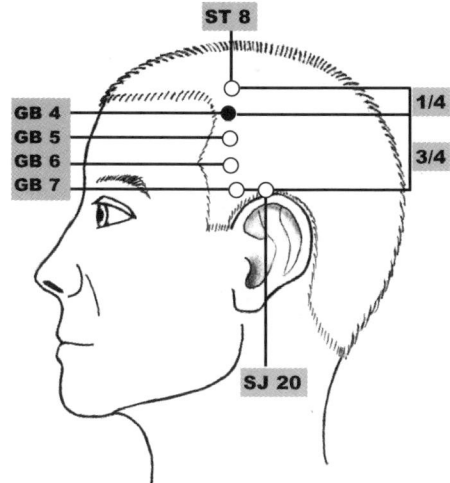

ST 8

GB 4
GB 5
GB 6
GB 7

1/4

3/4

SJ 20

LOCATION:
Within the hairline of the temporal region, at the junction of the upper 1/4 and lower 3/4 of the distance between ST 8 and GB 7.

INDICATIONS:
Migraine, vertigo, tinnitus, rhinitis, pain in the outer canthus, toothache, convulsions, epilepsy, seizures.

METHOD:
Puncture subcutaneously 0.3-0.5 cun.

NOTES:

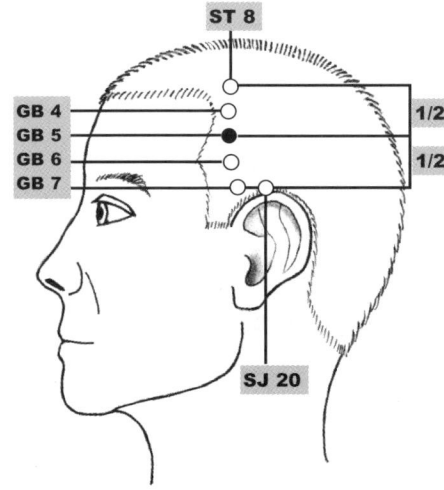

ST 8

GB 4
GB 5
GB 6
GB 7

1/2

1/2

SJ 20

LOCATION:
Within the hairline of the temporal region, midway of the border line connecting ST 8 and GB 7.

INDICATIONS:
Migraine, pain in the outer canthus, facial swelling, toothache, neurasthenia.

METHOD:
Puncture subcutaneously 0.3-0.5 cun.

NOTES:

310

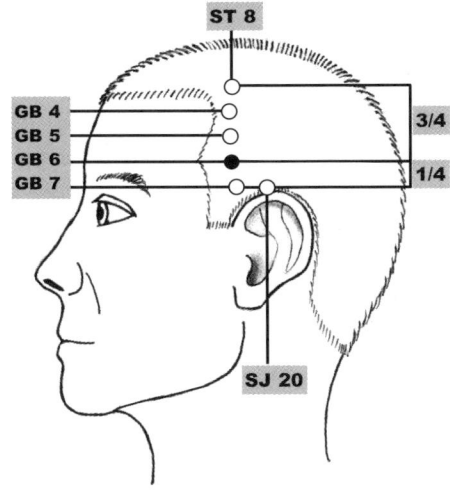

LOCATION:

Within the hairline, at the junction of the lower 1/4 and upper 3/4 of the distance between ST 8 and GB 7.

INDICATIONS:

Migraine, pain in the outer canthus, tinnitus, frequent sneezing, toothache, facial swelling, neurasthenia.

METHOD:

Puncture subcutaneously 0.3-0.5 cun.

NOTES:

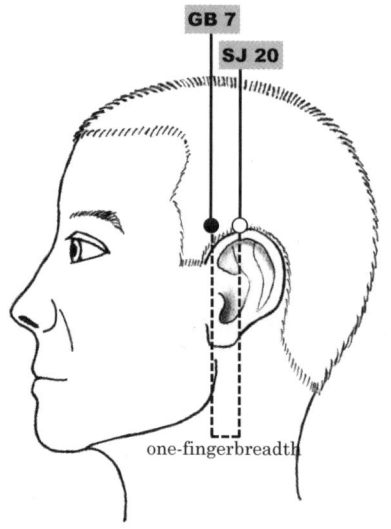

GB 7
SJ 20

one-fingerbreadth

LOCATION:
Directly above the posterior border of the pre-auricular hairline, about one finger-breadth anterior to SJ 20.

INDICATIONS:
Headache, migraine, swelling of the cheek, trismus, pain in the temporal region, spasms of the temporalis muscle, trigeminal neuralgia, infantile convulsion.

METHOD:
Puncture subcutaneously 0.3-0.5 cun.

NOTES:

312

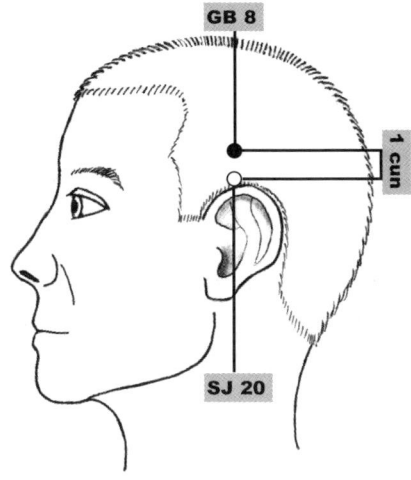

LOCATION:
Superior to the apex of the auricle, 1.5 cun within the hairline, and 1 cun directly above the apex of the ear.

INDICATIONS:
Migraine, vertigo, vomiting, infantile convulsion, eye diseases.

METHOD:
Puncture subcutaneously 0.3-0.5 cun.

NOTES:

313

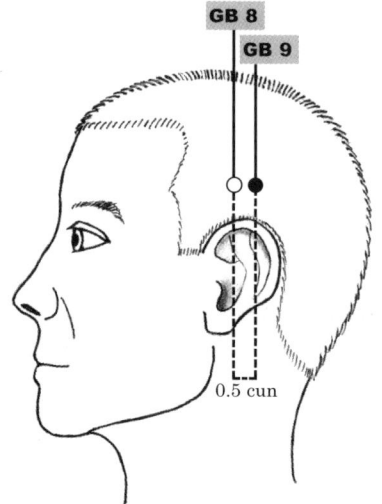

GB 8
GB 9

0.5 cun

LOCATION:
Directly above the posterior border of the auricle, 2 cun within the hairline, about 0.5 cun posterior to GB 8.

INDICATIONS:
Headache, epilepsy, swelling and pain of the gums, gingivitis, goiter, convulsion, seizures.

METHOD:
Puncture subcutaneously 0.3-0.5 cun.

NOTES:

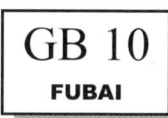

GB 10
FUBAI

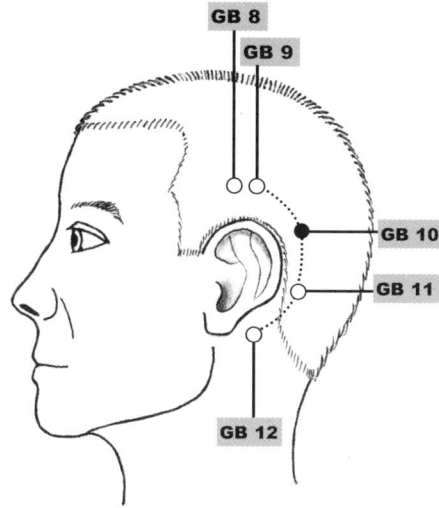

GB 8
GB 9
GB 10
GB 11
GB 12

LOCATION:
Posterior and superior to the mastoid process, midway of the curved line drawn from GB 9 to GB 11.

INDICATIONS:
Headache, tinnitus, deafness, toothache, bronchitis.

METHOD:
Puncture subcutaneously 0.3-0.5 cun.

NOTES:

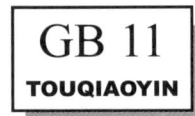

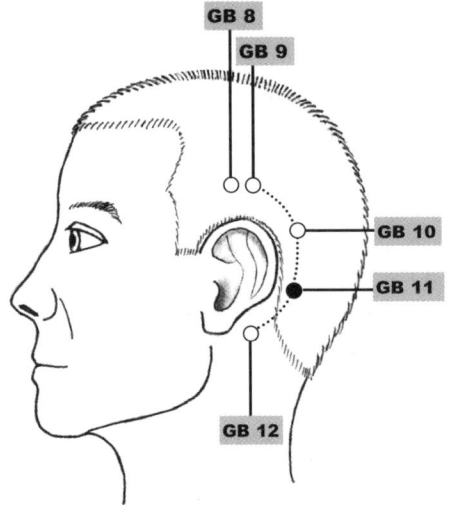

GB 8
GB 9
GB 10
GB 11
GB 12

LOCATION:
Posterior and superior to the mastoid process, on the line connecting GB 10 and GB 12.

INDICATIONS:
Pain of the head and neck, stiff neck, headache, tinnitus, deafness, pain in the ears, ear ache, bronchitis.

METHOD:
Puncture subcutaneously 0.3-0.5 cun.

NOTES:

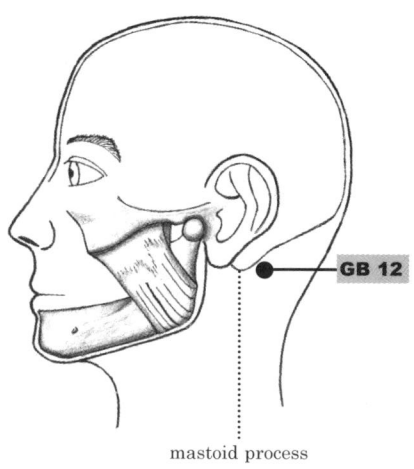

mastoid process

GB 12

LOCATION:
In the depression posterior and inferior to the mastoid process.

INDICATIONS:
Headache, insomnia, facial swelling, facial paralysis, swelling of the cheek, retroauricular pain, deviation of the eye and mouth, toothache, seizures, parotitis.

METHOD:
Puncture obliquely 0.3-0.5 cun.

NOTES:

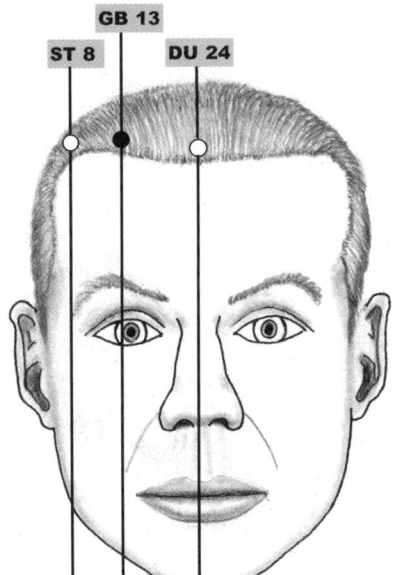

ST 8   GB 13   DU 24

one-third (1.5 cun)   two-thirds (3 cun)

LOCATION:

0.5 cun within the hairline of the fore-head, 3 cun lateral to DU 24.

INDICATIONS:

Headache, stiff neck, insomnia, vertigo, epilepsy, costalgia, seizures, hemiplegia.

METHOD:

Puncture subcutaneously 0.3-0.5 cun.

NOTES:

318

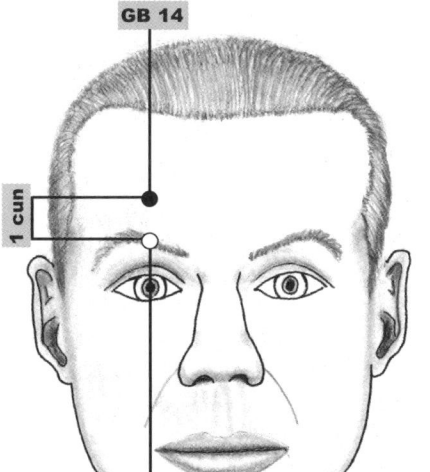

GB 14

1 cun

GB 14

Yuyao

LOCATION:
On the forehead, 1 cun directly above the mid-point of the eyebrow.

INDICATIONS:
Headache in the frontal region, supraorbital neuralgia, facial paralysis, pain of the orbital ridge, eye pain, eye diseases, vertigo, twitching of the eyelids, ptosis of the eyelids, lacrimation.

METHOD:
Puncture subcutaneously 0.3-0.5 cun.

NOTES:

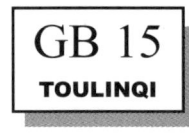

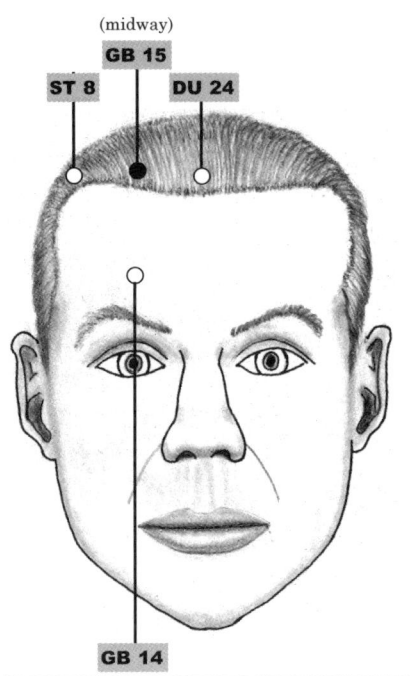

(midway)

GB 15

ST 8   DU 24

GB 14

LOCATION:
Directly above GB 14, 0.5 cun within the hairline, midway between DU 24 and ST 8.

INDICATIONS:
Headache, vertigo, lacrimation, pain in the outer canthus, acute & chronic conjunctivitis, rhinorrhea, nasal obstruction, panus, apoplectic coma, malaria, seizures.

METHOD:
Puncture subcutaneously 0.3-0.5 cun.

NOTES:

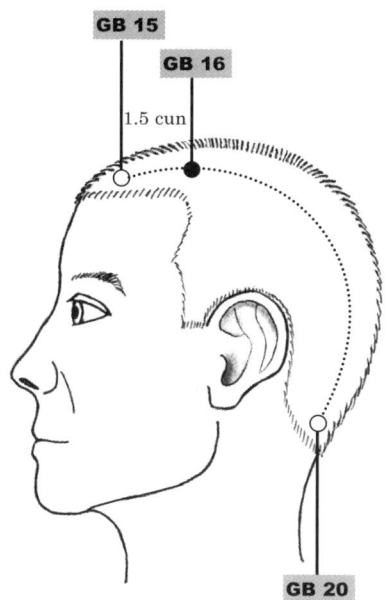

GB 15

GB 16

1.5 cun

GB 20

GB 16
MUCHUANG

LOCATION:
1.5 cun posterior to GB 15, on the line connecting GB 15 and GB 20.

INDICATIONS:
Headache, vertigo, facial edema, conjunctivitis, red and painful eyes, nasal obstruction, toothache, apoplectic coma.

METHOD:
Puncture subcutaneously 0.3-0.5 cun.

NOTES:

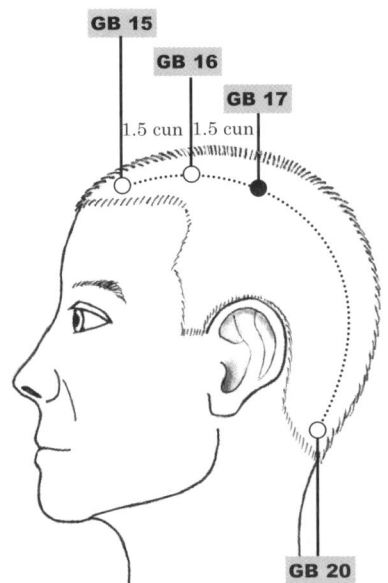

GB 15

GB 16

GB 17

1.5 cun 1.5 cun

GB 20

LOCATION:

1.5 cun posterior to GB 16, on the line joining GB 15 and GB 20.

INDICATIONS:

Migraine, headache, stiff neck, vertigo, toothache, vomiting.

METHOD:

Puncture subcutaneously 0.3-0.5 cun.

NOTES:

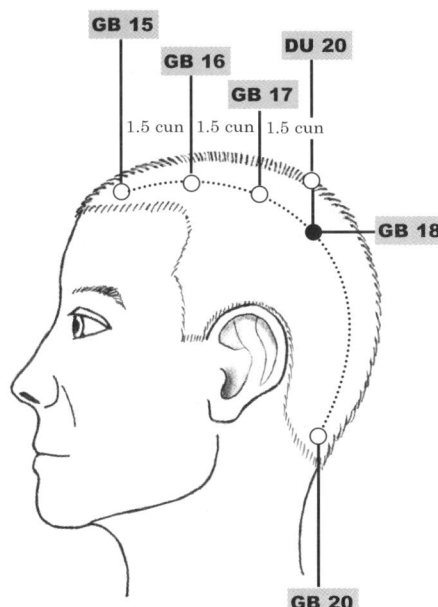

GB 15

GB 16

DU 20

GB 17

1.5 cun | 1.5 cun | 1.5 cun

GB 18

GB 20

LOCATION:
1.5 cun posterior to GB 17, on the line connecting GB 15 and GB 20.

INDICATIONS:
Headache, vertigo, epistaxis, rhinorrhea, occluded nose, common cold, bronchitis, eye diseases.

METHOD:
Puncture subcutaneously 0.3-0.5 cun.

NOTES:

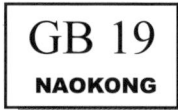

GB 19
NAOKONG

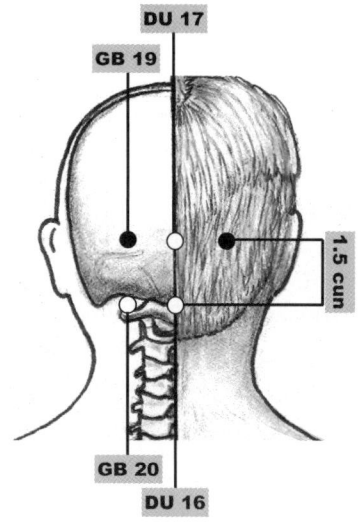

DU 17

GB 19

1.5 cun

GB 20

DU 16

LOCATION:
Directly above GB 20, at the level with DU 17, on the lateral side of the external occipital protuberance.

INDICATIONS:
Headache, common cold, asthma, stiffness of the neck, vertigo, painful eyes, tinnitus, epilepsy, seizures, mental illness, palpitations.

METHOD:
Puncture subcutaneously 0.3-0.5 cun.

NOTES:

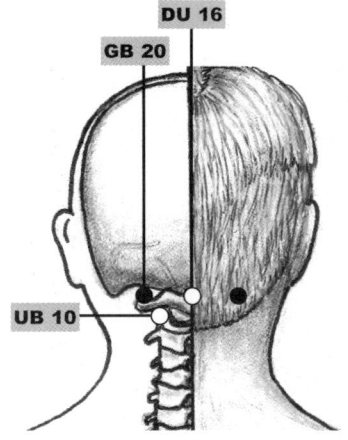

LOCATION:

In the depression between the upper portion of m.sternocleidomastoideus and m.trapezius, on the same level with DU 16.

INDICATIONS:

Headache, vertigo, insomnia, painful and stiff neck, blurred vision, glaucoma, red and painful eyes, eye diseases, tinnitus, deafness, convulsion, epilepsy, seizures, hemiplegia, brain diseases, infantile convulsion, febrile diseases, common cold, nasal obstruction, rhinnorhea, rhinitis, hypertension.

METHOD:

Puncture 0.5-0.8 cun towards the tip of the nose.

NOTES:

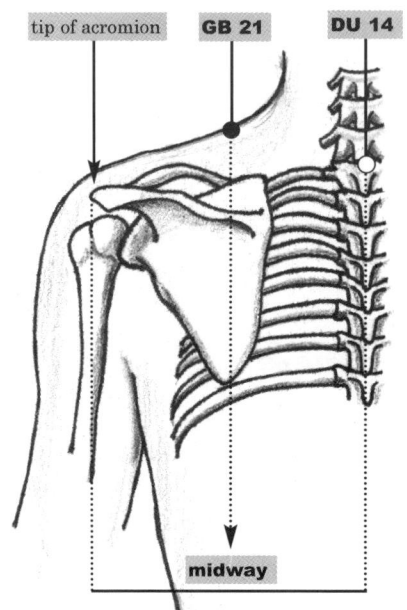

tip of acromion   GB 21   DU 14

midway

LOCATION:
Midway between DU 14 and the acromion, at the highest point of the shoulder.

INDICATIONS:
Pain and rigidity of the neck, pain in the shoulder and back, motor impairment of the arm, insufficient lactation, mastitis, functional uterine bleeding, scrofula, apoplexy, difficult labor, hemiplegia due to stroke.

METHOD:
Puncture perpendicularly 0.3-0.5 cun.

NOTES:

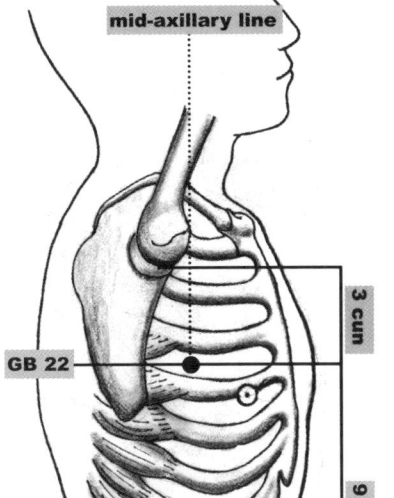

LOCATION:
On the mid-axillary line when the arm is raised, 3 cun below the axilla.

INDICATIONS:
Fullness of the chest, pleurisy, swelling of the axillary region, axillary lymphadenitis, pain in the hypochondriac region, interocostal neuralgia, pain and motor impairment of the arm & shoulders.

METHOD:
Puncture obliquely 0.3-0.5 cun.

NOTES:

327

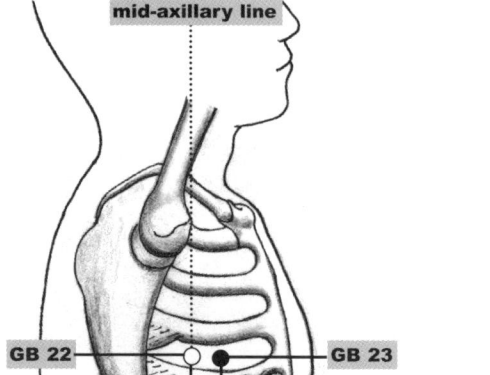

LOCATION:
1 cun anterior to GB 22, approximately at the level with the nipple.

INDICATIONS:
Fullness of the chest, pain in the hypochondriac region, asthma, pleurisy, vomiting, acidic belching.

METHOD:
Puncture obliquely 0.3-0.5 cun.

NOTES:

FRONT-MU POINT OF THE GALLBLADDER

GB 24
RIYUE

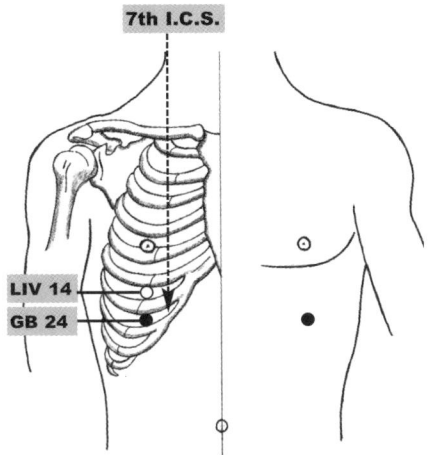

7th I.C.S.

LIV 14

GB 24

LOCATION:
One rib below LIV 14, directly below the nipple, in the 7th intercostal space.

INDICATIONS:
Pain in the hypochondriac region, intercostal neuralgia, cholecystitis, acute & chronic hepatitis, peptic ulcer, vomiting, acid regurgitation, hiccup, jaundice, mastitis.

METHOD:
Puncture obliquely 0.3-0.5 cun.

NOTES:

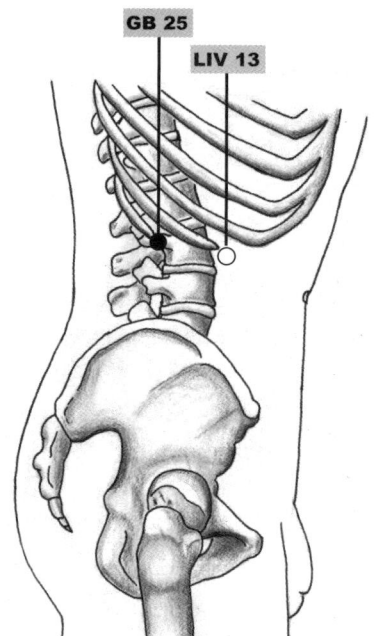

GB 25

LIV 13

LOCATION:
On the lateral side of the abdomen, on the lower border of the free end of the 12th rib.

INDICATIONS:
Abdominal distention, borborygmus, diarrhea, pain in the lumbar and hypochondriac region, intercostal neuralgia, pain of intestinal hernia, nephritis.

METHOD:
Puncture perpendicularly 0.3-0.5 cun.

NOTES:

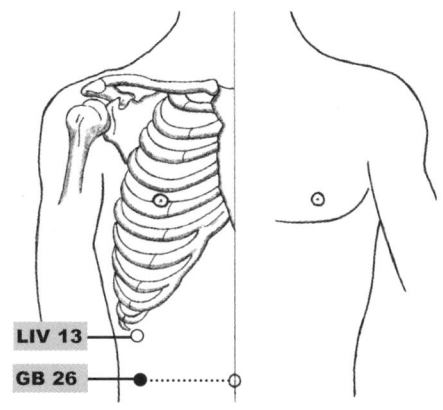

LIV 13

GB 26

LOCATION:
Directly below the free end of the 11th rib where LIV 13 is located, at the level with the umbilicus.

INDICATIONS:
Irregular menstruation, profuse blood & leukorrhea, amenorrhea, leukorrhea, endometritis, cystitis, abdominal pain, hernia, pain in the lumbar and hypochondriac region, paraplegia due to trauma.

METHOD:
Puncture perpendicularly 0.5-0.8 cun.

NOTES:

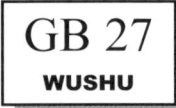

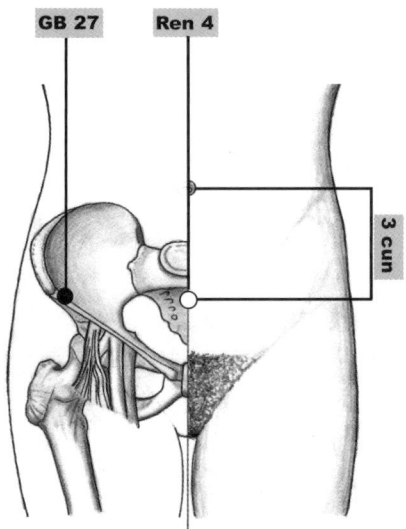

GB 27   Ren 4

3 cun

LOCATION:

On the lateral side of the abdomen, anterior to the superior iliac spine, approximately 3 cun below the level of the umbilicus.

INDICATIONS:

Leukorrhea, lower abdominal pain, endometritis, lumbar pain, hernia, orchitis, constipation.

METHOD:

Puncture perpendicularly 0.5-1.0 cun.

NOTES:

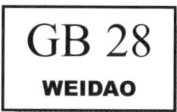

GB 28
WEIDAO

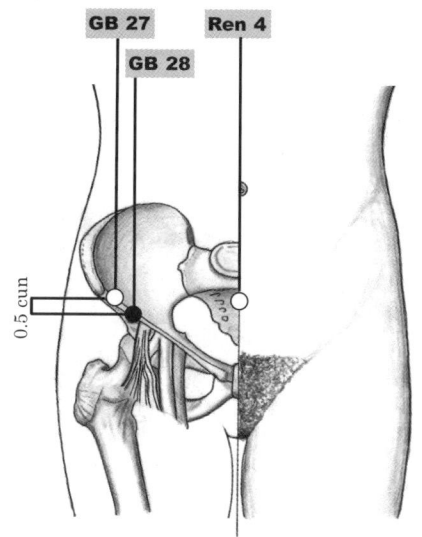

GB 27 GB 28 Ren 4

0.5 cun

LOCATION:
Anterior and inferior to the anterior superior iliac spine, 0.5 cun anterior and inferior to GB 27.

INDICATIONS:
Leukorrhea, lower abdominal pain, hernia, pain of intestinal hernia, prolapse of the uterus, adnexitis, endometritis, chronic constipation.

METHOD:
Puncture perpendicularly 0.5-1.0 cun.

NOTES:

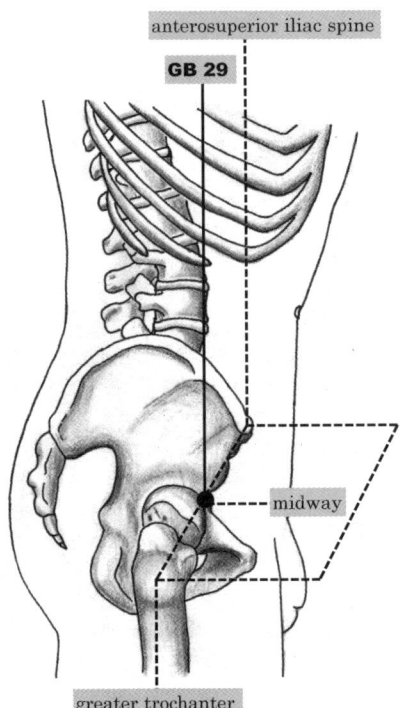

anterosuperior iliac spine

GB 29

midway

greater trochanter

LOCATION:

In the depression of the midpoint between the anterosuperior iliac spine and the greater trochanter.

INDICATIONS:

Pain and numbness in the thigh and lumbar region, lower abdominal pain, paralysis, muscular atrophy of the lower limbs, diseases of the hip joint & surrounding soft tissues, stomach ache, orchitis, endometritis, cystitis.

METHOD:

Puncture perpendicularly 0.5-1.0 cun.

NOTES:

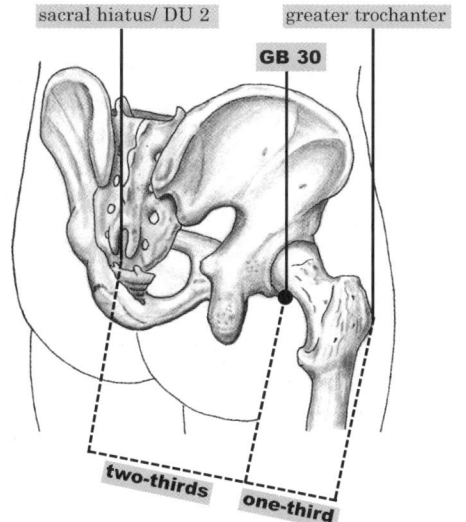

sacral hiatus/ DU 2   greater trochanter

GB 30

two-thirds   one-third

LOCATION:
At the junction of the lateral 1/3 and medial 2/3 of the distance between the greater trochanter and the hiatus of the sacrum (DU 2). When locating the point, put the patient in the lateral recumbent position with the thigh flexed.

INDICATIONS:
Pain of the lumbar region and thigh, numbness, paralysis & muscular atrophy of the lower limbs, hemiplegia, sciatica, diseases of the hip joint & surrounding soft tissues.

METHOD:
Puncture perpendicularly 1.5-2.5 cun.

NOTES:

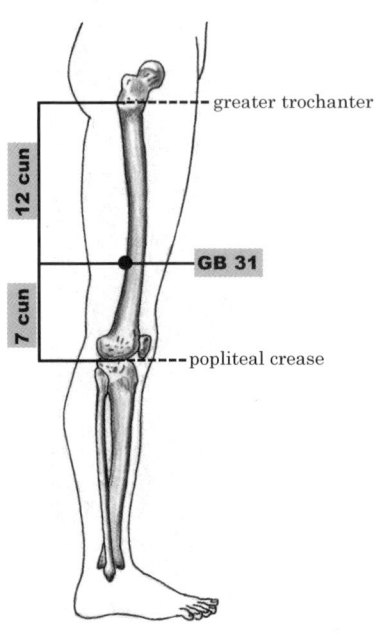

greater trochanter

12 cun

GB 31

7 cun

popliteal crease

LOCATION:

On the midline of the lateral aspect of the thigh, 7 cun above the transverse popliteal crease. When the patient is standing erect with the hands close to the sides, the point is where the tip of the middle finger touches.

INDICATIONS:

Pain and soreness in the thigh and lumbar region, paralysis of the lower limbs, neuritis of the lateral cutaneous nerve of the thigh & muscle branch of the femoral nerve, beriberi, general pruritis.

METHOD:

Puncture perpendicularly 0.7-1.2 cun.

NOTES:

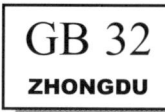

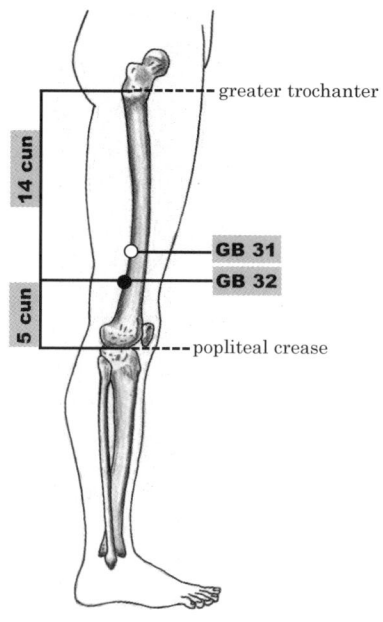

greater trochanter

14 cun

GB 31
GB 32

5 cun

popliteal crease

LOCATION:
On the lateral aspect of the thigh, 5 cun above the transverse popliteal crease, between m.vastus lateralis and m.biceps femoris.

INDICATIONS:
Pain and soreness of the thigh and knee, numbness, paralysis and weakness of the lower limbs, hemiplegia, beri beri, sciatica.

METHOD:
Puncture perpendicularly 0.7-1.0 cun.

NOTES:

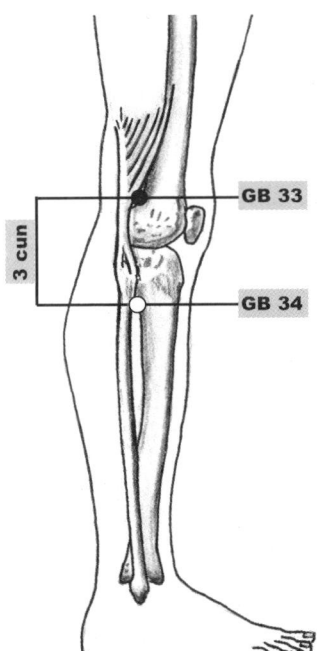

GB 33
XIYANGGUAN

LOCATION:
3 cun above GB 34, lateral to the knee joint, between the tendon of m.biceps femoris and the femur.

INDICATIONS:
Swelling and pain of the knee, contracture of the tendons in the popliteal fossa, diseases of the knee & surrounding soft tissues, numbness of the leg, paralysis of the lower limb.

METHOD:
Puncture perpendicularly 0.5-1.0 cun.

NOTES:

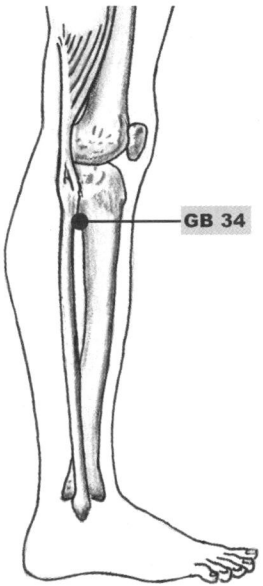

GB 34

LOCATION:
In the depression anterior and inferior to the head of the fibula.

INDICATIONS:
Hemiplegia, weakness, paralysis, numbness and pain of the lower extremities, swelling and pain of the knee, beriberi, hypochondriac pain, intercostal neuralgia, bitter taste in the mouth, vomiting, jaundice, hepatitis, cholecystitis, roundworm in the bile duct, habitual constipation, hypertension, infantile convulsion, perifocal inflammation of the shoulder.

METHOD:
Puncture perpendicularly 0.8-1.2 cun.

NOTES:

GB 35
YANGJIAO

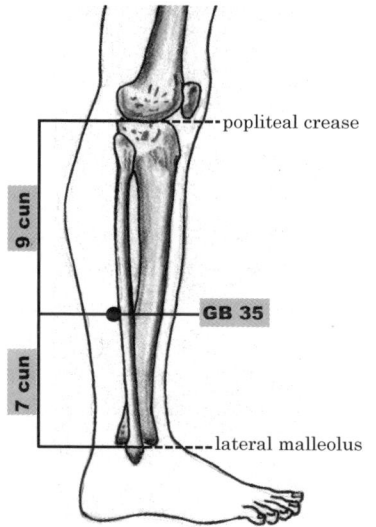

9 cun

7 cun

popliteal crease

GB 35

lateral malleolus

LOCATION:
7 cun above the tip of the external malleolus, on the posterior border of the fibula.

INDICATIONS:
Pain in the neck, chest, thigh and hypochondriac region, pain in the lateral aspect of the leg, sciatica, asthma, rabies.

METHOD:
Puncture perpendicularly 0.5-0.8 cun.

NOTES:

340

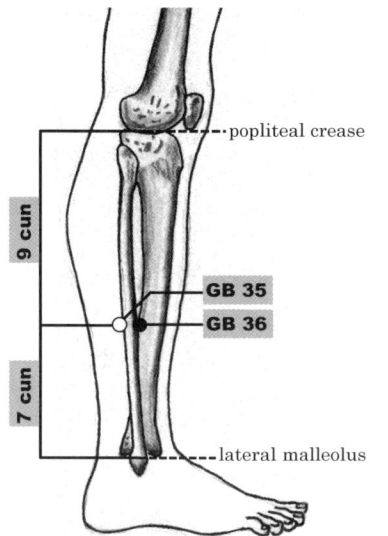

popliteal crease

9 cun

GB 35
GB 36

7 cun

lateral malleolus

LOCATION:
7 cun above the tip of the external malleolus, on the anterior border of the fibula.

INDICATIONS:
Pain in the neck, chest, thigh, and hypochondriac region, headache, hepatitis, paralysis of the lower limbs, rabies.

METHOD:
Puncture perpendicularly 0.5-0.8 cun.

NOTES:

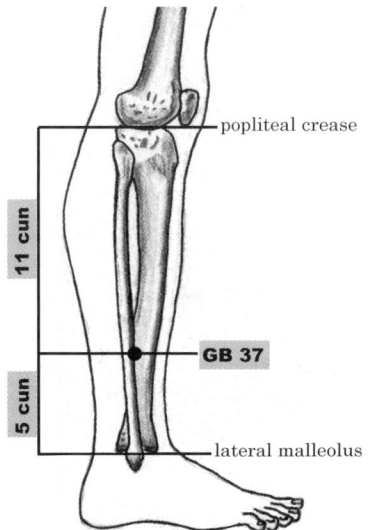

popliteal crease

11 cun

5 cun

GB 37

lateral malleolus

LOCATION:
5 cun directly above the tip of the external malleolus, on the anterior border of the fibula.

INDICATIONS:
Pain in the knee, muscular atrophy, motor impairment and pain of the lower extremities, pain along the lateral aspect of calf, blurry vision, atrophy of the optic nerve, ophthalmalgia, night blindness, cataract, migraine headache, breast distention.

METHOD:
Puncture perpendicularly 0.7-1.0 cun.

NOTES:

GB 38
YANGFU

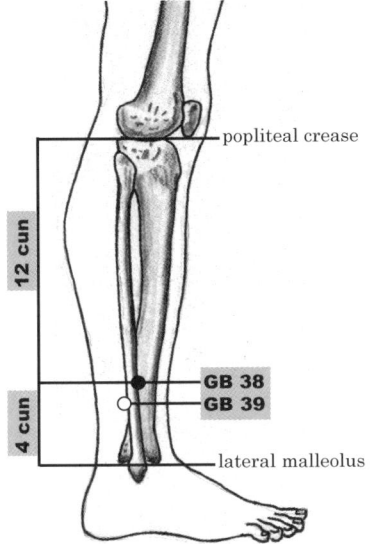

popliteal crease

12 cun

4 cun

GB 38
GB 39

lateral malleolus

LOCATION:
4 cun above and slightly anterior to the tip of the external malleolus, on the anterior border of the fibula, between m. extensor digitorum longus and m. peroneus brevis.

INDICATIONS:
Migraine, pain of the outer canthus, pain in the axillary region, scrofula, lumbar pain, pain in the chest, hypochondriac region and lateral aspect of the extremities, hemiplegia, paralysis of the lower limb, arthritis of knee, malaria.

METHOD:
Puncture perpendicularly 0.5-0.7 cun.

NOTES:

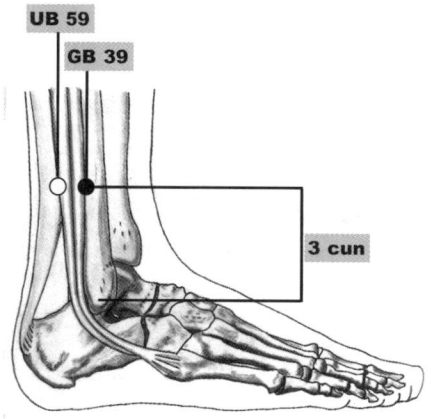

LOCATION:

3 cun above the tip of the external malleolus, in the depression between the posterior border of the fibula and the tendons of m.peroneus longus and brevis.

INDICATIONS:

Aploplexy, hemiplegia, stiffness & pain of the neck, migraine headache, scrofula, abdominal distention, pain in the hypochondriac region, muscular atrophy of the lower limbs, spastic pain of the leg, diseases of the knee & ankle joints & surrounding soft tissues, sciatica, beriberi.

METHOD:

Puncture perpendicularly 0.3-0.5 cun.

NOTES:

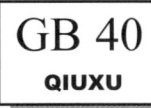

GB 40
QIUXU

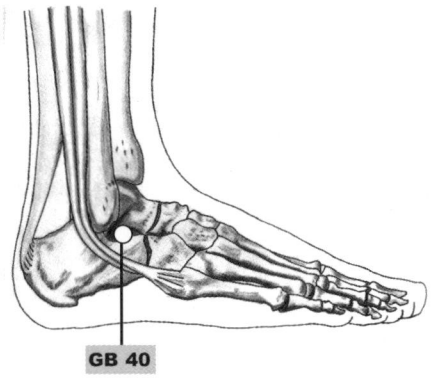

GB 40

LOCATION:
Anterior and inferior to the external malleo-lus, in the depression on the lateral side of m.extensor digitorum longus.

INDICATIONS:
Pain in the neck, pain in the chest & ribs, swelling of the axillary region, axillary lym-phadenitis, pain in the hypochondriac region, vomiting, acid regurgitation, cholecystitis, muscular atrophy of the lower limbs, sciatica, pain and swelling of the external malleolus, diseases of the ankle & surrounding soft tis-sues, malaria.

METHOD:
Puncture perpendicularly 0.5-0.8 cun.

NOTES:

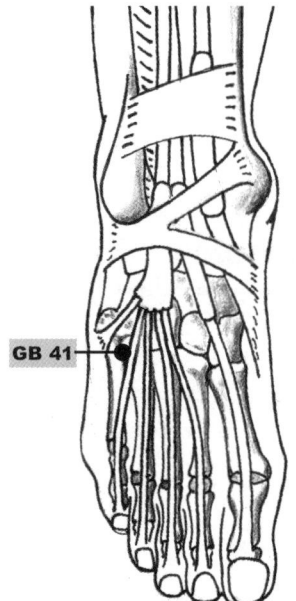

GB 41

LOCATION:

In the depression distal to the junction of the fourth and fifth metatarsal bones, on the lateral side of the tendon of m.extensor digiti minimi of the foot.

INDICATIONS:

Headache, vertigo, conjunctivitis, pain of the outer canthus, scrofula, pain in the hypochondriac region, rib pain, distending pain of the breast, mastitis, abscessed breast, irregular menstruation, Dampness, pain and swelling of the dorsum of the foot, spastic pain of the foot and toe.

METHOD:

Puncture perpendicularly 0.3-0.5 cun.

NOTES:

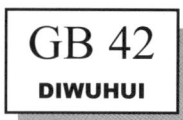

GB 42
DIWUHUI

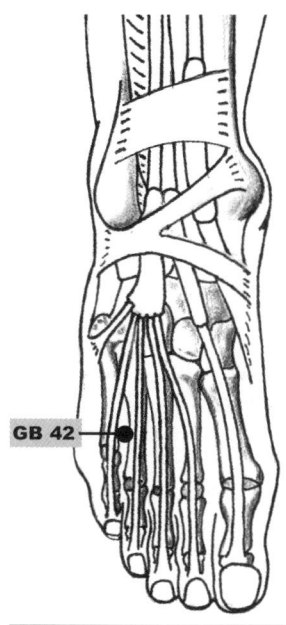

GB 42

LOCATION:
Between the fourth and fifth metatarsal bones, on the medial side of the tendon of m. extensor digiti minimi of the foot.

INDICATIONS:
Pain of the canthus, tinnitus, distending pain of the breast, mastitis, swelling, inflammation, and pain of the dorsum of the foot, low back pain.

METHOD:
Puncture perpendicularly 0.3-0.5 cun.

NOTES:

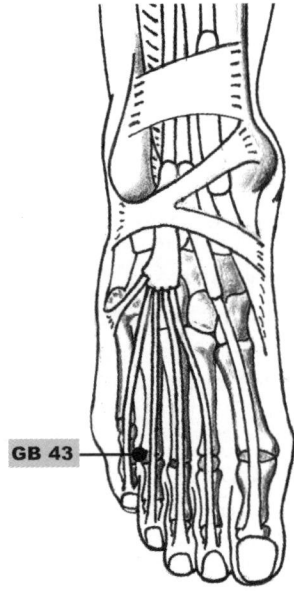

GB 43

LOCATION:
On the dorsum of the foot, between the fourth & fifth toe, proximal to the margin of the web.

INDICATIONS:
Headache, migraine, dizziness & vertigo, hypertension, pain of the outer canthus, tinnitus, deafness, swelling of the cheek, pain in the hypochondriac region, intercostal neuralgia, distending pain of the breast, febrile diseases.

METHOD:
Puncture perpendicularly 0.3-0.5 cun.

NOTES:

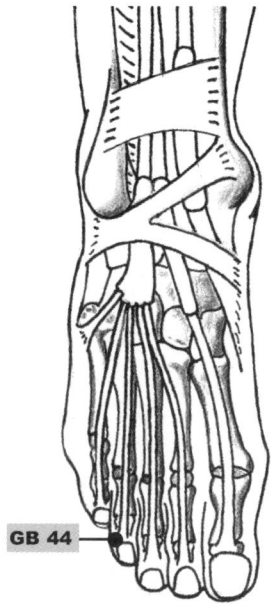

GB 44

LOCATION:
On the lateral side of the fourth toe, about 0.1 cun posterior to the corner of the nail.

INDICATIONS:
Migraine, headache, deafness, tinnitus, opthalmalgia, conjunctivitis, intercostal neuralgia, dream-disturbed sleep, febrile diseases, asthma, pleurisy, hypertension.

METHOD:
Puncture superficially about 0.1 cun.

NOTES:

NOTES

NOTES

LIVER
CHANNEL

LIVER MERIDIAN OF FOOT JUE-YIN

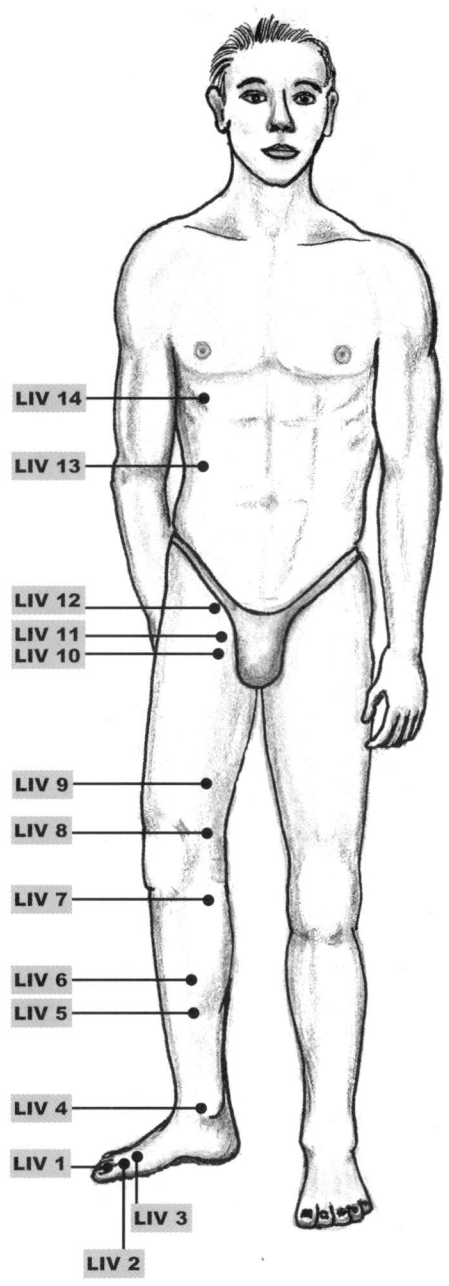

CHANNEL/ORGAN RELATIONSHIPS

- This channel is associated with the Liver and connects with the Gallbladder.

- It also joins directly with the Lungs, Stomach, Kidneys, and brain.

THERAPEUTIC INDICATIONS

- Liver diseases, gynecological diseases, diseases of the external genitalia, and other diseases of areas the meridian supplies.

PATHOLOGY

Channel: Chest fullness, lower abdominal pain, hernia, vertical headache, vertigo, blurred vision, tinnitus, dry throat, hiccups, fever, spasms in the extremities, low back pain, enuresis, dysuria, mental disturbance.

Organ: Fullness or pain in the costal region or chest, hard masses in the upper abdomen, lower abdominal pain, vomiting, jaundice, loose stool, hernia, enuresis, retention of urine, dark urine.

353

LIVER MERIDIAN OF FOOT JUE-YIN

GENERAL PATHWAY	●This channel begins on the dorsum of the big toe. ●Running upward along the dorsum of the foot, passing through LIV 4, 1 cun in front of the medial malleolus, it ascends to SP 6 where it intersects with the Spleen channel. ●From here, it continues up the medial aspect of the lower leg, re-crossing the Spleen channel 8 cun above the medial malleolus, and then runs posterior to the Spleen channel over the knee and thigh. ●Winding around the genitals, the channel enters the lower abdomen where it meets the Ren channel at Ren 2, Ren 3, and Ren 4, before curving around the Stomach & joining with its associated organ, the liver, and connecting with the gall bladder. ●Then the channel continues upward across the diaphragm & costal region, traverses the neck posterior to the pharynx, and enters the nasopharynx, connecting with the tissues around the eye. ●Finally, the channel ascends across the forehead & meets the DU channel at the vertex. **BRANCHES:** ●**BRANCH 1:** A branch separates below the eye & encircles the inside of the lips. ●**BRANCH 2:** A branch separates in the liver, crosses the diaphragm and reaches the lung.
CONNECTING CHANNEL	●After separating from the main channel at LIV 5 on the medial aspect of the lower leg, this channel connects with the Gall Bladder channel. ●**BRANCH:** A branch proceeds up the leg to the genitals.
DIVERGENT CHANNEL	●This channel separates from the main channel on the foot and continues upward to the pubic region, where it converges with the Gallbladder main channel.
MUSCULAR REGION	●This channel begins on the dorsum of the big toe, crosses in front of the medial malleolus and ascends along the medial aspect of the tibia, connecting at the inside of the knee. ●From here, it proceeds up the medial aspect of the thigh to the genitals, where it joins with other muscle channels.

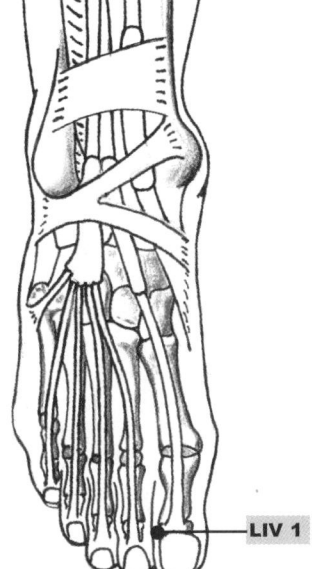

LIV 1

LOCATION:
On the lateral side of the dorsum of the terminal phalanx of the great toe, between the lateral corner of the nail and the interphalangeal joint.

INDICATIONS:
Hernia, enuresis, incontinence of urine, hematuria, orchitis, uterine bleeding, irregular menstruation, pain of hernia, prolapse of the uterus, epilepsy.

METHOD:
Puncture subcutaneously 0.1-0.2 cun.

NOTES:

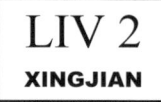
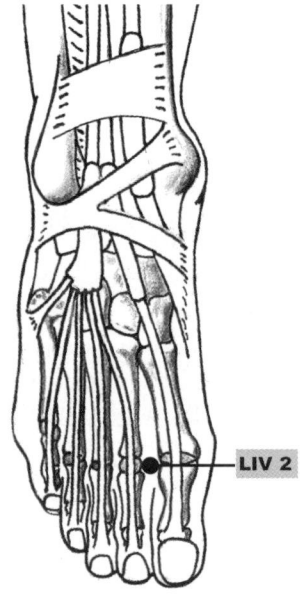

LIV 2

LOCATION:

On the dorsum of the foot between the first and second toe, proximal to the margin of the web.

INDICATIONS:

Pain in the hypochondrium, intercostal neuralgia, abdominal distention, headache, dizziness and vertigo, congestion, swelling and pain of the eye, glaucoma, deviation of the mouth, hernia & pain of hernia, painful urination, retention of urine, irregular menstruation, uterine bleeding, epilepsy, insomnia, convulsion, infantile convulsion, night sweats, orchitis.

METHOD:

Puncture obliquely 0.3-0.5 cun.

NOTES:

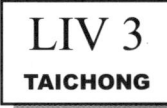
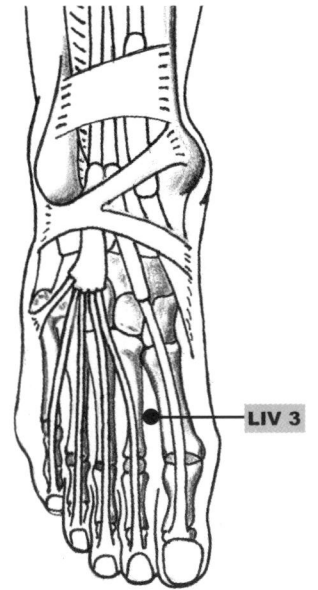

LIV 3

LOCATION:

On the dorsum of the foot, in the depression distal to the junction of the first and second metatarsal bones.

INDICATIONS:

Headache, dizziness and vertigo, insomnia, congestion, hypertension, thrombocytopenia, swelling, and pain of the eye, depression, infantile convulsion, deviation of the mouth, pain in the hypochondriac region, hepatitis, mastitis, uterine bleeding, irregular menstruation, hernia, enuresis, retention of urine, epilepsy, pain in the anterior aspect of the medial malleolus, soreness of the joints of the extremities.

METHOD:

Puncture perpendicularly 0.3-0.5 cun.

NOTES:

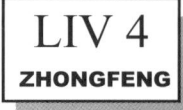
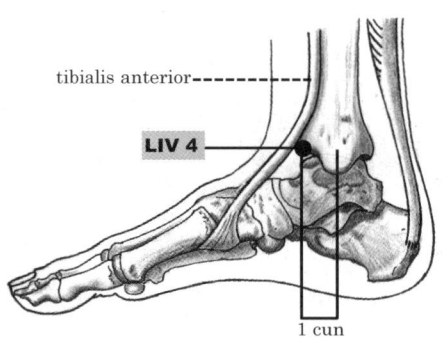

tibialis anterior

LIV 4

1 cun

LOCATION:
1 cun anterior to the medial malleolus, midway between SP 5 and ST 41, in the depression on the medial side of the tendon of m.tibialis anterior.

INDICATIONS:
Hernia & pain of hernia, pain in the external genitalia, nocturnal emission, retention of urine, distending pain in the hypochondrium, lower abdominal pain, diseases of the ankle & surrounding soft tissues, hepatitis.

METHOD:
Puncture perpendicularly 0.3-0.5 cun.

NOTES:

LIV 5
LIGOU

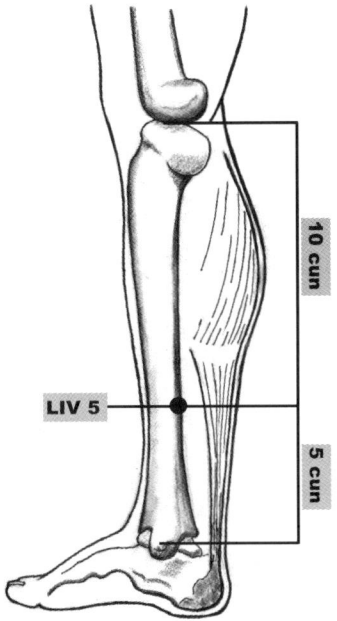

10 cun

LIV 5

5 cun

LOCATION:
5 cun above the tip of the medial malleolus, on the medial aspect and near the medial border of the tibia.

INDICATIONS:
Retention of urine, enuresis, hernia & pain of hernia, orchitis, irregular menstruation, endometritis, leukorrhea, pruritis vulvae, sexual dysfunction, weakness and atrophy of the leg.

METHOD:
Puncture subcutaneously 0.3-0.5 cun.

NOTES:

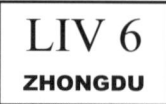
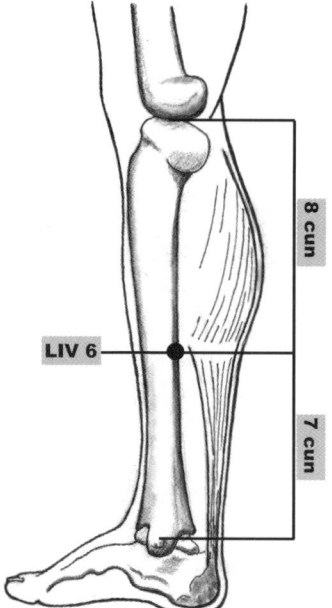

8 cun

LIV 6

7 cun

LOCATION:
7 cun above the tip of the medial malleo-lus, on the medial aspect and near the medial border of the tibia.

INDICATIONS:
Abdominal pain, hypochondriac pain, acute hepatitis, diarrhea, hernia, uterine bleeding, prolonged lochia, paralysis of the lower limb.

METHOD:
Puncture subcutaneously 0.5-0.8 cun.

NOTES:

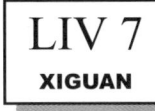

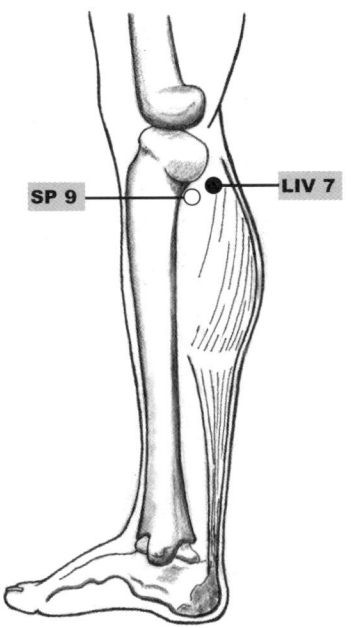

LOCATION:
Posterior and inferior to the medial condyle of the tibia, in the upper portion of the medial head of m. gastrocnemius, 1 cun posterior to SP 9.

INDICATIONS:
Pain of the knee, arthritis of the knees, strong recurrent headache.

METHOD:
Puncture subcutaneously 0.5-1.0 cun.

NOTES:

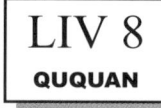
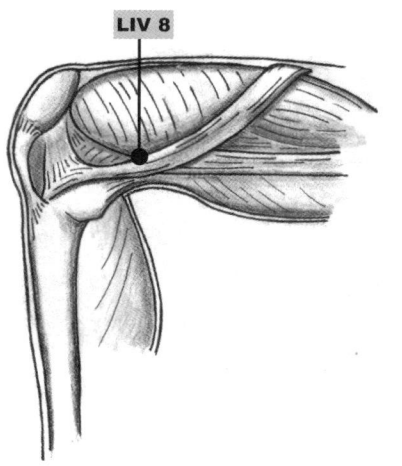

LIV 8

LOCATION:
When the knee is flexed, the point is in the depression above the medial end of the transverse popliteal crease, posterior to the medial epicondyle of the femur, on the anterior part of the insertion of m.semimembranosus and m.semitendinosus.

INDICATIONS:
Prolapse of the uterus, lower abdominal pain, pain of hernia, retention of urine, nephritis, nocturnal emission, impotence, prostatitis, pain in the external genitalia, vaginitis, pruritis vulvae, pain in the medial aspect of the knee and thigh, diseases of the knee & surrounding soft tissues.

METHOD:
Puncture perpendicularly 0.5-0.8 cun.

NOTES:

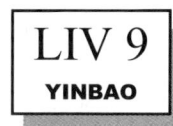

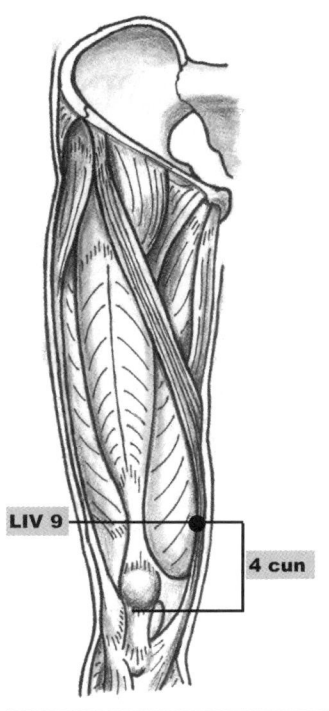

LIV 9

4 cun

LOCATION:
4 cun above the medial epicondyle of the femur, where LIV 8 is located, between m.vastus medialis and m.sartorius.

INDICATIONS:
Pain in the lumbosacral region, lower abdominal pain, enuresis, retention of urine, irregular menstruation.

METHOD:
Puncture perpendicularly 0.5-0.7 cun.

NOTES:

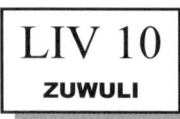

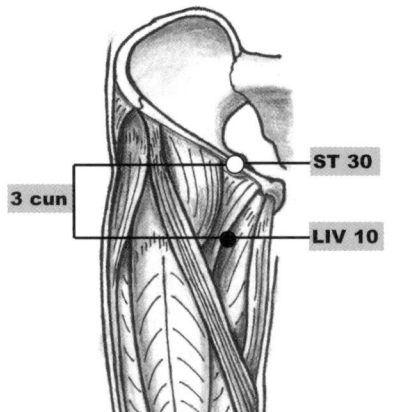

ST 30

3 cun

LIV 10

LOCATION:
3 cun directly below ST 30, on the lateral border of m.adductor longus.

INDICATIONS:
Lower abdominal distention and fullness, retention of urine, incontinence, eczema of the scrotum, pain in the medial side of the thigh, lassitude.

METHOD:
Puncture perpendicularly 0.5-1.0 cun.

NOTES:

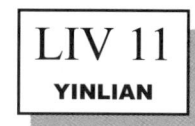

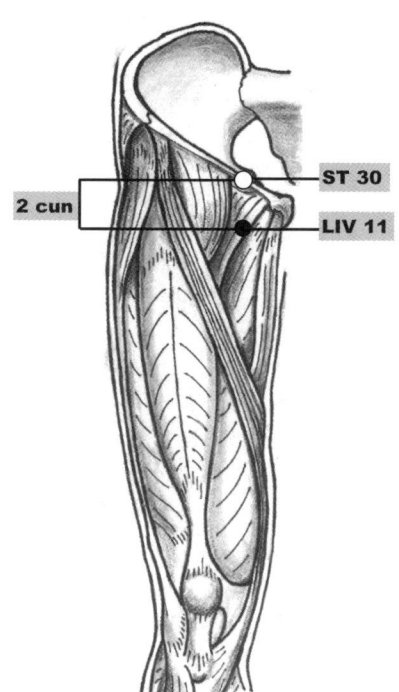

2 cun

ST 30

LIV 11

LOCATION:
2 cun directly below ST 30, on the lateral border of m.adductor longus.

INDICATIONS:
Irregular menstruation, leukorrhea, lower abdominal pain, pain of hernia, pain in the thigh and leg.

METHOD:
Puncture perpendicularly 0.5-1.0 cun.

NOTES:

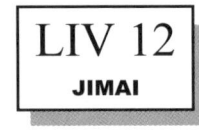

LIV 12
JIMAI

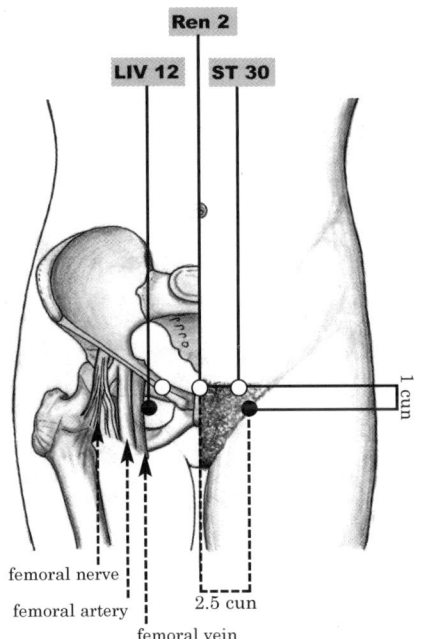

Ren 2

LIV 12 ST 30

1 cun

femoral nerve

femoral artery

2.5 cun

femoral vein

LOCATION:
2.5 cun lateral to the Ren meridian, at the inguinal groove lateral and 1 cun inferior to ST 30.

INDICATIONS:
Lower abdominal pain, hernia & pain of hernia, pain in the external genitalia, penile pain, prolapsed uterus.

METHOD:
Avoiding the artery, puncture medially and slightly obliquely, 0.5-0.8 cun.

NOTES:

FRONT-MU POINT OF THE SPLEEN
INFLUENTIAL POINT OF ZANG ORGANS

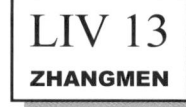

LIV 13
ZHANGMEN

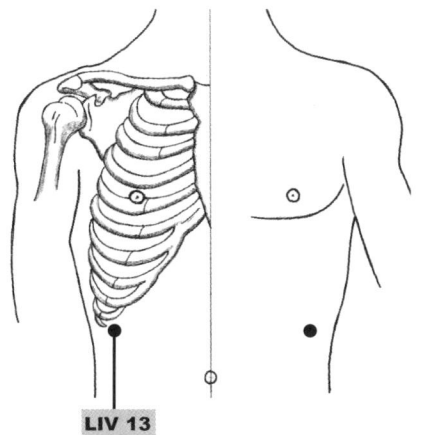

LIV 13

LOCATION:
On the lateral side of the abdomen, below the free end of the 11th floating rib.

INDICATIONS:
Abdominal distention, borborygmus, pain in the hypochondriac region & chest, enlargement of the liver & spleen, hepatitis, enteritis, vomiting, diarrhea, indigestion.

METHOD:
Puncture perpendicularly 0.5-0.8 cun.

NOTES:

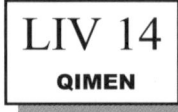
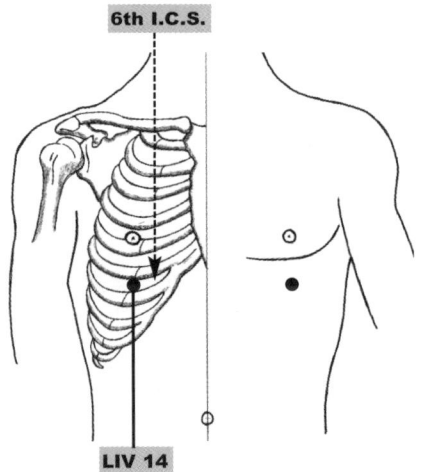

6th I.C.S.

LIV 14

LOCATION:
Directly below the nipple, in the 6th inter-costal space.

INDICATIONS:
Hypochondriac pain, intercostal neuralgia, abdominal distention, hiccup, acid regurgitation, mastitis, depression, febrile diseases, hepatitis, enlarged liver, cholecystitis, pleurisy, nervous dysfunction of the stomach.

METHOD:
Puncture obliquely 0.3-0.5 cun.

NOTES:

NOTES

NOTES

**DU
CHANNEL**

DU MERIDIAN

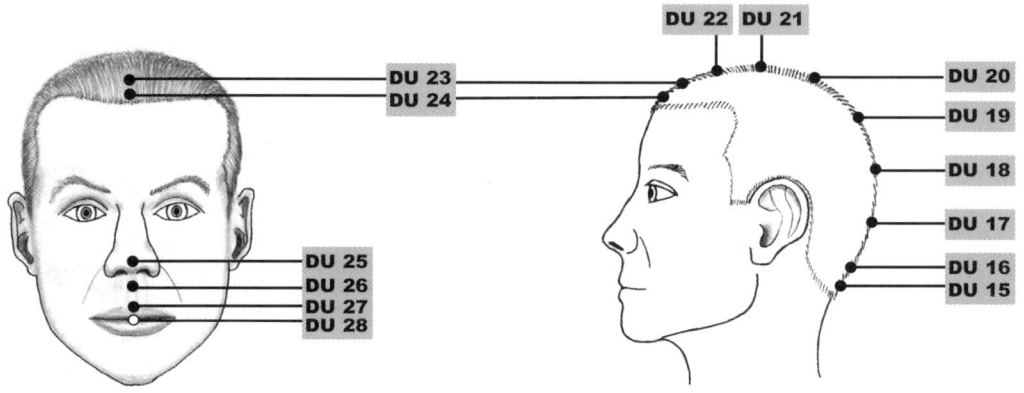

DU 22	DU 21	
DU 23		DU 20
DU 24		DU 19
		DU 18
DU 25		DU 17
DU 26		DU 16
DU 27		DU 15
DU 28		

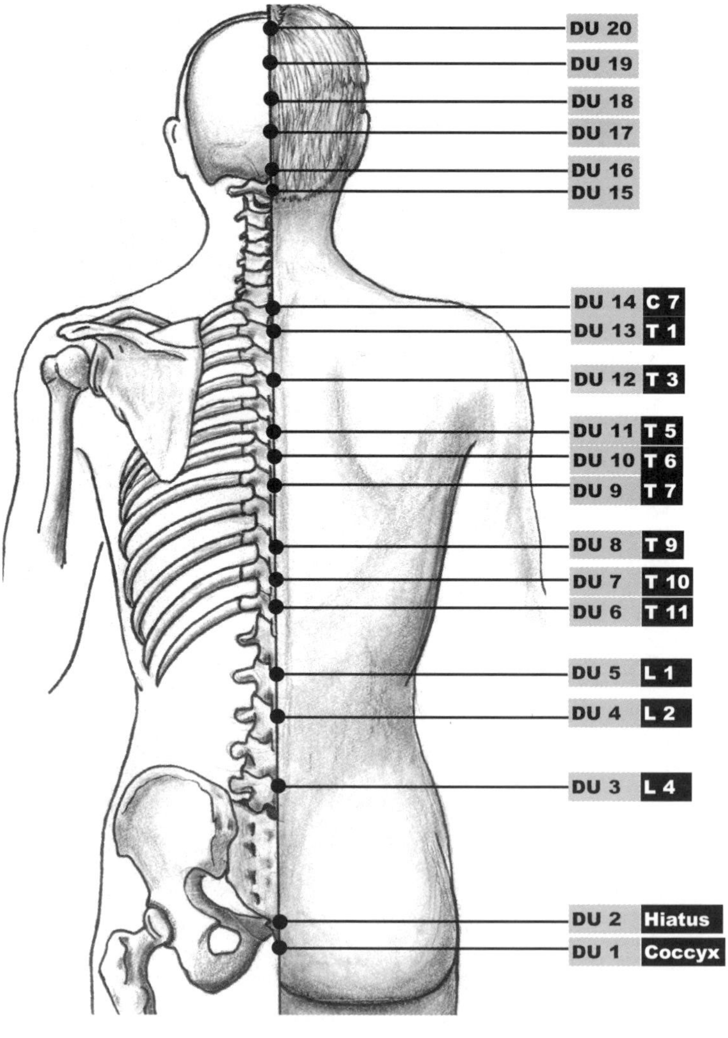

DU 20	
DU 19	
DU 18	
DU 17	
DU 16	
DU 15	
DU 14	C 7
DU 13	T 1
DU 12	T 3
DU 11	T 5
DU 10	T 6
DU 9	T 7
DU 8	T 9
DU 7	T 10
DU 6	T 11
DU 5	L 1
DU 4	L 2
DU 3	L 4
DU 2	Hiatus
DU 1	Coccyx

372

DU MERIDIAN

GENERAL PATHWAY	**PRIMARY COURSE:** Originates in the lower abdomen, emerges at the perineum, & ascends along the middle of the spine until it reaches DU 16 at the nape of the neck. ●It then enters the brain, ascends to the vertex (DU 20), and follows the midline of the forehead across the bridge of the nose and philtrum (DU 26), terminating at the upper lip. **BRANCH 1:** Begins in the pelvic region, descends to the genitals and perineum, and passes through the tip of the coccyx, winding around the anus. ●It then enters the gluteal region where it intersects the Kidney & Bladder channels before returning to the spinal column and then joining with the Kidneys. **BRANCH 2:** The origin of this course is the same as that of the Bladder channel at the inner canthus of the eye. ●The two bilateral branches from each of the inner canthi ascend across the forehead & meet at the vertex where the channel enters the brain. ●Emerging at the nape of the neck, the channel again divides into two branches which descends along opposite sides of the spine to the waist. Here they join with the Kidneys. **BRANCH 3:** Begins in the lower abdomen, winds around the genitalia, ascends directly across the navel, passes through the Heart and enters the trachea. ●Continuing upward, the channel crosses the cheek and encircles the mouth, before terminating at a point below the middle of the eye. ●The DU channel intersects the Bladder channel at UB 12 and the Ren channel at Ren 1.
CONNECTING CHANNEL	●Arises from DU 1 in the perineum, ascends along both sides of the spine to the nape, and spreads over the top of the head. ●When it gets to the scapular regions, it connects with the Bladder meridian and enters the spine.
THERAPEUTIC INDICATIONS	●Mental disorders, febrile diseases, disorders of the spine, diseases of the anus, rectum, intestines, genitals, urinary system, uterus, and zang-fu organs.
PATHOLOGY	●This channel supplies the brain and spine & intersects the Liver channel at the vertex, therefore its pathology is associated with these areas. ●Qi Stagnation may cause such symptoms as stiffness and pain along the spine. ●Qi Deficiency in the channel may cause a heavy sensation in the head, shaking, and vertigo. ●Mental disorders may be caused by Wind entering the brain through the DU channel. ●Febrile diseases are often associated with the DU channel. ●Because one branch of the channel ascends through the abdomen, when the channel is imbalanced, its Qi may rush upward toward the Heart. ●This may cause symptoms such as colic, constipation, enuresis, hemorrhoids and functional infertility. ●Other symptoms of the DU channel include opisthotonos, headache, and epilepsy.

373

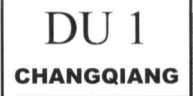
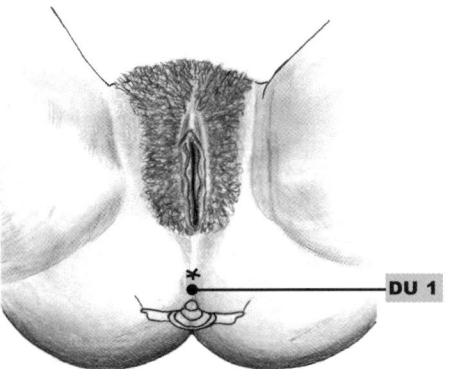

DU 1

LOCATION:
Midway between the tip of the coccyx and the anus, locating the point in the prone position.

INDICATIONS:
Diarrhea, bloody stools, hemorrhoids, prolapse of the rectum & anus, constipation, pain in the lower back, epilepsy, eczema of the scrotum, inducing labor, impotence, psychosis.

METHOD:
Puncture perpendicularly 0.5-1.0 cun.

NOTES:

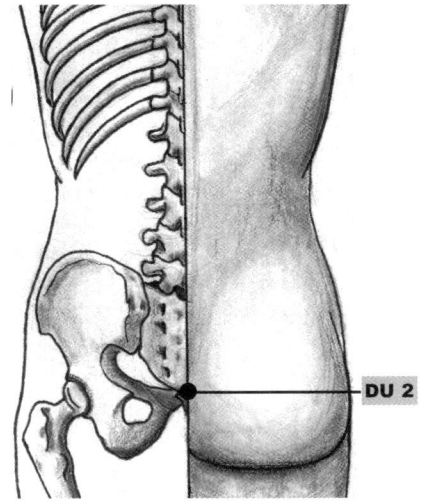

DU 2

LOCATION:
In the hiatus of the sacrum.

INDICATIONS:
Irregular menstruation, pain and stiffness of the lower back, hemorrhoids, enuresis, muscular atrophy & paralysis of the lower extremities, incontinence due to paraplegia, epilepsy, seizures.

METHOD:
Puncture obliquely upward 0.5-1.0 cun.

NOTES:

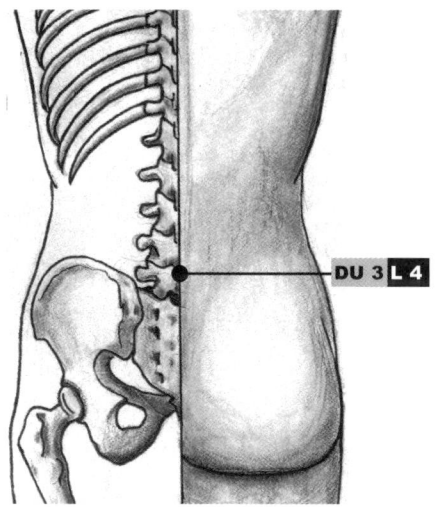

DU 3 L 4

LOCATION:
Below the spinous process of the 4th lumbar vertebra, at the level with the crista iliaca.

INDICATIONS:
Irregular menstruation, nocturnal emission, spermatorrhea, impotence, pain in the lumbosacral region, muscular atrophy, motor impairment, numbness, paralysis and pain of the lower extremities, chronic enteritis.

METHOD:
Puncture perpendicularly 0.5-1.0 cun.

NOTES:

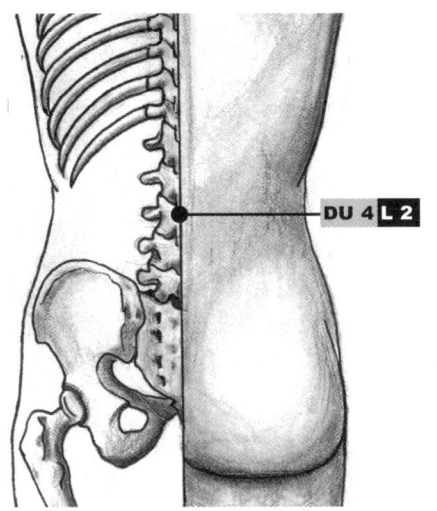

DU 4 **L 2**

LOCATION:

Below the spinous process of the 2nd lumbar vertebra.

INDICATIONS:

Stiffness of the back, lumbago, sciatica, low back sprain or pain, impotence, nocturnal emission, spermatorrhea, enuresis, nephritis, irregular menstruation, diarrhea, indigestion, leukorrhea, endometritis, peritonitis, spinal myelitis, sequelae of infantile paralysis.

METHOD:

Puncture perpendicularly 0.5-1.0 cun.

NOTES:

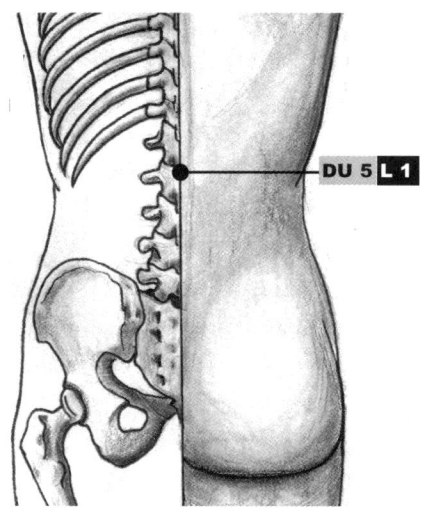

DU 5 L 1

LOCATION:

Below the spinous process of the 1st lumbar vertebra.

INDICATIONS:

Pain and stiffness of the lower back, diarrhea, indigestion, dysentery, abdominal pain, prolapsed anus.

METHOD:

Puncture perpendicularly 0.5-1.0 cun.

NOTES:

378

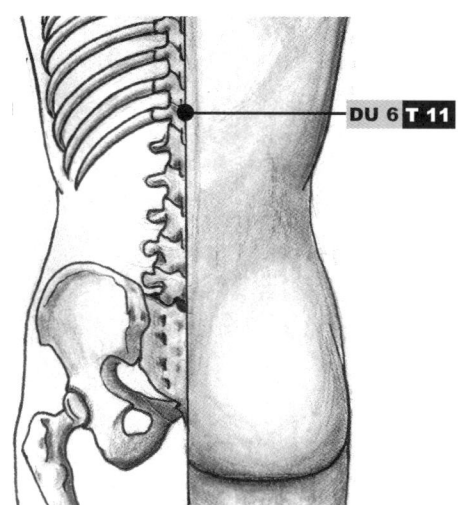

DU 6 T 11

LOCATION:
Below the spinous process of the 11th thoracic vertebra.

INDICATIONS:
Pain in the epigastric region, diarrhea, jaundice, hepatitis, epilepsy, seizures, stiffness and pain of the low back, paralysis of the lower limbs.

METHOD:
Puncture perpendicularly 0.5-1.0 cun.

NOTES:

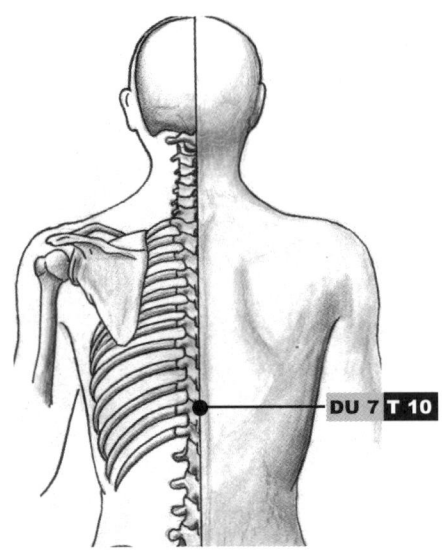

DU 7
ZHONGSHU

LOCATION:
Below the spinous process of the 10th thoracic vertebra.

INDICATIONS:
Pain in the epigastric region, low back pain, stiffness of the back, stomach ache, cholecystitis, diminishing vision.

METHOD:
Puncture perpendicularly 0.5-1.0 cun.

NOTES:

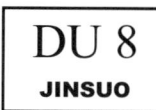

DU 8
JINSUO

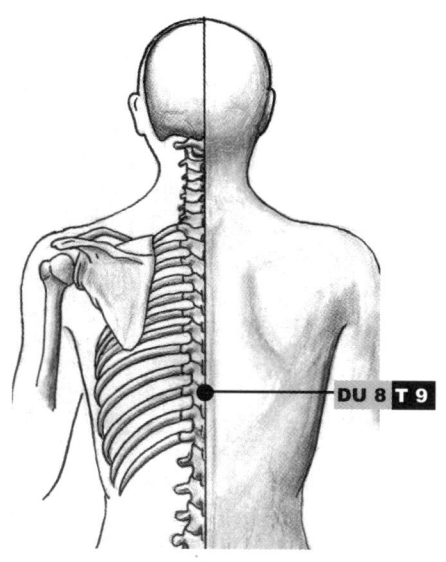

DU 8 T 9

LOCATION:
Below the spinous process of the 9th thoracic vertebra.

INDICATIONS:
Epilepsy, seizures, stiffness of the back, gastric pain, hepatitis, cholecystitis, pleurisy, hysteria, intercostal neuralgia.

METHOD:
Puncture perpendicularly 0.5-1.0 cun.

NOTES:

381

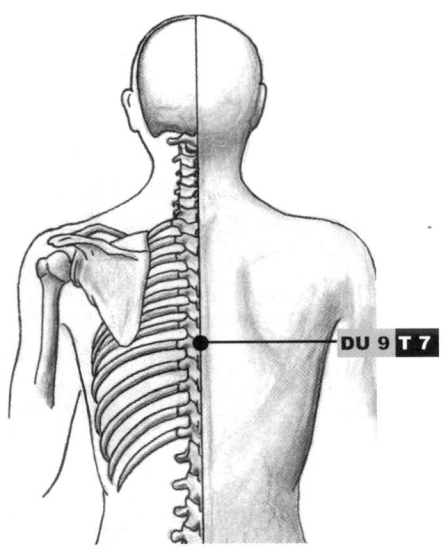

DU 9 T 7

DU 9
ZHIYANG

LOCATION:
Below the spinous process of the 7th thoracic vertebra, approximately at the level with the inferior angle of the scapula.

INDICATIONS:
Jaundice, hepatitis, cholecystitis, malaria, bronchial asthma, pleurisy, cough, asthma, stiffness of the back, pain in the chest and back, intercostal neuralgia, roundworm in the bile duct, stomach ache.

METHOD:
Puncture obliquely upward 0.5-1.0 cun.

NOTES:

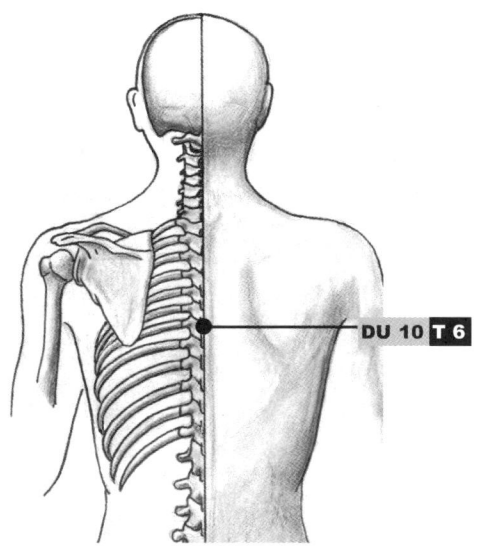

DU 10 T 6

LOCATION:
Below the spinous process of the 6th thoracic vertebra.

INDICATIONS:
Cough, bronchitis, asthma, furuncles, boils, stomach ache, back pain, neck rigidity, roundworm in the bile duct, malaria.

METHOD:
Puncture obliquely upward 0.5-1.0 cun.

NOTES:

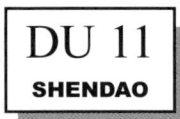

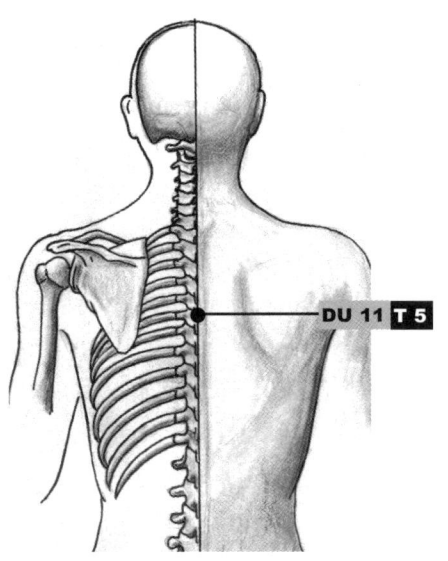

DU 11 T 5

LOCATION:
Below the spinous process of the 5th thoracic vertebra.

INDICATIONS:
Poor memory, anxiety, palpitation, heart disease, cardiac pain, pain and stiffness of the back, cough, fever, malaria, seizures, intercostal neuralgia.

METHOD:
Puncture obliquely upward 0.5-1.0 cun.

NOTES:

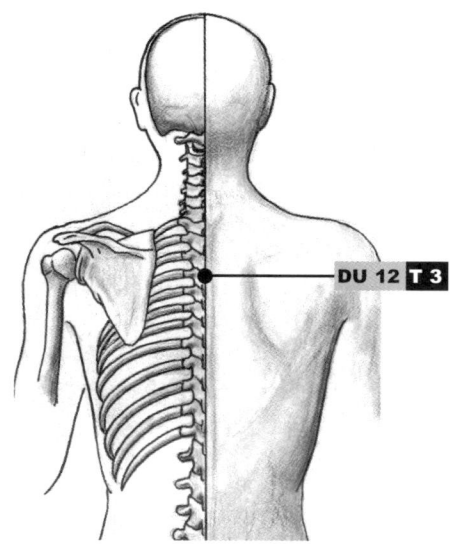

DU 12 T 3

LOCATION:
Below the spinous process of the 3rd thoracic vertebra.

INDICATIONS:
Cough, asthma, bronchitis, pneumonia, pulmonary tuberculosis, chest pain, epilepsy, pain and stiffness of the back, furuncles, mental diseases, hysteria.

METHOD:
Puncture obliquely upward 0.5-1.0 cun.

NOTES:

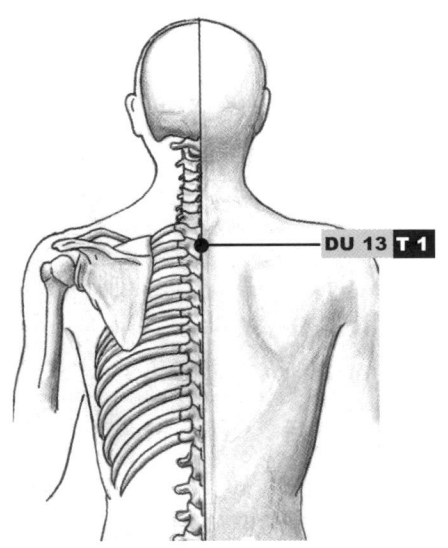

DU 13 **T 1**

LOCATION:
Below the spinous process of the 1st thoracic vertebra.

INDICATIONS:
Stiffness of the back, head & neck, muscle spasms, headache, malaria, febrile diseases, fever, seizures, psychosis, pulmonary tuberculosis.

METHOD:
Puncture obliquely upward 0.5-1.0 cun.

NOTES:

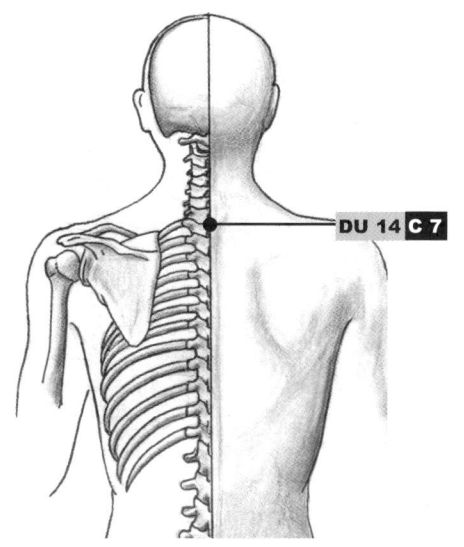

DU 14 C 7

LOCATION:
Below the spinous process of the 7th cervical vertebra, approximately at the level of the shoulders.

INDICATIONS:
Neck pain and rigidity, malaria, hepatitis, blood diseases, eczema, febrile diseases, fever, heat stroke, epilepsy, seizures, afternoon fever, cough, bronchitis, asthma, pulmonary tuberculosis, emphysema, common cold, back stiffness, hemiplegia, pain in the back of the shoulder, psychosis.

METHOD:
Puncture obliquely upward 0.5-1.0 cun.

NOTES:

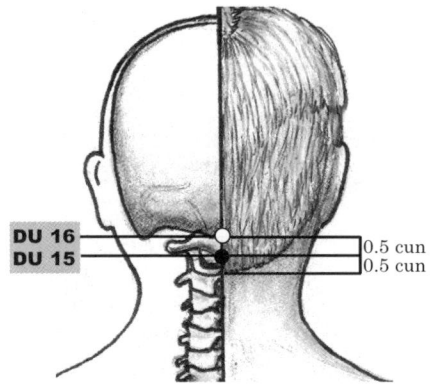

DU 16 ——
DU 15 ——

0.5 cun
0.5 cun

LOCATION:

0.5 cun directly above the midpoint of the posterior hairline, in the depression below the spinous process of the 1st cervical vertebra.

INDICATIONS:

Mental disorders, hysteria, convulsions, epilepsy, seizures, deafness and mute, cerebral palsy, incomplete maturation of the brain, sudden hoarseness of voice, apoplexy, stiffness of the tongue and aphasia, occipital headache, neck rigidity.

METHOD:

Puncture perpendicularly 0.5-0.8 cun. Upward oblique or deep puncture is forbidden.

NOTES:

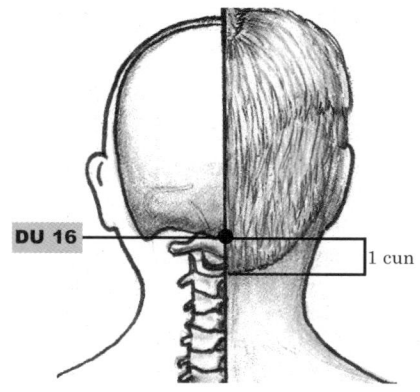

DU 16 — 1 cun

LOCATION:
1 cun directly above the midpoint of the posterior hairline, directly below the external occipital protuberance, in the depression between m.trapezius of both sides.

INDICATIONS:
Headache, neck rigidity, blurry vision, epistaxis, common cold, sore throat, post-apoplexy aphasia, hemiplegia, stroke, numbness of the limbs, mental disorders.

METHOD:
Puncture perpendicularly 0.5-0.8 cun. Upward oblique or deep puncture is forbidden.

NOTES:

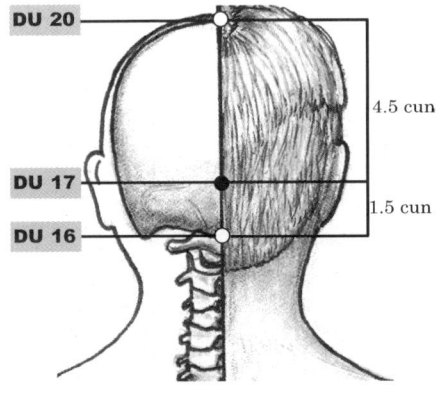

DU 20

4.5 cun

DU 17

1.5 cun

DU 16

LOCATION:
On the midline of the head, 1.5 cun directly above DU 16, superior to the external occipital protuberance.

INDICATIONS:
Epilepsy, seizures, dizziness, pain and stiffness of the neck, headache, insomnia.

METHOD:
Puncture subcutaneously 0.3-0.5 cun.

NOTES:

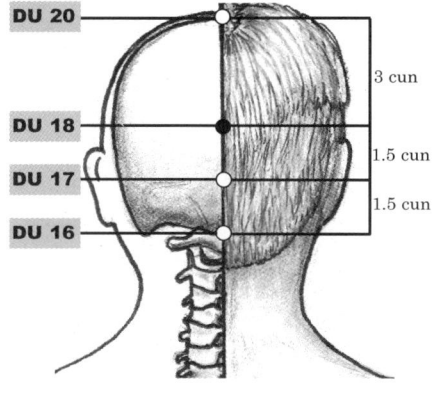

DU 20

3 cun

DU 18

1.5 cun

DU 17

1.5 cun

DU 16

LOCATION:
On the midline of the head, 1.5 cun directly above DU 17, midway between DU 16 and DU 20.

INDICATIONS:
Headache, neck rigidity, blurry vision, mania, insomnia, seizures.

METHOD:
Puncture subcutaneously 0.3-0.5 cun.

NOTES:

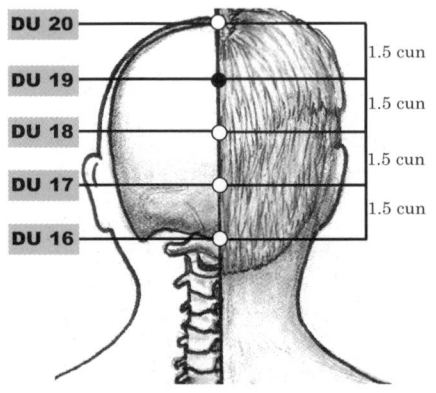

DU 20

DU 19

DU 18

DU 17

DU 16

1.5 cun

1.5 cun

1.5 cun

1.5 cun

LOCATION:
On the midline of the head, 1.5 cun directly above DU 18.

INDICATIONS:
Headache, migraine, common cold, insomnia, vertigo, mania, epilepsy, seizures.

METHOD:
Puncture subcutaneously 0.3-0.5 cun.

NOTES:

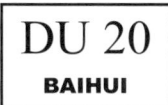

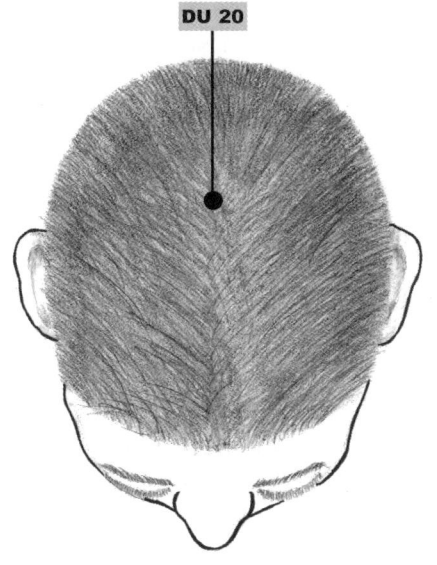

DU 20

LOCATION:
On the midline of the head, 7 cun directly above the posterior hairline, approximately on the midpoint of the line connecting the apexes of the two auricles.

INDICATIONS:
Headache, vertigo, dizziness, tinnitus, hypertension, nasal obstruction, aphasia by apoplexy, shock, coma, mental disorders, insomnia, seizures, prolapse of the rectum and uterus.

METHOD:
Puncture subcutaneously 0.3-0.5 cun.

NOTES:

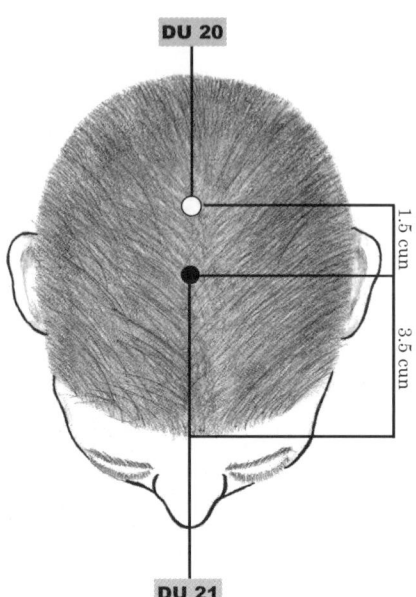

DU 20

1.5 cun

3.5 cun

DU 21

LOCATION:
On the midline of the head, 1.5 cun anterior to DU 20.

INDICATIONS:
Epilepsy, infantile convulsions, dizziness, vertigo, blurry vision, vertex headache, rhinorrhea, rhinitis, rhinopolypus.

METHOD:
Puncture subcutaneously 0.3-0.5 cun.

NOTES:

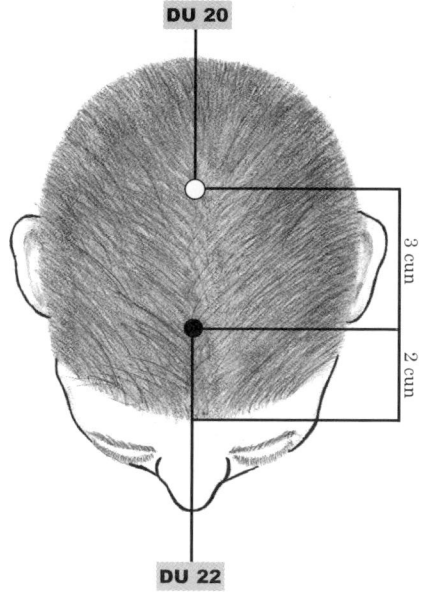

DU 20

3 cun

2 cun

DU 22

LOCATION:
2 cun posterior to the midpoint of the anterior hairline, 3 cun anterior to DU 20.

INDICATIONS:
Headache, vertigo, blurry vision, rhinorrhea, rhinitis, rhinopolypus, infantile convulsion.

METHOD:
Puncture subcutaneously 0.3-0.5 cun. This point is prohibited in infants with a patent frontal suture.

NOTES:

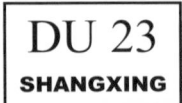

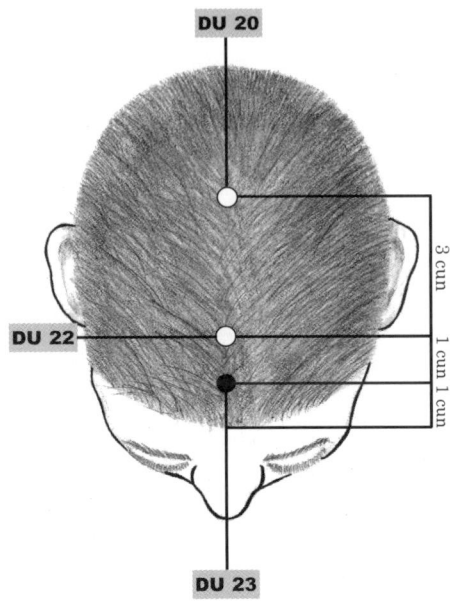

DU 20

DU 22

DU 23

3 cun

1 cun 1 cun

LOCATION:
1 cun directly above the midpoint of the anterior hairline.

INDICATIONS:
Headache, ophthalmalgia, keratitis, sore eyes, epistaxis, rhinorrhea, rhinitis, rhinopolypus, mental disorders.

METHOD:
Puncture subcutaneously 0.3-0.5 cun or prick to cause bleeding. This point is prohibited in infants with a patent frontal suture.

NOTES:

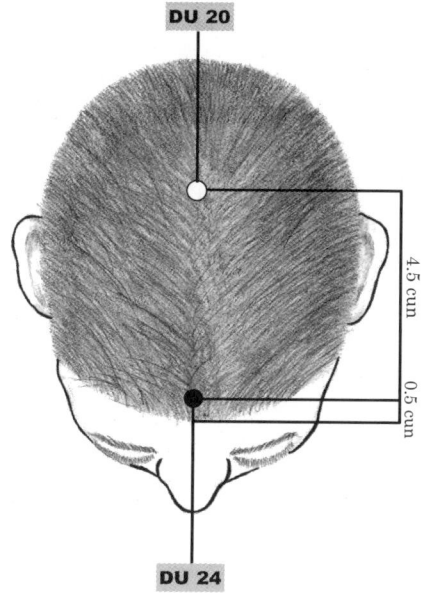

DU 20

4.5 cun

0.5 cun

DU 24

LOCATION:

0.5 cun directly above the midpoint of the anterior hairline.

INDICATIONS:

Epilepsy, seizures, stomatitis, anxiety, palpitation, insomnia, headache, vertigo, rhinorrhea, rhinitis, rhinopolypus.

METHOD:

Puncture subcutaneously 0.3-0.5 cun or prick to cause bleeding.

NOTES:

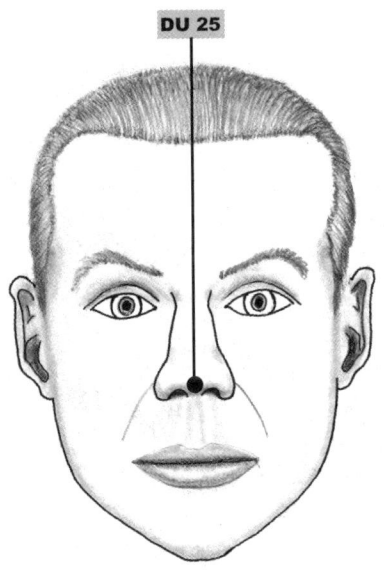

DU 25

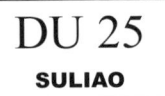

DU 25
SULIAO

LOCATION:
On the tip of the nose.

INDICATIONS:
Loss of consciousness, shock, low blood pressure, bradycardia, nasal obstruction, epistaxis, rhinorrhea, rhinitis, rosacea, brandy nose.

METHOD:
Puncture perpendicularly 0.2-0.3 cun, or prick to cause bleeding.

NOTES:

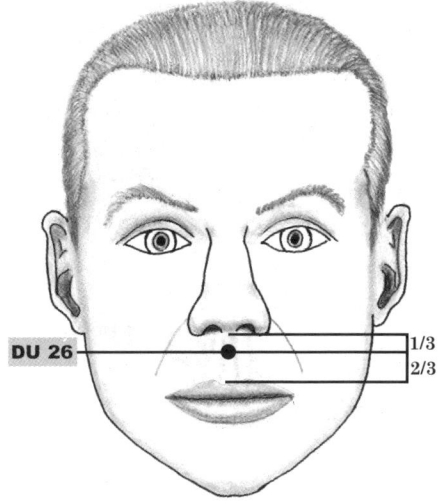

DU 26 — 1/3 2/3

LOCATION:
In the philtrum, approximately 1/3 of the distance from the bottom of the nose to the top of the lip.

INDICATIONS:
Mental disorders, psychosis, epilepsy, seizures, hysteria, infantile convulsion, coma, shock, fainting, heat exhaustion, motion sickness, trismus, deviation of the mouth and eyes, puffiness of the face, facial edema, nose diseases, halitosis, spasm of the muscles in the region of the mouth or eyes, pain and stiffness of the lower back, acute lower back sprain.

METHOD:
Puncture obliquely upward 0.3-0.5 cun.

NOTES:

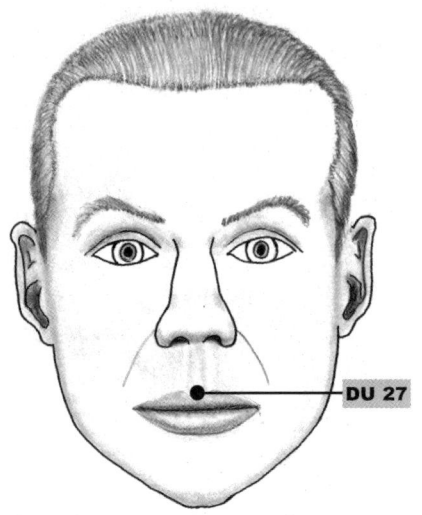

DU 27

LOCATION:
On the median tubercle of the upper lip, at the junction of the skin and upper lip.

INDICATIONS:
Mental disorders, lip twitching, lip stiffness, pain and swelling of the gums, stomatitis, vomiting, occluded nose, rhinopolypus, seizures.

METHOD:
Puncture obliquely upward 0.2-0.3 cun.

NOTES:

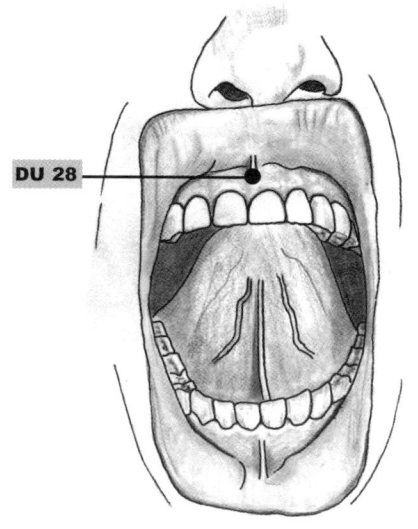

DU 28

LOCATION:
At the junction of the gum and the frenulum of the upper lip.

INDICATIONS:
Mental disorders, pain and swelling of the gums, pain & bleeding around the teeth, rhinnorhea, rhinopolypus, acute wrist pain.

METHOD:
Puncture obliquely upward 0.1-0.2 cun, or prick to cause bleeding.

NOTES:

NOTES

402

NOTES

REN
CHANNEL

REN MERIDIAN

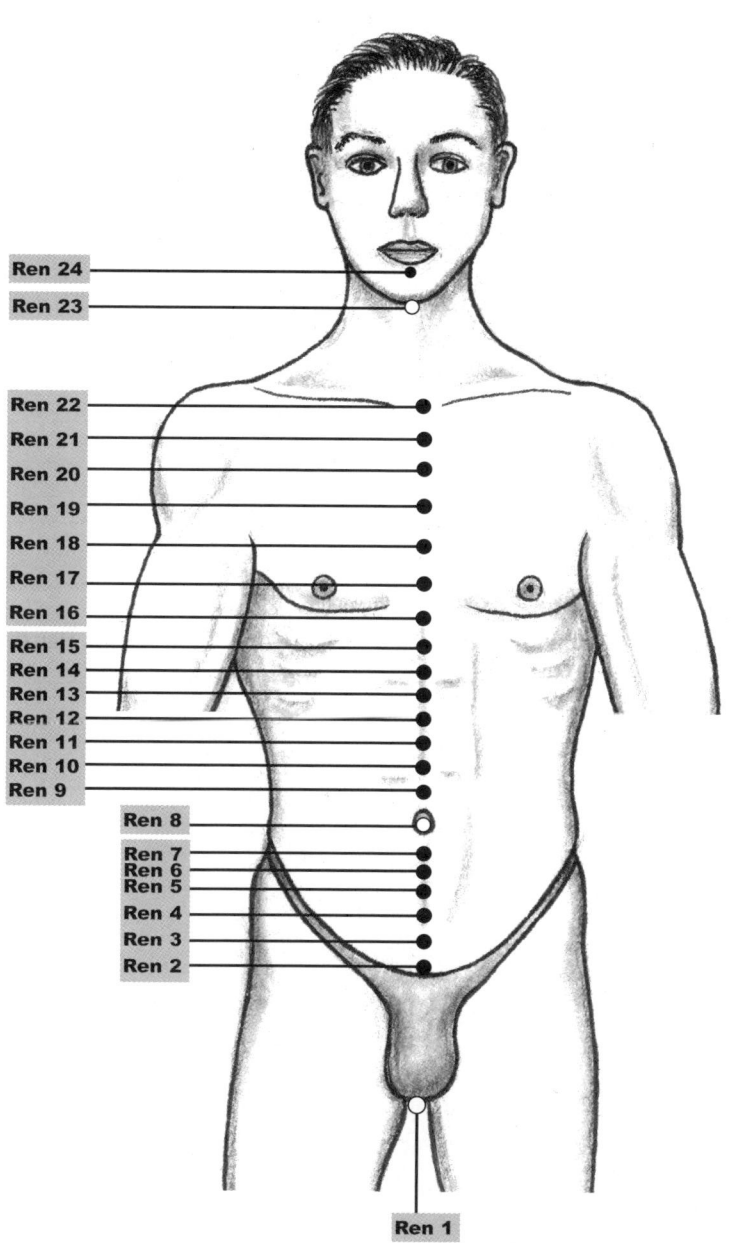

Ren 24
Ren 23
Ren 22
Ren 21
Ren 20
Ren 19
Ren 18
Ren 17
Ren 16
Ren 15
Ren 14
Ren 13
Ren 12
Ren 11
Ren 10
Ren 9
Ren 8
Ren 7
Ren 6
Ren 5
Ren 4
Ren 3
Ren 2
Ren 1

REN MERIDIAN

GENERAL PATHWAY	**COURSE 1:** Arises in the lower abdomen below Ren 3, ascends along the midline of the abdomen and chest, crosses the throat & jaw, and finally winds around the mouth (connects with DU 28), terminating in the region of the eye (connects with ST 1). **COURSE 2:** Arises in the pelvic cavity, enters the spine and ascends along the back.
CONNECTING CHANNEL	• Separates from the DU channel at the lower end of the sternum. • From Ren 15, it spreads over the abdomen.

THERAPEUTIC INDICATIONS	• Local diseases of the abdomen, chest, neck, head and face and their related internal organs. A few points have tonic functions or can be used in treating mental disorders.
PATHOLOGY	• Pathology will appear primarily in pathological symptoms of the Yin channels, especially symptoms associated with the Liver and Kidneys. • Its function is closely related with pregnancy and therefore has intimate links with the Kidneys and uterus. • If there is Qi Deficiency, infertility or other disorders of the urogenital system may result. • Leukorrhea, irregular menstruation, colic, etc. are all symtoms associated with the Ren channel.

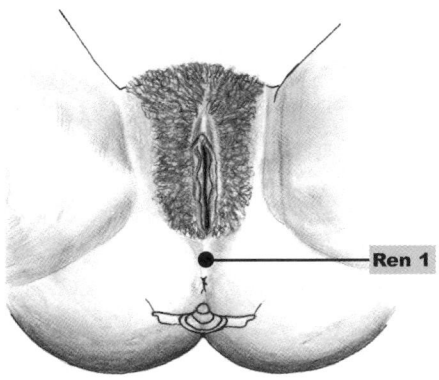

Ren 1

LOCATION:
Between the anus and the root of the scrotum in males and between the anus and the posterior labial commissure in females.

INDICATIONS:
Vaginitis, retention of urine, hemorrhoids, nocturnal emission, enuresis, urethritis, prostatitis, irregular menstruation, mental disorders, to revive from drowning.

METHOD:
Puncture perpendicularly 0.5-1.0 cun.

NOTES:

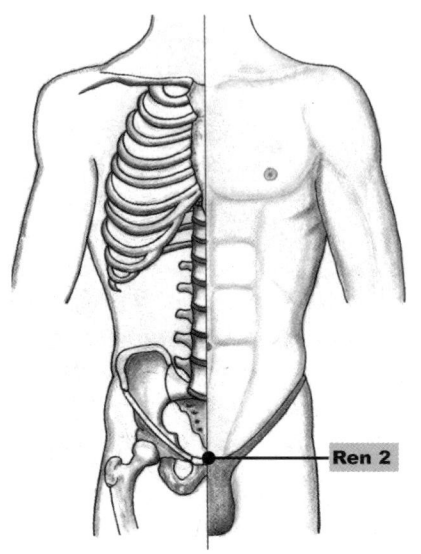

Ren 2

LOCATION:
On the midpoint of the upper border of the symphysis pubis.

INDICATIONS:
Retention and dribbling of urine, cystitis, enuresis, nocturnal emission, impotence, orchitis, morbid leukorrhea, irregular menstruation, dysmenorrhea, prolapsed uterus, hernia.

METHOD:
Puncture perpendicularly 0.5-1.0 cun.

NOTES:

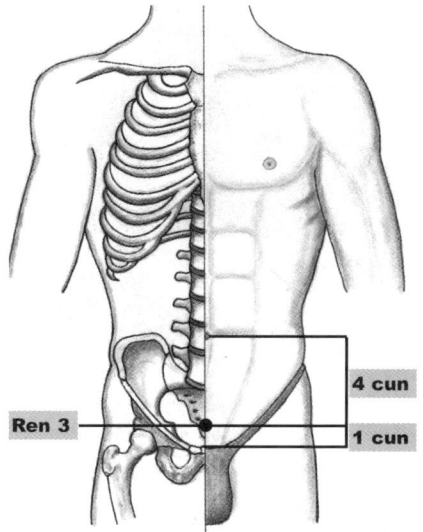

4 cun

Ren 3

1 cun

LOCATION:
On the midline of the abdomen, 4 cun below the umbilicus.

INDICATIONS:
Enuresis, nocturnal emission, spermatorrhea, impotence, premature ejaculation, hernia, uterine bleeding, irregular menstruation, dysmenorrhea, female sterility, morbid leukorrhea, frequency of urination, retention of urine, nephritis, urethritis, pelveoperitonitis, pain in the lower abdomen, prolapse of the uterus, vaginitis, sciatica.

METHOD:
Puncture perpendicularly 0.5-1.0 cun.

NOTES:

Ren 4
GUANYUAN

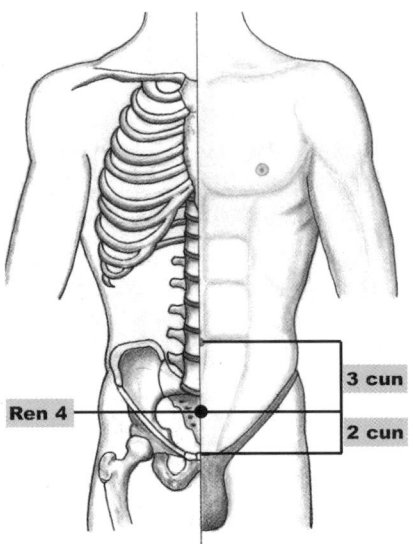

Ren 4

3 cun

2 cun

LOCATION:
On the midline of the abdomen, 3 cun below the umbilicus.

INDICATIONS:
Enuresis, nocturnal emission, spermatorrhea, impotence, frequency of urination, urinary tract infections, nephritis, retention of urine, hernia, irregular menstruation, pelveoperitonitis, morbid leukorrhea, dysmennorhea, uterine bleeding, postpartum hemorrhage, prolapsed uterus, lower abdominal pain, indigestion, diarrhea, dysentery, roundworms in the intestinal tract, prolapse of the rectum, flaccid type of aploplexy.

METHOD:
Puncture perpendicularly 0.8-1.2 cun. This is one of the most important points for tonification.

NOTES:

410

FRONT-MU POINT OF THE SAN JIAO

Ren 5
SHIMEN

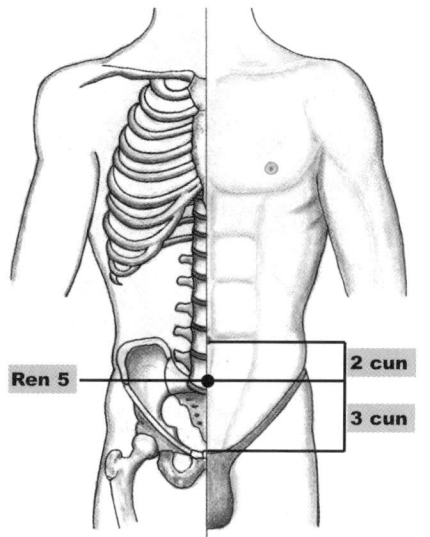

Ren 5

2 cun

3 cun

LOCATION:
On the midline of the abdomen, 2 cun below the umbilicus.

INDICATIONS:
Abdominal pain, diarrhea, edema, hernia, anuria, enuresis, retention of urine, mastitis, amenorrhea, morbid leukorrhea, uterine bleeding, postpartum hemorrhage.

METHOD:
Puncture perpendicularly 0.5-1.0 cun.

NOTES:

411

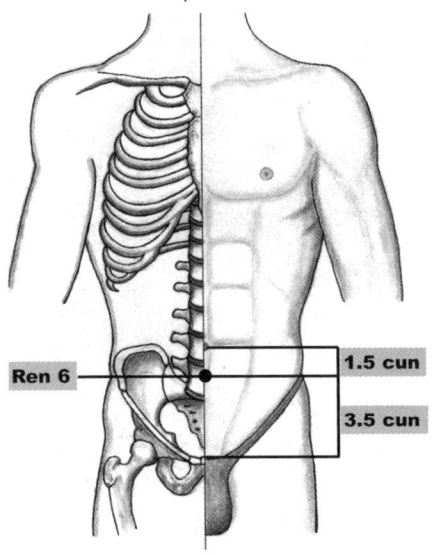

Ren 6

1.5 cun

3.5 cun

LOCATION:
On the midline of the abdomen, 1.5 cun below the umbilicus.

INDICATIONS:
Abdominal distention & pain, enuresis, nocturnal emission, incontinence, polyuria, urinary retention, spermatorrhea, impotence, hernia, edema, diarrhea, dysentery, intestinal paralysis, uterine bleeding, irregular menstruation, dysmenorrhea, amenorrhea, morbid leukorrhea, post-partum hemorrhage, constipation, flaccid type of apoplexy, asthma, neurasthenia.

METHOD:
Puncture perpendicularly 0.8-1.2 cun. This is one of the important points for tonification.

NOTES:

412

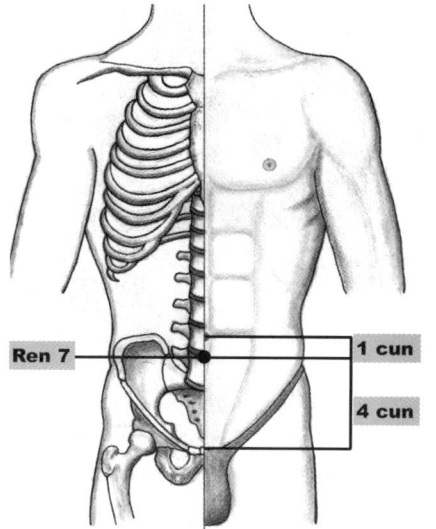

Ren 7

1 cun

4 cun

LOCATION:
On the midline of the abdomen, 1 cun below the umbilicus.

INDICATIONS:
Abdominal distention, edema, hernia & hernia pain, irregular menstruation, uterine bleeding, morbid leukorrhea, pruritus vulvae, postpartum hemorrhage, prolapsed uterus, abdominal pain around the umbilicus.

METHOD:
Puncture perpendicularly 0.8-1.2 cun.

NOTES:

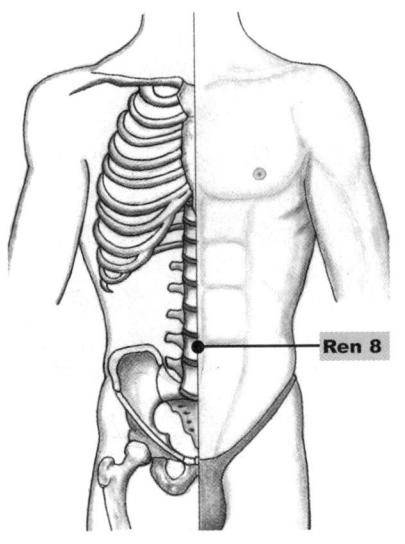

LOCATION:
In the center of the umbilicus.

INDICATIONS:
Abdominal pain, borborygmus, flaccid type of apoplexy, prolapse of the rectum & anus, chronic diarrhea, acute & chronic enteritis, intestinal tuberculosis, shock resulting from intestinal adhesions, edema.

METHOD:
Needling is not done at this point. Moxibustion with moxa stick or cones, over a layer of salt, is applicable.

NOTES:

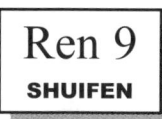

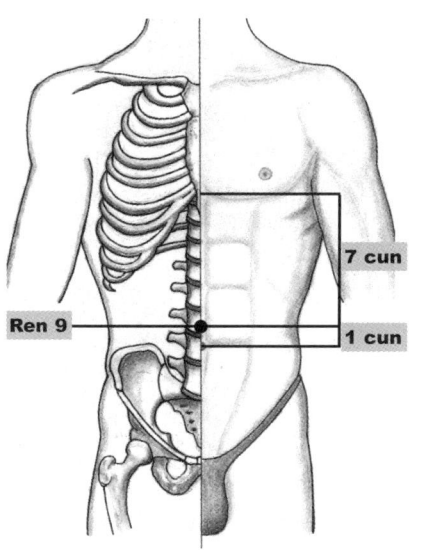

7 cun

Ren 9

1 cun

LOCATION:
On the midline of the abdomen, 1 cun above the umbilicus.

INDICATIONS:
Abdominal pain, borborygmus, edema, ascites, retention of urine, nephritis, diarrhea, vomiting.

METHOD:
Puncture perpendicularly 0.5-1.0 cun.

NOTES:

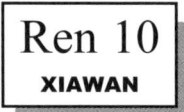

Ren 10
XIAWAN

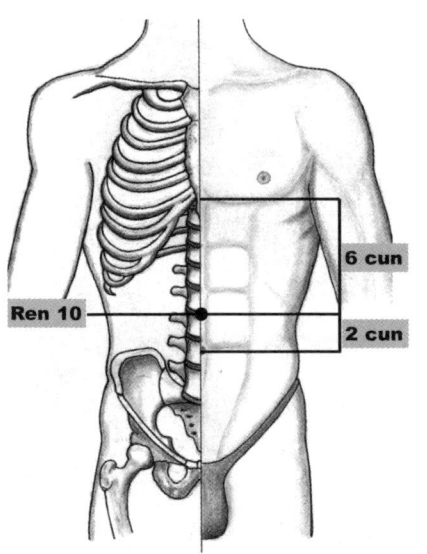

Ren 10

6 cun

2 cun

LOCATION:
On the midline of the abdomen, 2 cun above the umbilicus.

INDICATIONS:
Epigastric pain, abdominal pain, stomach ache, prolapsed stomach, borborygmus, indigestion, vomiting, diarrhea.

METHOD:
Puncture perpendicularly 0.5-1.2 cun.

NOTES:

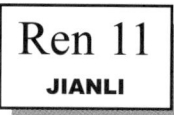

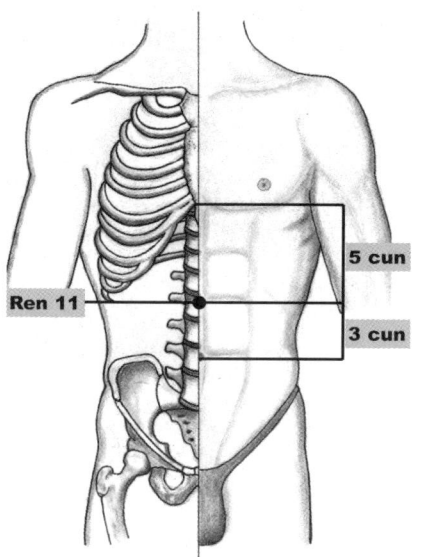

Ren 11

5 cun

3 cun

LOCATION:
On the midline of the abdomen, 3 cun above the umbilicus.

INDICATIONS:
Stomachache, acute & chronic gastritis, vomiting, abdominal distention & pain, borborygmus, edema, ascites, anorexia, angina pectoris.

METHOD:
Puncture perpendicularly 0.5-1.2 cun.

NOTES:

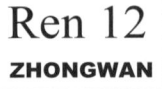
Ren 12
ZHONGWAN

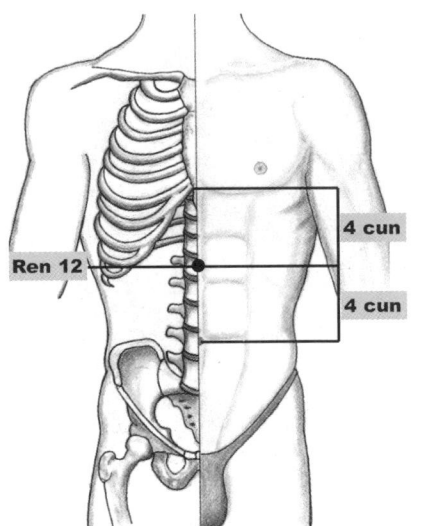

Ren 12

4 cun

4 cun

LOCATION:
On the midline of the abdomen, 4 cun above the umbilicus.

INDICATIONS:
Stomach ache, abdominal distention, borborygmus, nausea, vomiting, acid regurgitation, diarrhea, constipation, dysentery, acute or chronic gastritis, gastric ulcers, prolapsed stomach, acute intestinal obstruction, jaundice, indigestion, insomnia, hypertension, neurasthenia, mental diseases.

METHOD:
Puncture perpendicularly 0.5-1.2 cun.

NOTES:

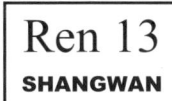

Ren 13
SHANGWAN

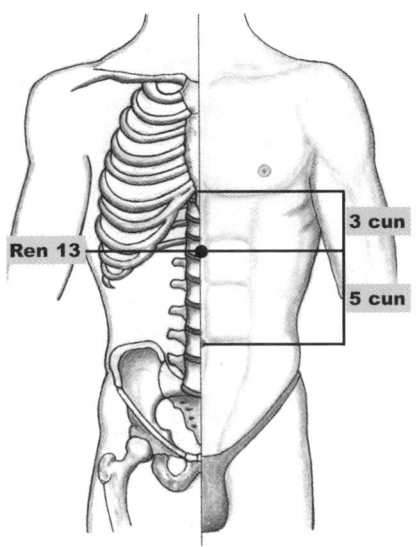

Ren 13

3 cun

5 cun

LOCATION:
On the midline of the abdomen, 5 cun above the umbilicus.

INDICATIONS:
Stomach ache, abdominal distention, acute & chronic gastritis, dilated stomach, stomach spasms, cardiac spasms, nausea, vomiting, epilepsy, insomnia.

METHOD:
Puncture perpendicularly 0.5-1.2 cun.

NOTES:

FRONT-MU POINT OF THE HEART

Ren 14
JUQUE

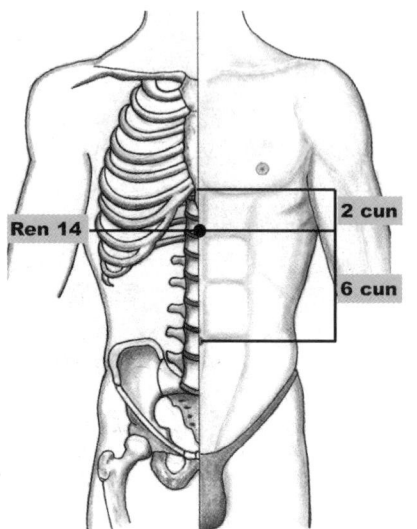

LOCATION:
On the midline of the abdomen, 6 cun above the umbilicus.

INDICATIONS:
Pain in the cardiac region and the chest, angina pectoris, stomach ache, nausea, acid regurgitation, difficulty in swallowing, vomiting, hiccup, roundworms in the bile duct, chronic hepatitis, mental disorders, epilepsy, seizures, palpitation.

METHOD:
Puncture perpendicularly 0.3-0.8 cun.

NOTES:

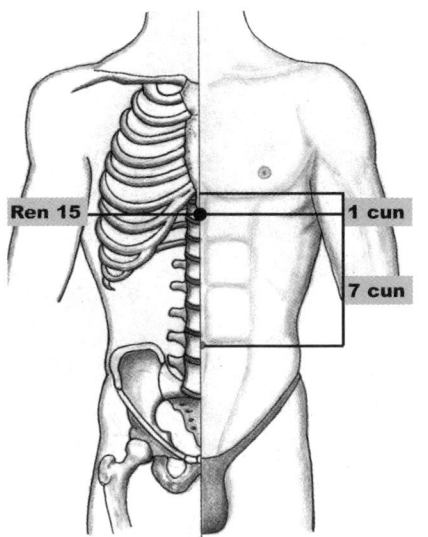

Ren 15

1 cun

7 cun

LOCATION:
Below the xiphoid process, 7 cun above the umbilicus; locate the point in the supine position with the arms uplifted.

INDICATIONS:
Pain in the cardiac region and the chest, angina pectoris, nausea, hiccups, asthma, mental disorders, epilepsy, seizures.

METHOD:
Puncture obliquely downward 0.4-0.6 cun.

NOTES:

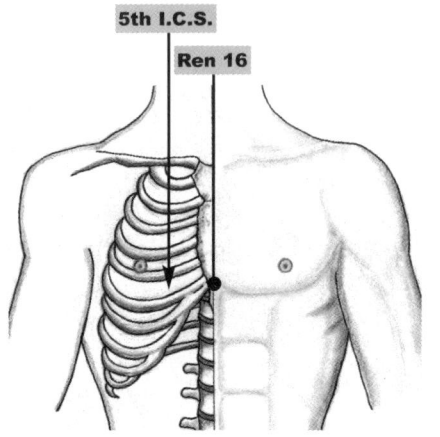

5th I.C.S.

Ren 16

LOCATION:
On the midline of the sternum, at the level with the 5th intercostal space.

INDICATIONS:
Distention and fullness in the chest and intercostal region, asthma, vomiting, food stuck in throat, hiccup, nausea, anorexia.

METHOD:
Puncture subcutaneously 0.3-0.5 cun.

NOTES:

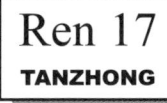
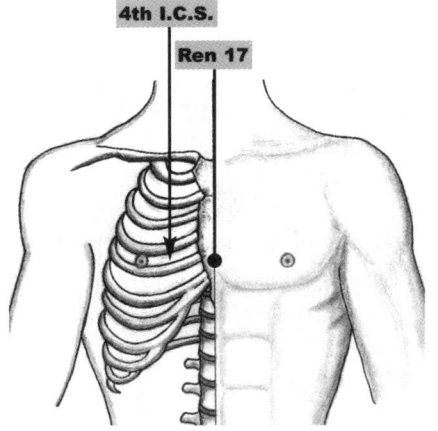

4th I.C.S.

Ren 17

LOCATION:

On the anterior midline, at the level with the 4th intercostal space, midway between the nipples.

INDICATIONS:

Asthma, bronchial asthma, bronchitis, pain in the chest, intercostal neuralgia, fullness in the chest, palpitation, insufficient lactation, mastitis, hiccup, difficulty in swallowing.

METHOD:

Puncture subcutaneously 0.3-0.5 cun.

NOTES:

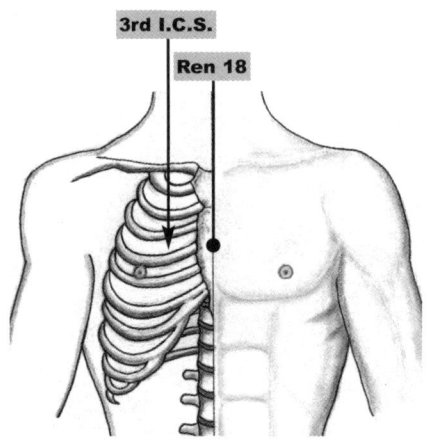

3rd I.C.S.

Ren 18

LOCATION:
On the anterior midline, at the level with the 3rd intercostal space.

INDICATIONS:
Pain in the chest, intercostal neuralgia, cough, bronchitis, emphysema, asthma, vomiting.

METHOD:
Puncture subcutaneously 0.3-0.5 cun.

NOTES:

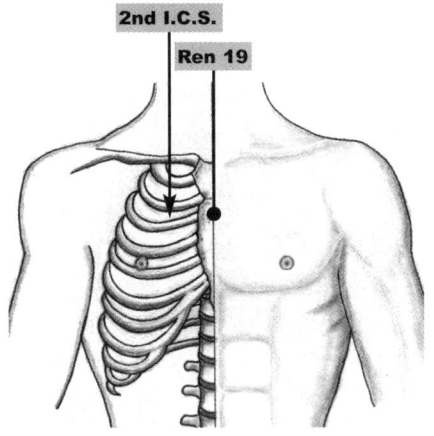

2nd I.C.S.

Ren 19

LOCATION:
On the anterior midline, at the level with the 2nd intercostal space.

INDICATIONS:
Pain in the chest, asthma, cough, bronchiectasis, pulmonary tuberculosis.

METHOD:
Puncture subcutaneously 0.3-0.5 cun.

NOTES:

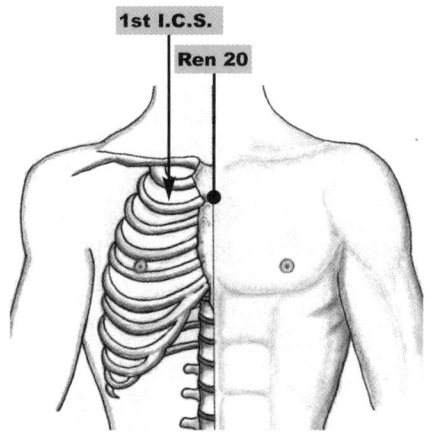

1st I.C.S.

Ren 20

LOCATION:
On the anterior midline, at the midpoint of the sternal angle, at the level with the 1st intercostal space.

INDICATIONS:
Pain in the chest and intercostal regions, intercostal neuralgia, asthma, cough, bronchitis, pharyngitis.

METHOD:
Puncture subcutaneously 0.3-0.5 cun.

NOTES:

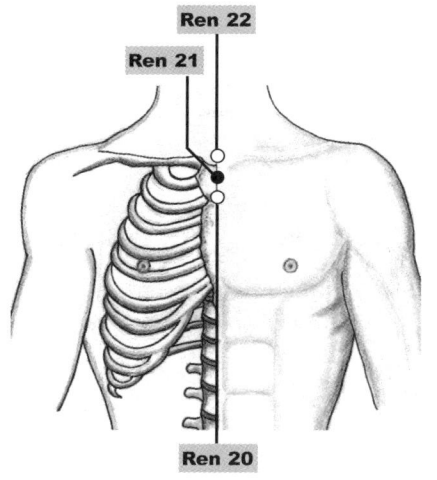

LOCATION:
On the anterior midline, in the center of the sternal manubrium, 1 cun below Ren 22.

INDICATIONS:
Pain in the chest, cough, bronchial asthma, chronic bronchitis, asthma, spasms of the esophagus, cardiac spasms.

METHOD:
Puncture subcutaneously 0.3-0.5 cun.

NOTES:

427

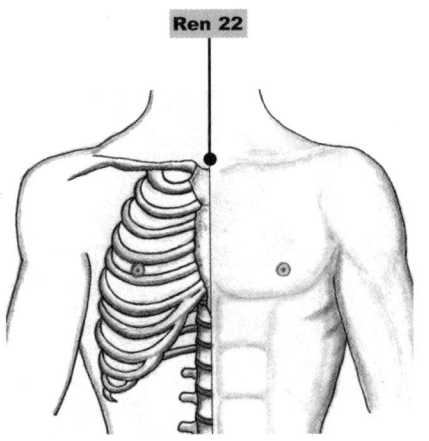

Ren 22

LOCATION:
In the center of the suprasternal fossa.

INDICATIONS:
Asthma, cough, bronchial asthma, bronchitis, sore throat, dry throat, hiccup, sudden hoarseness of the voice, difficulty in swallowing, goiter, nervous vomiting, spasms of the esophagus, diseases of the vocal cords.

METHOD:
First puncture perpendicularly 0.2 cun and then insert the needle tip downward along the posterior aspect of the sternum 0.5-1.0 cun.

NOTES:

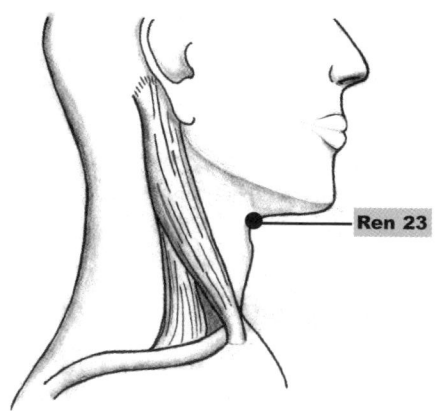

LOCATION:

Above the Adam's apple, in the depression of the upper border of the hyoid bone.

INDICATIONS:

Swelling and pain of the subglossal region, paralysis of the hypoglossal muscle, salivation with glossoplegia, aphasia with stiffness of the tongue by apoplexy, sudden hoarseness of the voice, bronchitis, pharyngitis, tonsillitis, loss of voice, difficulty in swallowing.

METHOD:

Puncture obliquely 0.5-1.0 cun toward the tongue root.

NOTES:

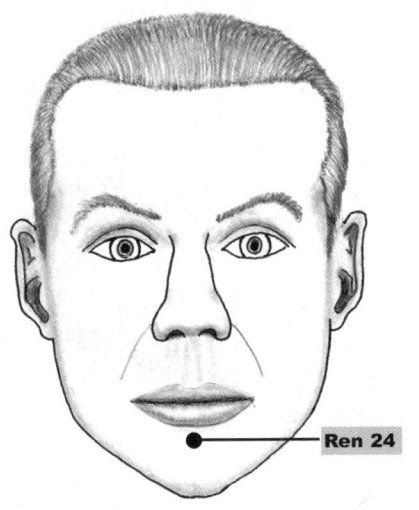

Ren 24
CHENGJIANG

LOCATION:

In the depression in the center of the mentolabial groove.

INDICATIONS:

Facial puffiness, swelling of the gums, ulcers of the mouth, toothache, excessive salivation, mental disorders, deviation of the eyes and mouth, facial paralysis, hemiplegia.

METHOD:

Puncture obliquely upward 0.2-0.3 cun.

NOTES:

NOTES

NOTES

EXTRA POINTS

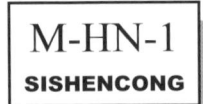

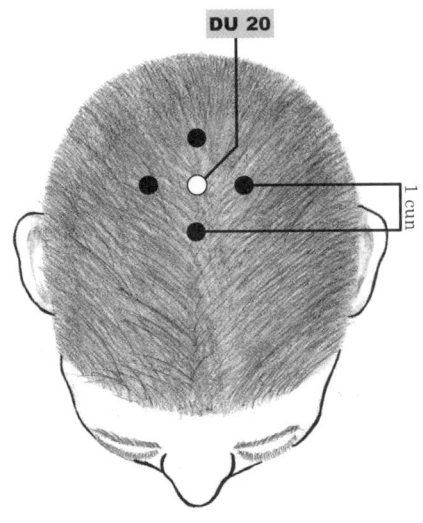

DU 20

1 cun

LOCATION:

A group of 4 points at the vertex, 1 cun respectively posterior, anterior and lateral to DU 20.

INDICATIONS:

Headache, swollen sensation at the vertex, vertigo, insomnia, poor memory, epilepsy, neurasthenia, seizures.

METHOD:

Puncture subcutaneously 0.5-1.0 cun.

NOTES:

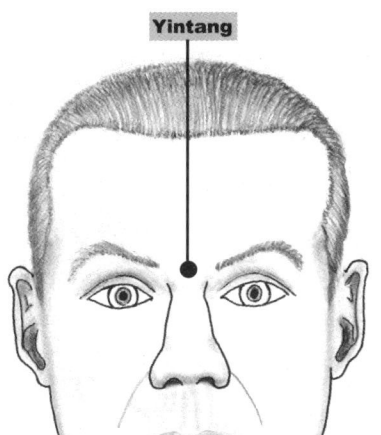

Yintang

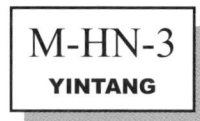

M-HN-3
YINTANG

LOCATION:
Midway between the medial ends of the two eyebrows.

INDICATIONS:
Headache, frontal headache, vertigo, heavy head, epistaxis, rhinorrhea, rhinitis, common cold, hypertension, infantile convulsion, insomnia.

METHOD:
Puncture subcutaneously 0.3-0.5 cun.

NOTES:

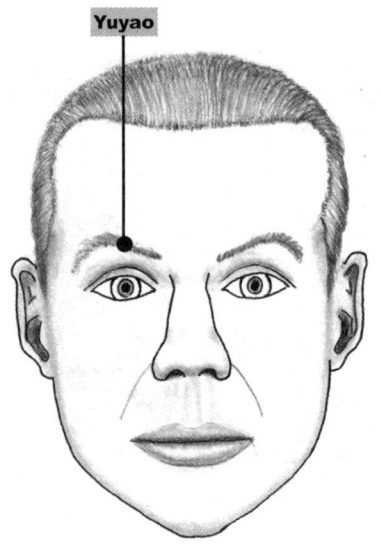

Yuyao

LOCATION:
At the midpoint of the eyebrow, directly above the pupil when the eyes are looking forward.

INDICATIONS:
Pain in the supraorbital region, supraorbital neuralgia, twitching of the eyelids, ptosis, myopia, cloudiness of the cornea, redness, swelling and pain of the eyes, acute conjunctivitis, ophthalmoplegia, facial paralysis.

METHOD:
Puncture subcutaneously 0.3-0.5 cun or prick to cause bleeding.

NOTES:

436

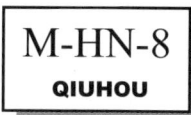
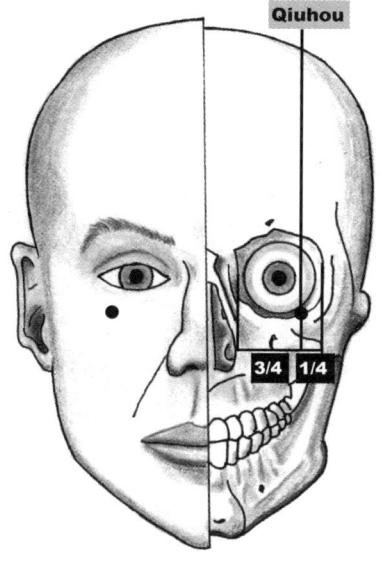

Qiuhou

3/4 1/4

LOCATION:

At the junction of the lateral 1/4 and the medial 3/4 of the infraorbital margin.

INDICATIONS:

Eye diseases, myopia, inflammation or atrophy of the optic nerve, glaucoma, retinitis pigmentosa, opacity of the vitreous body, convergent squint (esotropia).

METHOD:

Push the eyeball upward gently, then puncture perpendicularly 0.5-1.2 cun along the orbital region slowly without movements of lifing, thrusting, twisting and rotating.

NOTES:

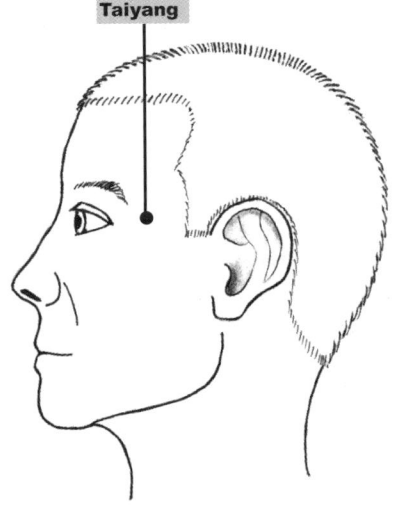

Taiyang

LOCATION:
In the depression about 1 cun posterior to the midpoint between the lateral end of the eyebrow and the outer canthus.

INDICATIONS:
Headache, migraine, common cold, facial paralysis, trigeminal neuralgia, eye diseases, deviation of the eyes and mouth.

METHOD:
Puncture perpendicularly 0.3-0.5 cun, or prick to cause bleeding.

NOTES:

438

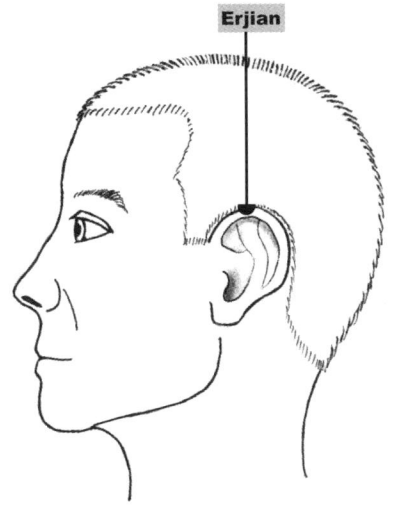

Erjian

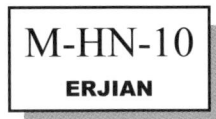

LOCATION:
Fold the auricle, the point is at the apex of the auricle.

INDICATIONS:
Redness, swelling and pain of the eyes, febrile disease, nebula.

METHOD:
Puncture perpendicularly 0.1-0.2 cun or prick to cause bleeding.

NOTES:

439

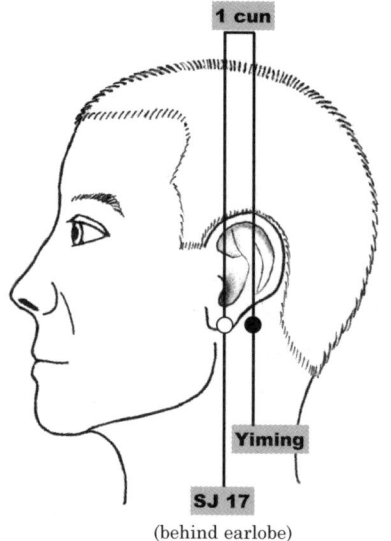

1 cun

SJ 17
(behind earlobe)

Yiming

LOCATION:
1 cun posterior to SJ 17.

INDICATIONS:
Eye diseases, myopia, hypermetropia, night blindness, atrophy of the optic nerve, cataract, vertigo, parotitis, headache, tinnitus, insomnia, mental illness.

METHOD:
Puncture perpendicularly 0.5-0.8 cun.

NOTES:

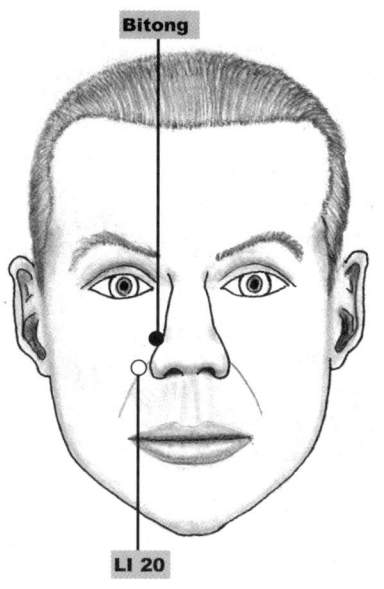

Bitong

LI 20

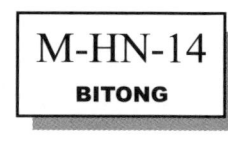

LOCATION:
At the highest point of the nasolabial groove.

INDICATIONS:
Allergic rhinitis, hypertrophic rhinitis, atrophic rhinitis, rhinopolypus, nasosinusitis, nasal obstruction, nasal boils.

METHOD:
Puncture subcutaneously upward 0.3-0.5 cun.

NOTES:

441

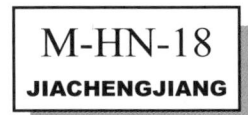

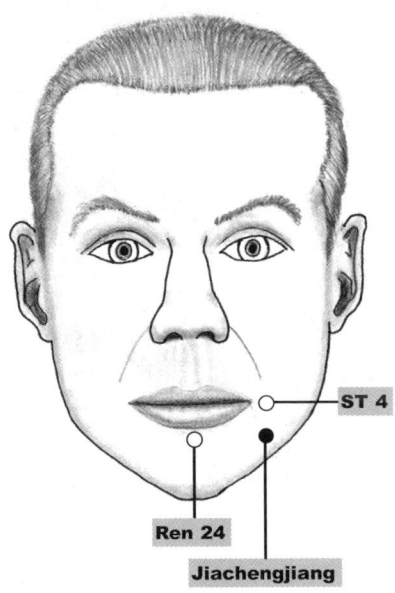

ST 4

Ren 24

Jiachengjiang

LOCATION:
1 cun lateral to Ren 24, directly below ST 4, where the mental foramen of the mandible can be felt.

INDICATIONS:
Pain in the face, deviation of the eyes and mouth, spasm of the facial muscle, trigeminal neuralgia, facial paralysis or spasm.

METHOD:
Puncture obliquely 0.5-1.0 cun.

NOTES:

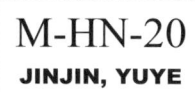

M-HN-20
JINJIN, YUYE

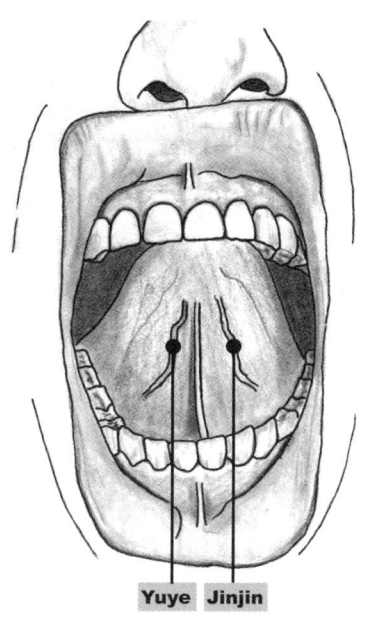

Yuye   Jinjin

LOCATION:

On the veins on both sides of the frenulum of the tongue, Jinjin is on the left,
Yuye on the right.

INDICATIONS:

Swelling of the tongue, vomiting, aphasia
with stiffness of the tongue, stomatitis,
glossitis, tonsillitis, acute gastritis, symp-
toms of emaciation & thirst.

METHOD:

Prick to cause bleeding.

NOTES:

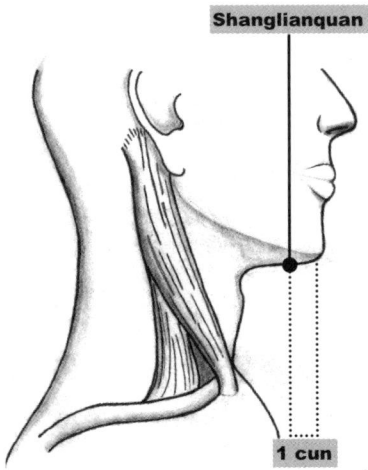

Shanglianquan

1 cun

LOCATION:
1 cun below the midpoint of the lower jaw, in the depression between the hyoid bone and the lower border of the jaw.

INDICATIONS:
Salivation with stiff tongue, stomatitis, acute or chronic pharyngitis, sore throat, difficulty in swallowing, slurred speech, mutism, loss of voice.

METHOD:
Puncture obliquely 0.8-1.2 cun towards the tongue root.

NOTES:

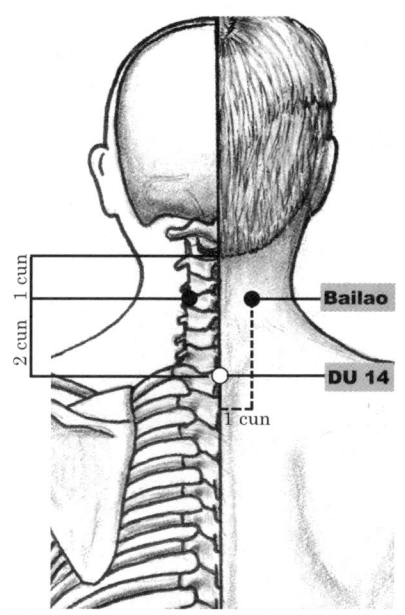

Bailao

DU 14

2 cun 1 cun

1 cun

LOCATION:
2 cun above DU 14, 1 cun lateral to the midline.

INDICATIONS:
Scrofula, cough, asthma, whooping cough, neck rigidity.

METHOD:
Puncture perpendicularly 0.3-0.5 cun.

NOTES:

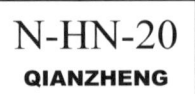

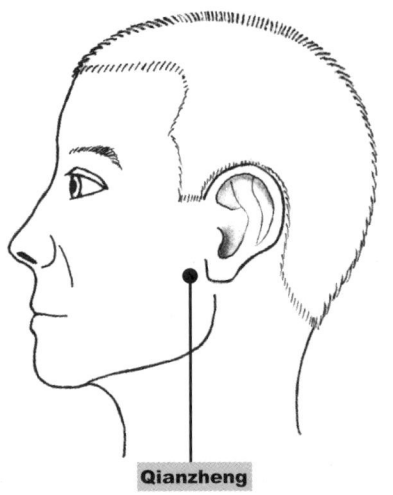

Qianzheng

LOCATION:
0.5-1.0 cun anterior to the auricular lobe.

INDICATIONS:
Deviation of the eyes and mouth, facial paralysis, parotitis, ulceration on tongue and mouth.

METHOD:
Puncture obliquely 0.5-1.0 cun.

NOTES:

446

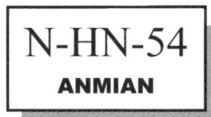

N-HN-54
ANMIAN

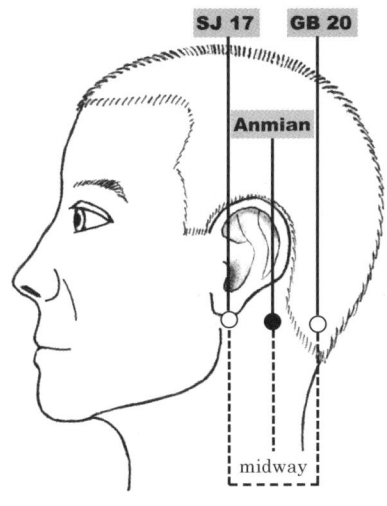

SJ 17   GB 20

Anmian

midway

LOCATION:
Midway between SJ 17 and GB 20.

INDICATIONS:
Insomnia, vertigo, headache, palpitation, mental disorders, hysteria.

METHOD:
Puncture perpendicularly 0.5-0.8 cun.

NOTES:

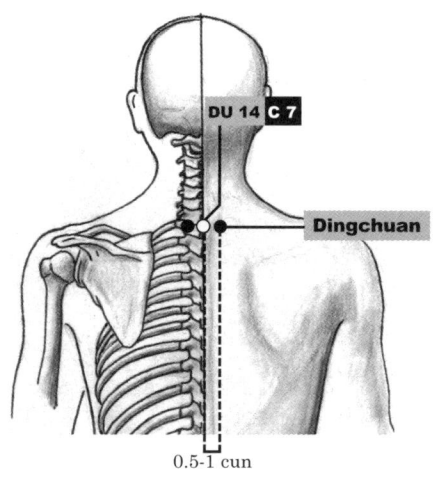

DU 14 C 7

Dingchuan

0.5-1 cun

LOCATION:
0.5-1.0 cun lateral to the lower border of the spinous process of the 7th cervical vertebra where DU 14 is located.

INDICATIONS:
Asthma, cough, bronchitis, urticaria, neck rigidity, pain in the shoulder and back, rubella.

METHOD:
Puncture perpendicularly 0.5-0.8 cun.

NOTES:

448

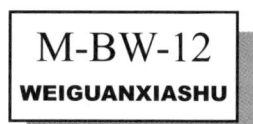

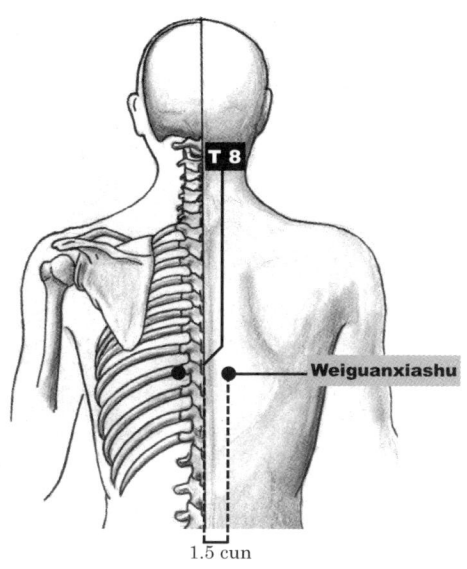

Weiguanxiashu

1.5 cun

LOCATION:
1.5 cun lateral to the lower border of the spinous process of the 8th thoracic vertebra.

INDICATIONS:
Diabetes, vomiting, abdominal pain, pain in the chest and hypochondriac region.

METHOD:
Puncture obliquely 0.5-0.7 cun.

NOTES:

449

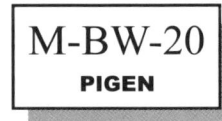

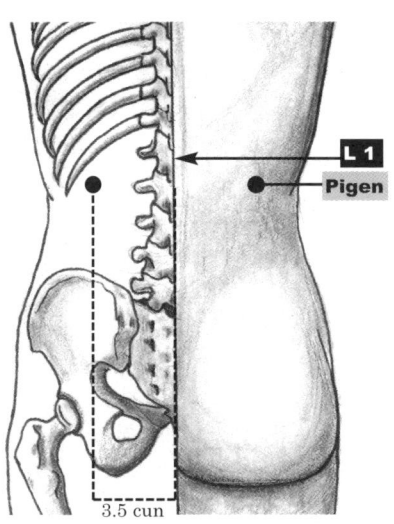

L 1
Pigen

3.5 cun

LOCATION:
3.5 cun lateral to the lower border of the spinous process of L1.

INDICATIONS:
Hepatosplenomegaly, gastritis, enteritis, prolapsed kidney, lumbar pain.

METHOD:
Puncture perpendicularly 0.5-0.8 cun.

NOTES:

450

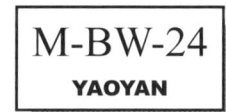

M-BW-24
YAOYAN

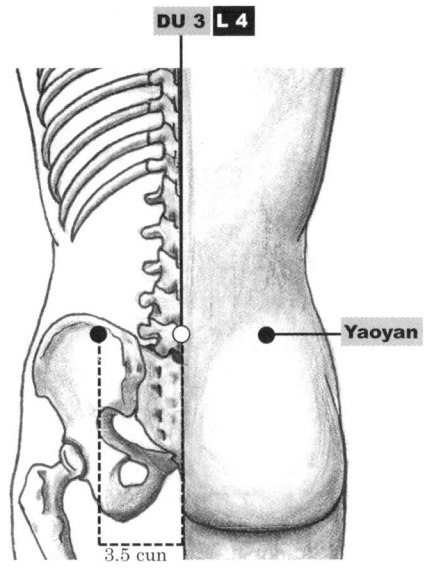

DU 3 L 4

Yaoyan

3.5 cun

LOCATION:
About 3.5 cun lateral to the lower border of the spinous process of L4. The point is in the depression appearing in the prone position.

INDICATIONS:
Lumbar pain, injury to soft tissues of the lumbar region, nephroptosis, frequency of urine, irregular menstruation, gynecological diseases, orchitis.

METHOD:
Puncture perpendicularly 0.8-1.2 cun.

NOTES:

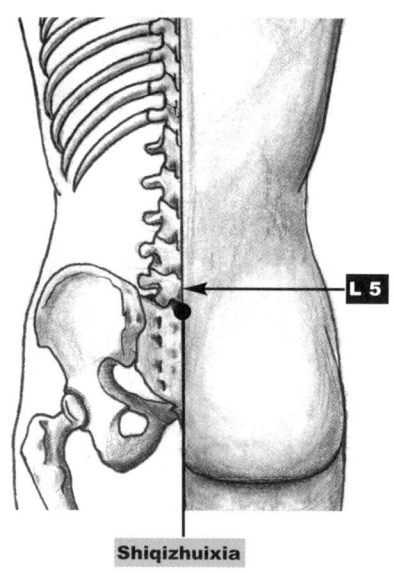

Shiqizhuixia

LOCATION:
Below the spinous process of L5.

INDICATIONS:
Pain in lumbar-sacral region, sciatica, thigh pain, paralysis of the lower extremities, traumatic paraplegia, irregular menstruation, functional uterine bleeding, dysmenorrhea, anal diseases, sequelae of infantile paralysis.

METHOD:
Puncture perpendicularly 0.8-1.2 cun.

NOTES:

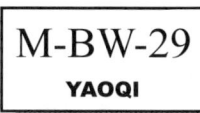

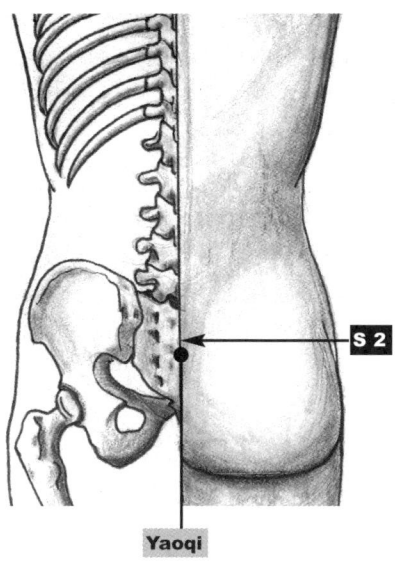

S 2

Yaoqi

LOCATION:

Below the spinous process of the 2nd sacral vertebra.

INDICATIONS:

Epilepsy, seizures, headache, insomnia, constipation.

METHOD:

Puncture subcutaneously upward 1.0-2.0 cun.

NOTES:

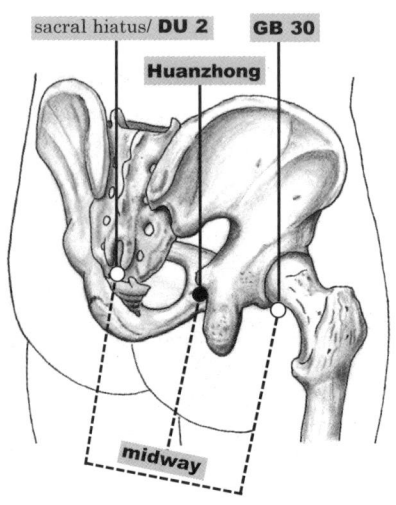

sacral hiatus/ **DU 2**   **GB 30**

Huanzhong

midway

LOCATION:
Midway between GB 30 and DU 2.

INDICATIONS:
Lumbar pain, thigh pain, sciatica, pain in the leg.

METHOD:
Puncture perpendicularly 1.5-2.0 cun.

NOTES:

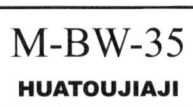

M-BW-35
HUATOUJIAJI

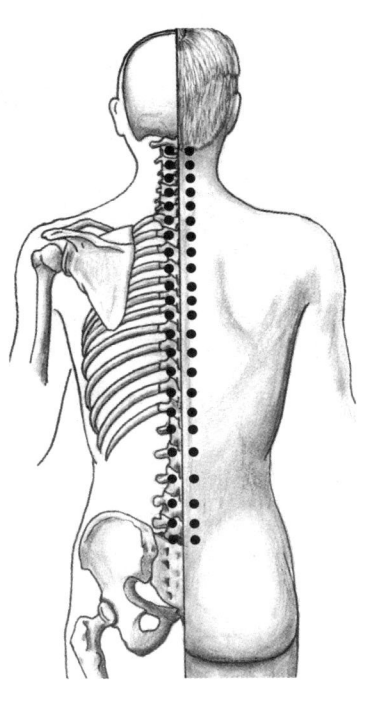

LOCATION:
A group of 48 points on both sides of each of the 24 cervical, thoracic, & lumbar vertebrae, 0.5-1.0 cun lateral to the lower border of each spinous process.

INDICATIONS:
T1-T3: Diseases in the upper limbs
T1-T8: Diseases in the chest region
T6-L5: Diseases in the abdominal region
L1-L5: Diseases in the lower limbs

METHOD:
Puncture perpendicular-oblique 0.5-1.0 cun in the cervical and thoracic regions, puncture perpendicular-oblique 1.0-1.5 cun in the lumbar region.

NOTES:

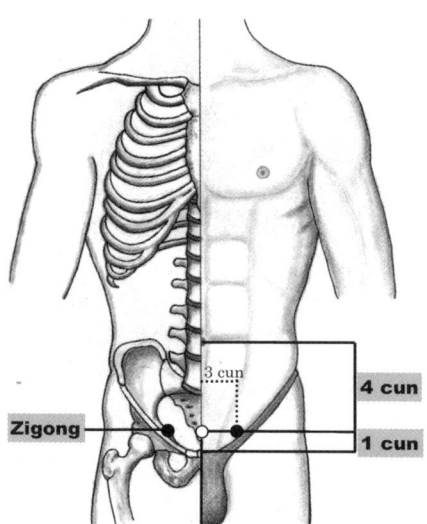

Zigong

3 cun

4 cun

1 cun

Ren 3

LOCATION:
3 cun lateral to Ren 3.

INDICATIONS:
Prolapse of the uterus, irregular menstruation, dysmenorrhea, pelvioperitonitis, female sterility, pyelonephritis, cystitis, orchitis, appendicitis.

METHOD:
Puncture perpendicularly 0.8-1.2 cun.

NOTES:

456

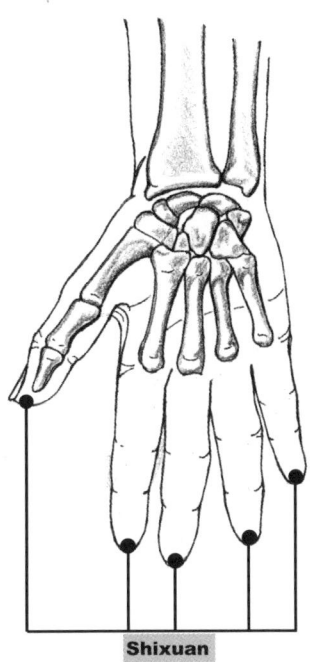

Shixuan

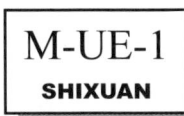

LOCATION:
On the tips of the ten fingers, about 0.1 cun distal to the nails.

INDICATIONS:
Apoplexy, coma, shock, fainting, epilepsy, seizures, hysteria, high fever, heat exhaustion, acute tonsillitis, infantile convulsion, infantile fainting due to fright, numbness of the finger tips.

METHOD:
Puncture 0.1-0.2 cun superficially, or prick to cause bleeding.

NOTES:

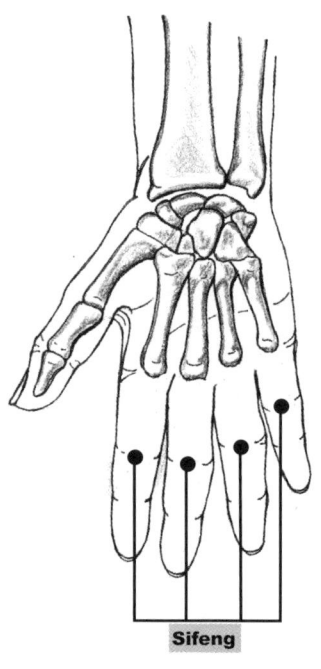

Sifeng

LOCATION:
On the palmar surface, in the midpoint of the transverse creases of the proximal interphalangeal joints of the index, middle, ring, and little fingers.

INDICATIONS:
Malnutrition and indigestion syndrome in children, whooping cough, pertussis, arthritis of the fingers, roundworm in the intestines.

METHOD:
Prick to cause bleeding, or squeeze out a small amount of yellowish viscous fluid locally.

NOTES:

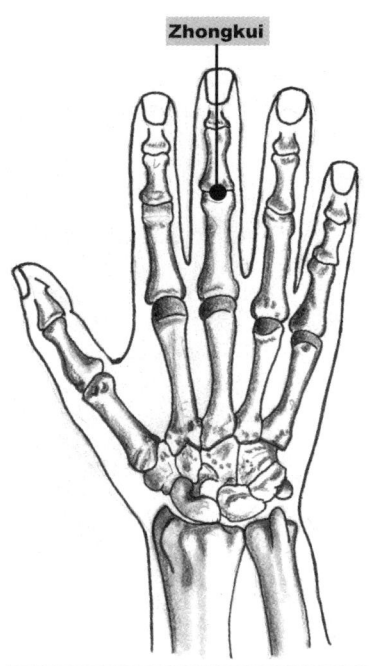

Zhongkui

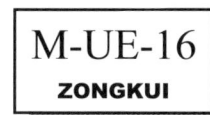
LOCATION:
On the midpoint of the proximal inter-phalangeal joint of the middle finger at the dorsal aspect.

INDICATIONS:
Nausea, vomiting, hiccup, spasm of the esophagus, nose bleed.

METHOD:
Moxibustion is applied with three moxa cones.

NOTES:

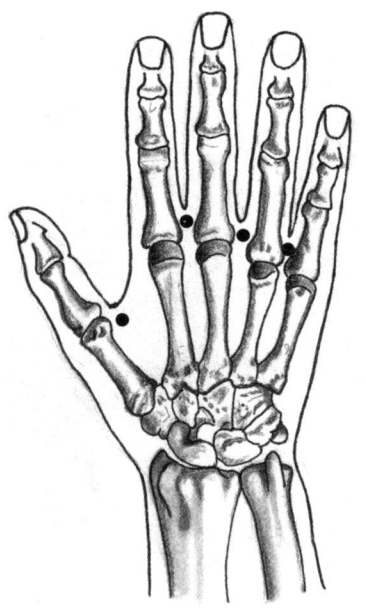

LOCATION:

On the dorsum of the hand, at the junction of the white and red skin of the hand webs, eight in all, making a loose fist to locate the points.

INDICATIONS:

Excessive heat, finger numbness, spasm and contracture of the fingers, diseases of the finger joints, redness and swelling of the dorsum of the hand, headache, stiff neck, toothache, sore throat, snakebite.

METHOD:

Puncture obliquely 0.3-0.5 cun, or prick to cause bleeding.

NOTES:

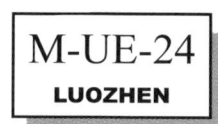

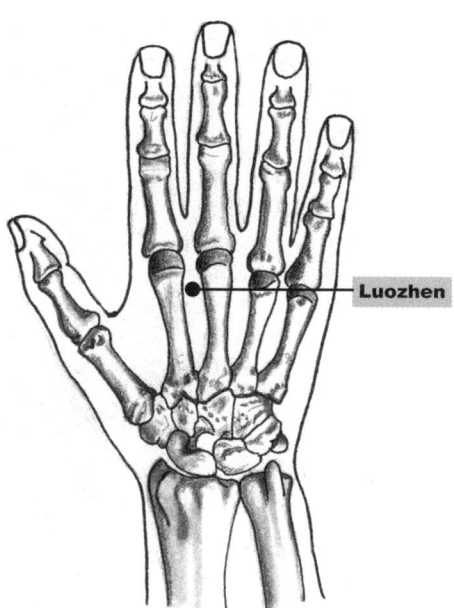

Luozhen

LOCATION:

On the dorsum of the hand, between the 2nd and 3rd metacarpal bones, about 0.5 cun posterior to the metacarpophalangeal joint.

INDICATIONS:

Sore neck, stiff neck, migraine headache, stomach ache, sore throat, pain in the shoulder and arm.

METHOD:

Puncture perpendicularly 0.5-0.8 cun.

NOTES:

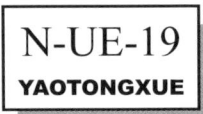

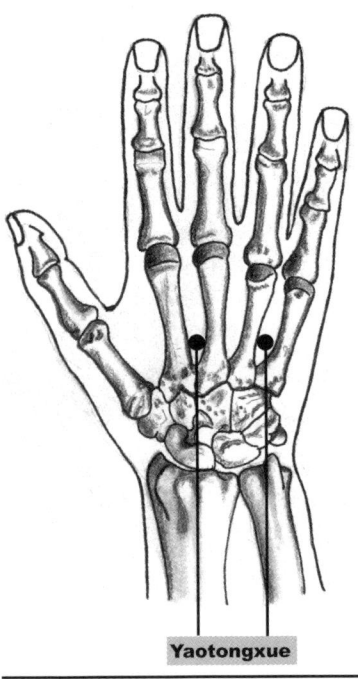

Yaotongxue

LOCATION:

On the dorsum of the hand, midway between the transverse wrist crease and metacarpophalangeal joint, between the 2nd and 3rd metacarpal bones, and between the 4th and 5th metacarpal bones, four points in all on both hands.

INDICATIONS:

Acute lumbar sprain.

METHOD:

Puncture obliquely 0.5-1.0 cun towards the center of the metacarpus from both sides.

NOTES:

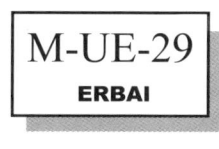

M-UE-29
ERBAI

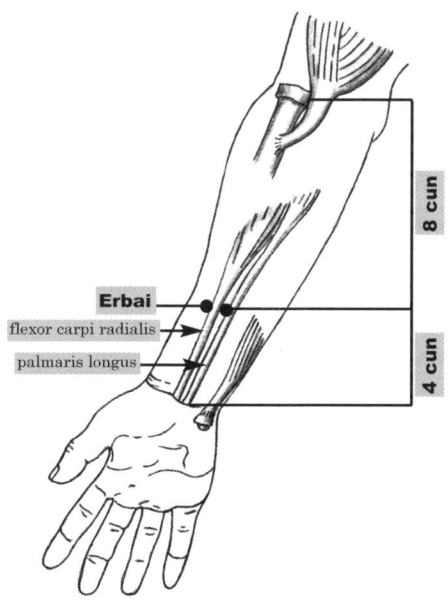

Erbai

flexor carpi radialis

palmaris longus

8 cun

4 cun

LOCATION:
On the metacarpal aspect of the forearm, 4 cun above the transverse wrist crease, on both sides of the tendon of m.flexor carpi radialis, two points on one hand.

INDICATIONS:
Hemorrhoids, prolapse of the rectum & anus, neuralgia of the forearm.

METHOD:
Puncture perpendicularly 0.5-1.0 cun.

NOTES:

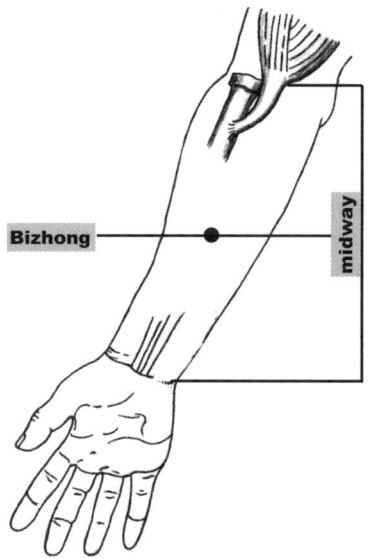

Bizhong | midway

LOCATION:

On the lateral aspect of the forearm, midway between the transverse wrist crease and elbow crease, between the radius and the ulna.

INDICATIONS:

Paralysis, spasm and contracture of the upper extremities, hemiplegia of the upper limb, neuralgia of forearm, pain of the forearm, hysteria.

METHOD:

Puncture perpendicularly 1.0-1.2 cun.

NOTES:

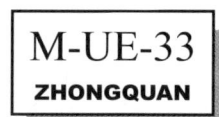

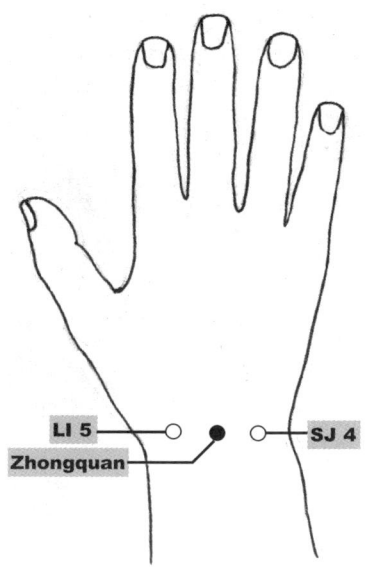

LI 5
Zhongquan

SJ 4

LOCATION:
In the depression between LI 5 and SJ 4.

INDICATIONS:
Stuffy chest, bronchitis, asthma, opacity of the cornea, stomach ache, gastric pain, spitting of blood, diseases of the wrist & surrounding soft tissues.

METHOD:
Puncture perpendicularly 0.3-0.5 cun.

NOTES:

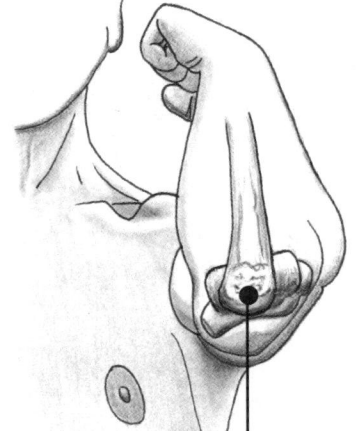

Zhoujian

LOCATION:
On the tip of the ulnar olecrenon when the elbow is flexed.

INDICATIONS:
Scrofula, abscessed carbuncle.

METHOD:
Moxibustion is applied with 7-14 cones.

NOTES:

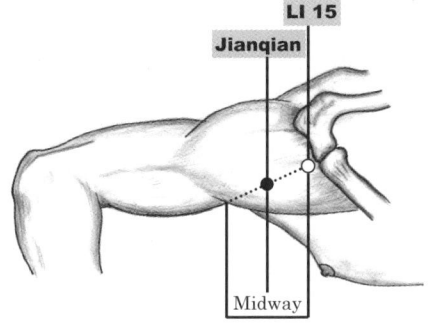

LOCATION:
Midway between the end of the anterior axillary fold and LI 15.

INDICATIONS:
Pain in the shoulder and arm, perifocal inflammation of the shoulder joint, paralysis of the upper extremities, hemiplegia, hypertension, excessive sweating.

METHOD:
Puncture perpendicularly 0.8-1.2 cun.

NOTES:

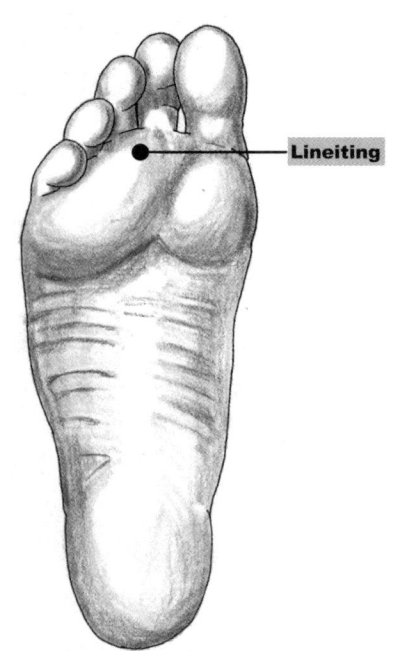
Lineiting

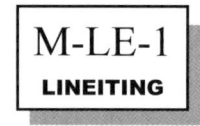

LOCATION:
On the sole, between the 2nd and 3rd toes, on the site just opposite to Neiting (ST 44).

INDICATIONS:
Pain in the toes, infantile convulsions, seizures, acute gastric pain.

METHOD:
Puncture perpendicularly 0.3-0.5 cun.

NOTES:

468

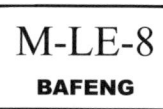

M-LE-8
BAFENG

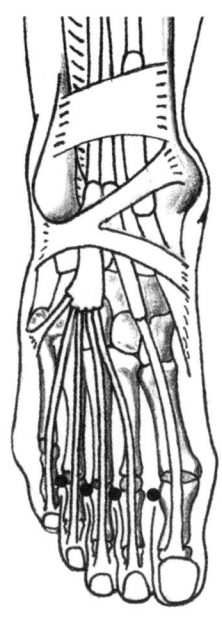

LOCATION:
On the dorsum of the foot, in the depressions on the webs between the toes, proximal to the margins of the webs, eight points in all.

INDICATIONS:
Beriberi, toe pain, redness and swelling of the dorsum of the foot, headache, toothache, stomach ache, irregular menstruation.

METHOD:
Puncture obliquely 0.5-0.8 cun.

NOTES:

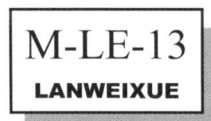

M-LE-13
LANWEIXUE

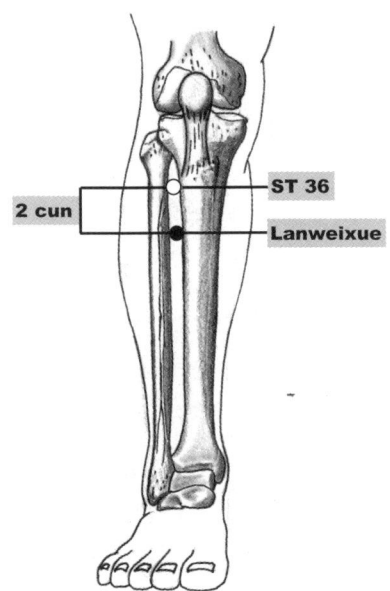

2 cun

ST 36

Lanweixue

LOCATION:
The tender spot about 2 cun below ST 36.

INDICATIONS:
Acute and chronic appendicitis, indigestion, paralysis of the lower extremities, drop foot, indigestion.

METHOD:
Puncture perpendicularly 1.0-1.2 cun.

NOTES:

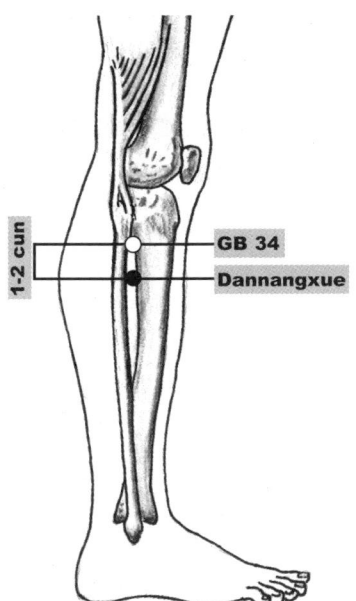

1-2 cun

GB 34

Dannangxue

LOCATION:
The tender spot 1-2 cun below GB 34.

INDICATIONS:
Acute and chronic cholecystitis, cholelithiasis, biliary ascariasis, diseases of the bile duct, muscular atrophy and numbness of the lower extremities, diseases of the lower limb.

METHOD:
Puncture perpendicularly 0.8-1.2 cun.

NOTES:

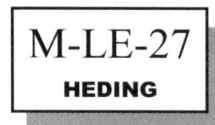

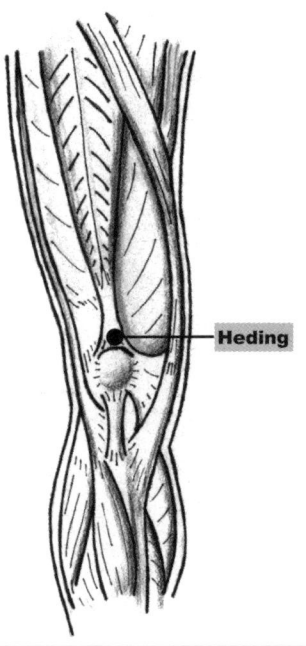

Heding

LOCATION:
In the depression of the midpoint of the superior patellar border.

INDICATIONS:
Knee pain, diseases of the knee joint & surrounding soft tissues, weakness of the foot and leg, paralysis.

METHOD:
Puncture perpendicularly 0.3-0.5 cun.

NOTES:

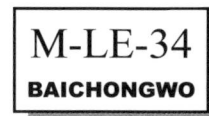

M-LE-34
BAICHONGWO

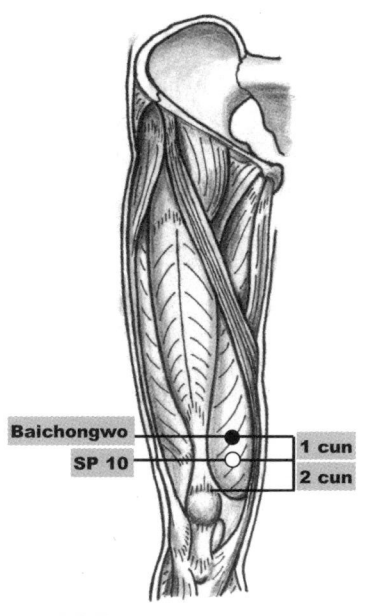

Baichongwo
SP 10
1 cun
2 cun

LOCATION:
1 cun above SP 10.

INDICATIONS:
Rubella, eczema, urticaria, gastrointestinal parasitic diseases.

METHOD:
Puncture perpendicularly 1.0-1.2 cun.

NOTES:

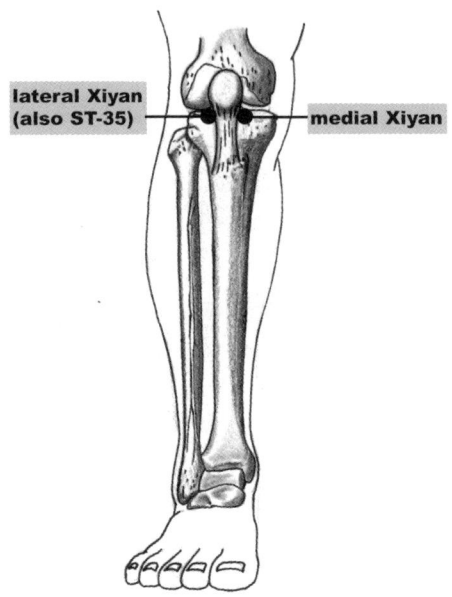

lateral Xiyan (also ST-35) — medial Xiyan

LOCATION:

A pair of points in the two depressions, medial and lateral to the patellar ligament, locating the point with the knee flexed. These two points are also termed medial and lateral Xiyan respectively. Lateral Xiyan overlaps with ST 35.

INDICATIONS:

Knee pain, diseases of the knee & surrounding soft tissue, weakness of the lower extremities.

METHOD:

Puncture perpendicularly 0.5-1.0 cun.

NOTES:

SCALP ACUPUNCTURE

SCALP ACUPUNCTURE

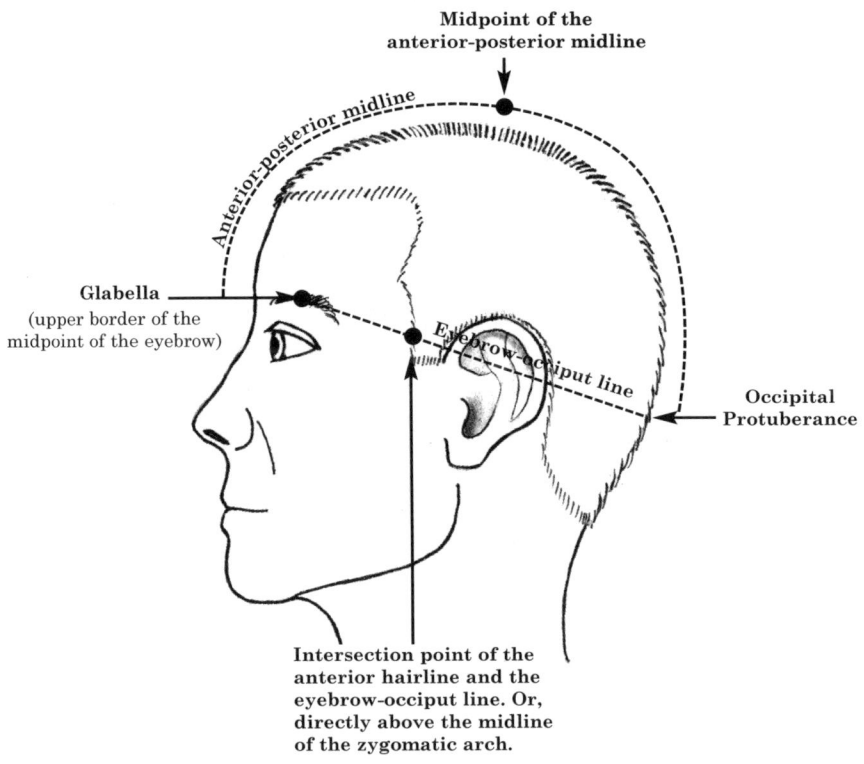

Midpoint of the anterior-posterior midline

Anterior-posterior midline

Glabella
(upper border of the midpoint of the eyebrow)

Eyebrow-occiput line

Occipital Protuberance

Intersection point of the anterior hairline and the eyebrow-occiput line. Or, directly above the midline of the zygomatic arch.

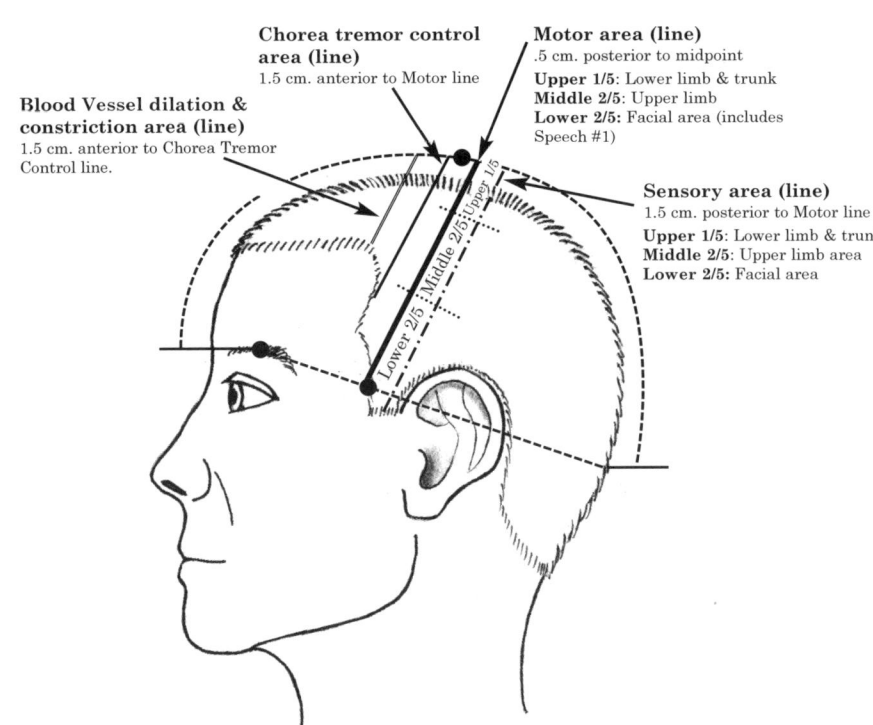

Chorea tremor control area (line)
1.5 cm. anterior to Motor line

Motor area (line)
.5 cm. posterior to midpoint
Upper 1/5: Lower limb & trunk
Middle 2/5: Upper limb
Lower 2/5: Facial area (includes Speech #1)

Blood Vessel dilation & constriction area (line)
1.5 cm. anterior to Chorea Tremor Control line.

Sensory area (line)
1.5 cm. posterior to Motor line
Upper 1/5: Lower limb & trunk
Middle 2/5: Upper limb area
Lower 2/5: Facial area

Upper 1/5 : Middle 2/5 : Lower 2/5

SCALP ACUPUNCTURE

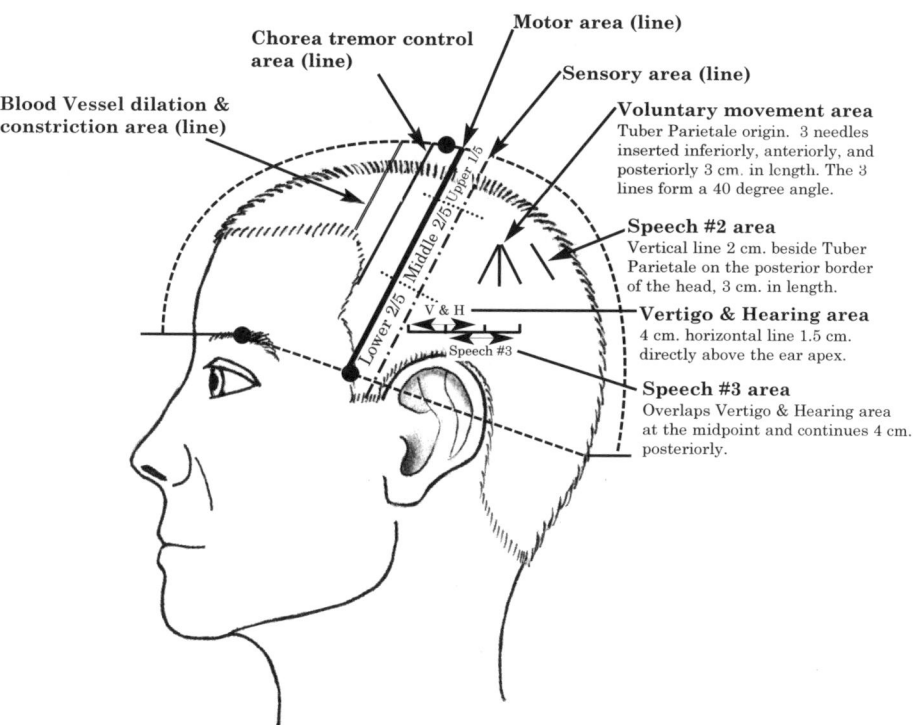

Chorea tremor control area (line)

Motor area (line)

Blood Vessel dilation & constriction area (line)

Sensory area (line)

Voluntary movement area
Tuber Parietale origin. 3 needles inserted inferiorly, anteriorly, and posteriorly 3 cm. in length. The 3 lines form a 40 degree angle.

Speech #2 area
Vertical line 2 cm. beside Tuber Parietale on the posterior border of the head, 3 cm. in length.

Vertigo & Hearing area
4 cm. horizontal line 1.5 cm. directly above the ear apex.

Speech #3 area
Overlaps Vertigo & Hearing area at the midpoint and continues 4 cm. posteriorly.

Lower 2/5 Middle 2/5 Upper 1/5

V & H

Speech #3

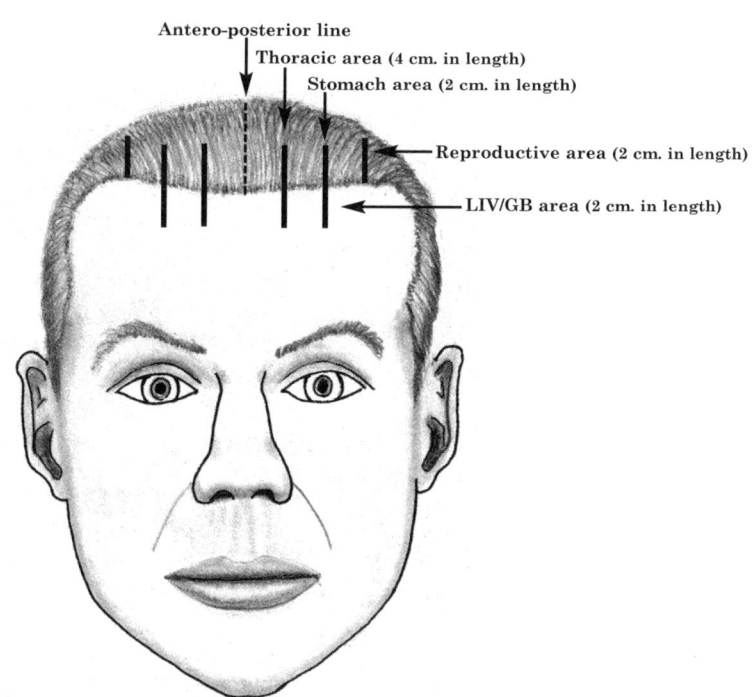

Antero-posterior line

Thoracic area (4 cm. in length)

Stomach area (2 cm. in length)

Reproductive area (2 cm. in length)

LIV/GB area (2 cm. in length)

SCALP ACUPUNCTURE

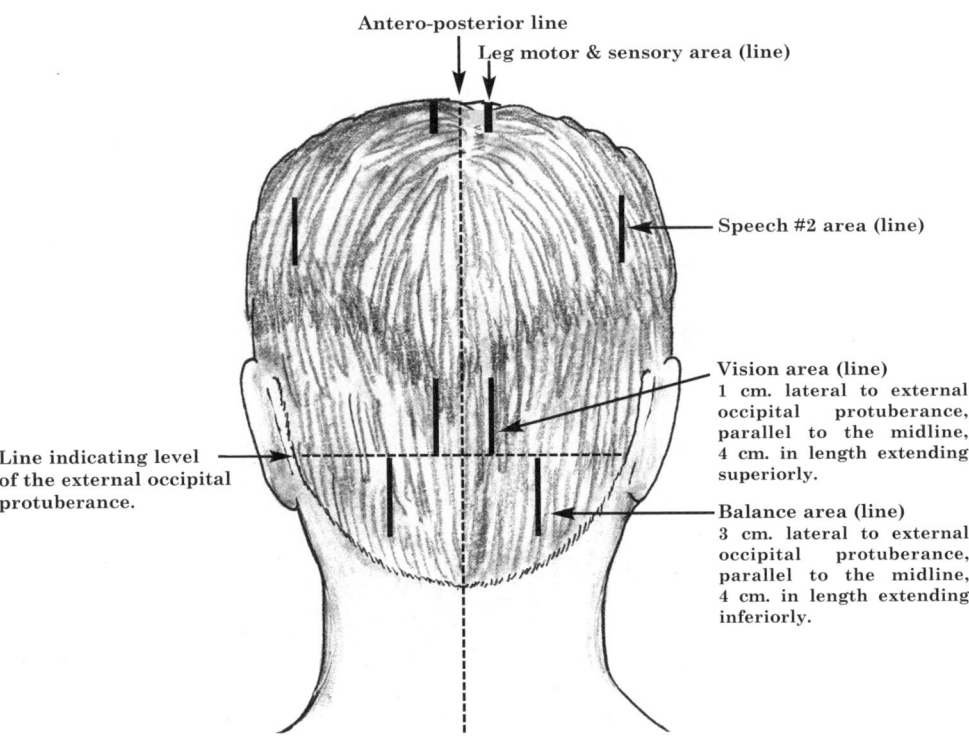

Antero-posterior line

Leg motor & sensory area (line)

Speech #2 area (line)

Vision area (line)
1 cm. lateral to external occipital protuberance, parallel to the midline, 4 cm. in length extending superiorly.

Line indicating level of the external occipital protuberance.

Balance area (line)
3 cm. lateral to external occipital protuberance, parallel to the midline, 4 cm. in length extending inferiorly.

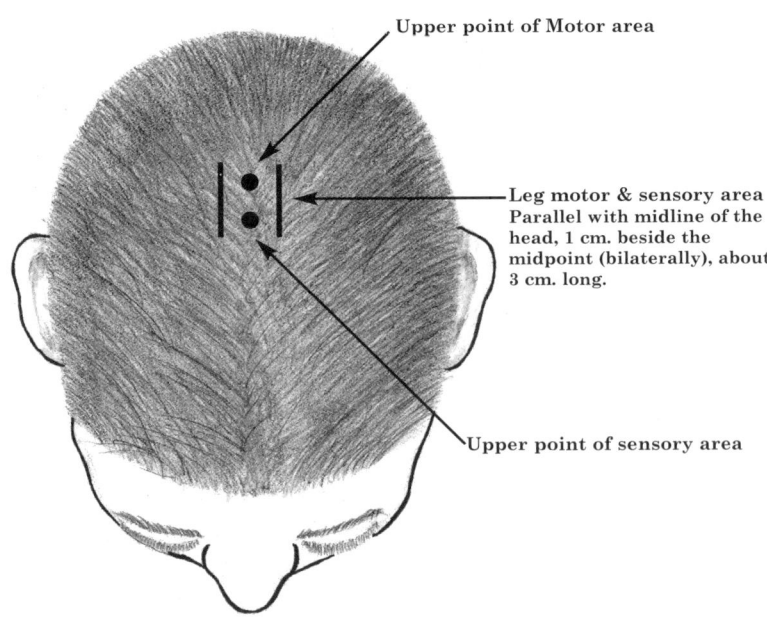

Upper point of Motor area

Leg motor & sensory area
Parallel with midline of the head, 1 cm. beside the midpoint (bilaterally), about 3 cm. long.

Upper point of sensory area

Area	Location	Indications
Motor Area	A line starting from a point .5 cm. posterior to the midpoint of anterio-posterior plane that goes diagonally across the head to a point at the intersection of the zygomatic arch (superior margin) and the hairline at the temple.	
Lower Limb and trunk area	Upper 1/5 of Motor area line	Paralysis of the lower limbs on the opposite side.
Upper Limb area	Middle 2/5 of Motor area line	Paralysis of the upper limbs on the opposite side.
Facial area (includes Speech #1 area)	Lower 2/5 of Motor area line	Upper motor neuron paralysis of face (opposite side), motor aphasia, dribbling saliva, impaired speech.
Sensory Area	A line parallel and 1.5 cm. posterior to Motor area line	
Lower limb, head, and trunk area	Upper 1/5 of Sensory area line	Pain, numbness, and abnormal sensation in the lower extremities on opposite side; neck pain, occipital headache, tinnitus, vertigo.
Upper limb area	Middle 2/5 of Sensory area line	Pain, numbness, tingling in upper extremities on opposite side.
Facial area	Lower 2/5 of Sensory area line	Migraine headache, facial paralysis, trigeminal neuralgia, arthritis of temporomandibular joint, toothache (opposite side).
Vertigo & hearing area	Horizontal line 1.5 cm. superior and centered on the apex of the ear, 4 cm. in length	Meniere's syndrome, tinnitus, diminished hearing, vertigo.
Blood vessel dilation & constriction area	Parallel with and 1.5 cm. anterior to Chorea and tremor control area	Hypertension, superficial edema.
Chorea and tremor control area	Parallel with and 1.5 cm. anterior to Motor area line	Syndenham's chorea, tremors, palsy, Parkinson's.
Leg Motor & Sensory area	Parallel with midline of head, 1 cm. lateral to midpoint, approximately 3 cm. in length (bilateral)	Paralysis, pain or numbness of lower limbs, acute low back sprain, prolapsed uterus, nocturnal urination.

Area	Location	Indications
Stomach area	Beginning at the hairline directly above the pupil of the eye, parallel with the midline of the head, extending posteriorly 2 cm. (bilateral)	Upper abdominal pain or discomfort.
Liver & Gallbladder area	Beginning at the hairline it extends anteriorly from the Stomach area line 2 cm. in length. (bilateral)	Pain in the upper right abdomen and/or right rib cage, chronic hepatitis.
Thoracic Area	Beginning at the hairline midway between and parallel with the Stomach area line and midline of the head, extending posteriorly and anteriorly 2 cm. in each direction.	Asthma, chest discomfort or pain, tachycardia.
Reproductive area	Beginning at the hairline parallel and lateral to the Stomach area line at a distance equal to that between the Stomach area and Thoracic area line, extending posteriorly 2 cm. in length. (bilateral)	Menstrual disorders, combined with the Leg Motor area line for uterine prolapse.
Vision area	1 cm. lateral to the EOP, parallel to the midline of the head, 4 cm. in length extending superiorly.	Cortical visual disturbances.
Balance area	3 cm. lateral to the EOP, parallel to the midline of the head, 4 cm. in length extending inferiorly.	Loss of balance due to cerebellar disturbances.
Voluntary movement area	Tuber Parietale origin. 3 needles inserted inferiorly, anteriorly, and posteriorly 3 cm. in length. The 3 lines will form a 40 degree angle.	Apraxia (nerve injury in which unable to carry out purposeful movement despite normal muscle power & coordination.)
Speech #1	Lower 1/5 of the Motor area line.	Motor aphasia, impaired speech, dribbling saliva.
Speech #2	Vertical line 2 cm. beside tuber parietale on back of head, 3 cm. in length.	Nominal aphasia.
Speech #3	Overlaps Vertigo & Hearing area line at midpoint & continues 4 cm. posteriorly.	Receptive aphasia.

EAR
ACUPUNCTURE

EAR ACUPUNCTURE

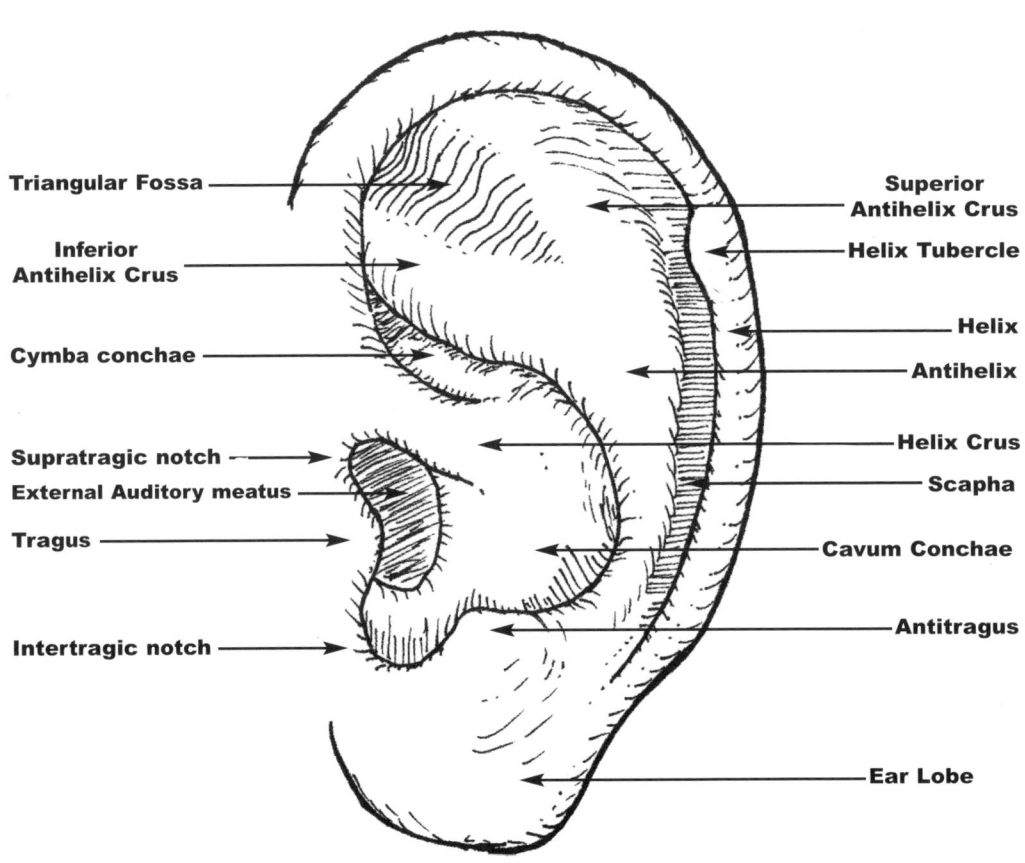

Triangular Fossa

Inferior Antihelix Crus

Cymba conchae

Supratragic notch

External Auditory meatus

Tragus

Intertragic notch

Superior Antihelix Crus

Helix Tubercle

Helix

Antihelix

Helix Crus

Scapha

Cavum Conchae

Antitragus

Ear Lobe

NOTES:

EAR ACUPUNCTURE

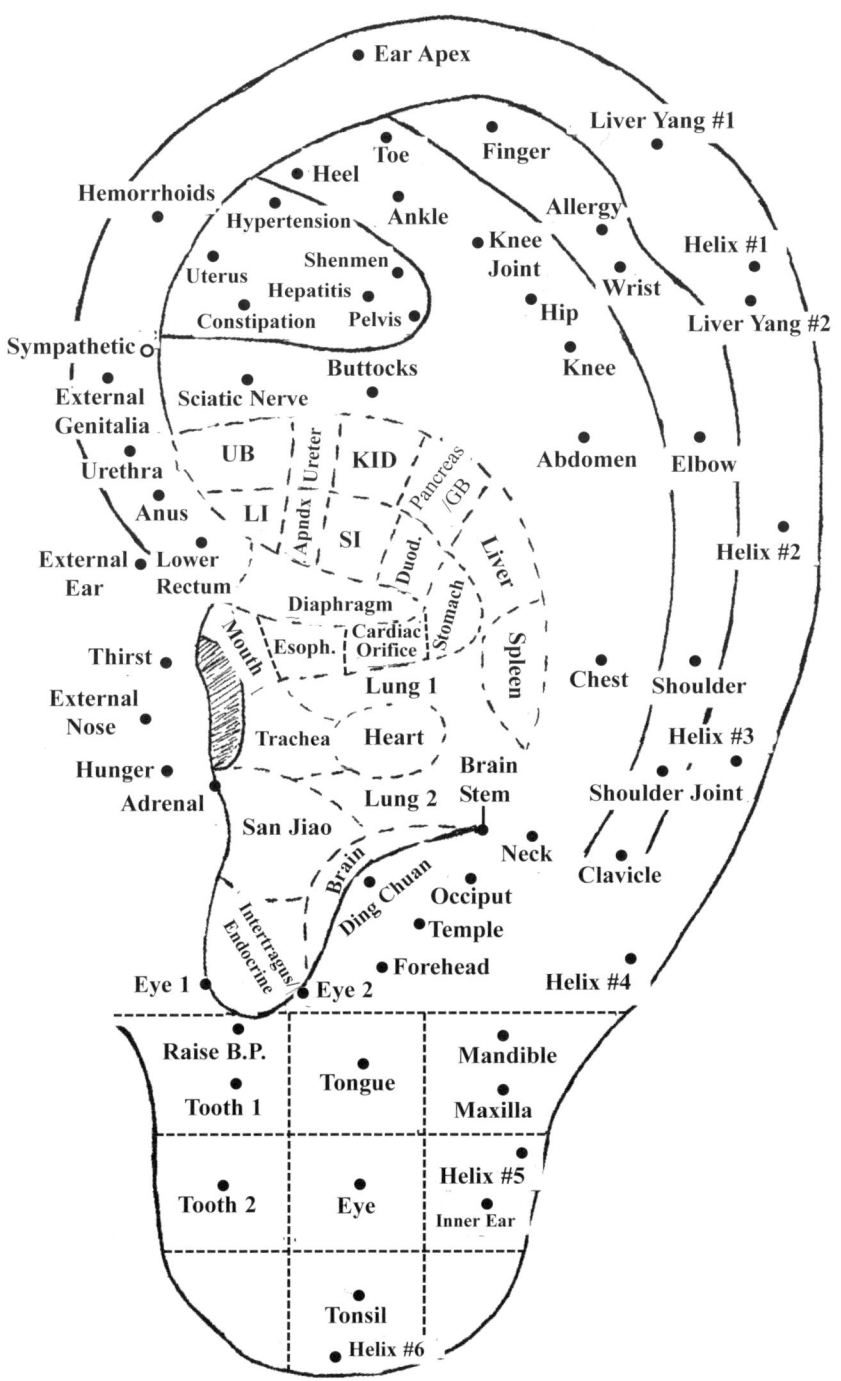

NOTES

CUN MEASUREMENTS

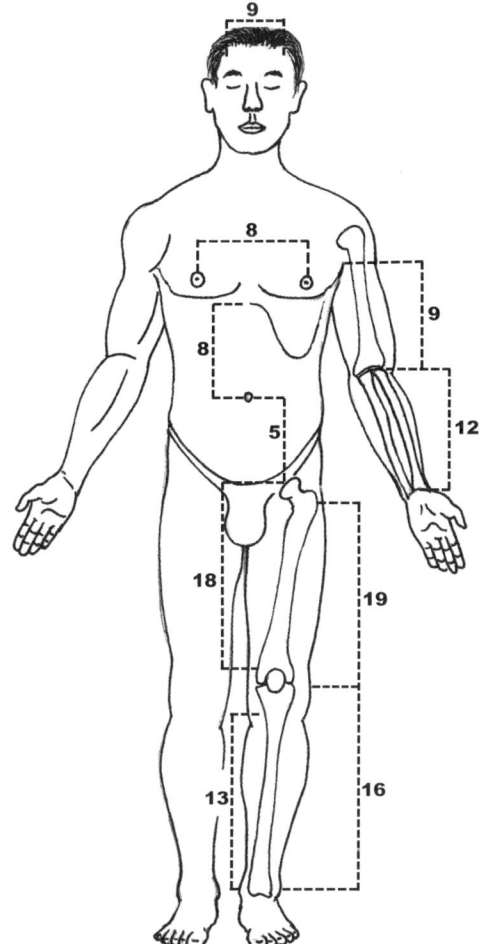

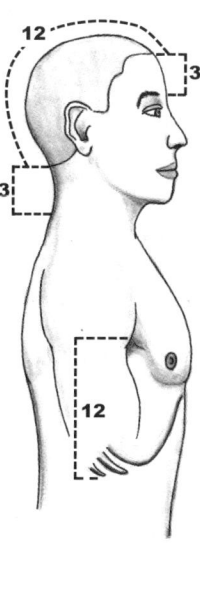

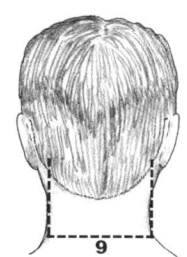

AREA	CUN MEASUREMENT
HEAD	• Between anterior and posterior hairlines: **12 cun** • Between the two mastoid processes: **9 cun**
CHEST & ABDOMEN	• Between sternocostal angle and umbilicus: **8 cun** • Between umbilicus and upper border of pubic symphysis: **5 cun** • Between the nipples: **8 cun** • Between the tip of the acromion process and the midline of the body: **8 cun**
BACK	• Between the medial border of the scapula and the posterior midline: **3 cun** • Between the posterior hairline and the inferior border of C7 spinous process: **3 cun**
LATERAL CHEST	• Between end of axillary fold on the lateral side of chest to the tip of the 11th rib: **12 cun**
UPPER EXTREMITIES	• Between the end of the axillary fold and the cubital crease: **9 cun** • Between the cubital crease and wrist crease: **12 cun**
LOWER EXTREMITIES	• Between upper border of pubic symphysis and the medial epicondyle of the femur: **18 cun** • Between the prominence of the greater trochanter and the popliteal crease: **19 cun** • Between lower border of the medial condyle of the tibia to the tip of the medial malleolus: **13 cun** • Between the popliteal crease and the lateral malleolus: **16 cun** • Between the popliteal crease and the medial malleolus: **15 cun**

ACUPUNCTURE TABLES

5 SHU POINTS OF THE YIN MERIDIANS & LUO, XI, YUAN POINTS

WOOD Jing Well	FIRE Ying Spring	EARTH Shu Stream	METAL Jing River	WATER He Sea	LUO	XI-CLEFT	YUAN
LU 11	LU 10	LU 9	LU 8	LU 5	LU 7	LU 6	LU 9
P 9	P 8	P 7	P 5	P 3	P 6	P 4	P 7
H 9	H 8	H 7	H 4	H 3	H 5	H 6	H 7
SP 1	SP 2	SP 3	SP 5	SP 9	SP 4	SP 8	SP 3
LIV 1	LIV 2	LIV 3	LIV 4	LIV 8	LIV 5	LIV 6	LIV 3
K 1	K 2	K 3	K 7	K 10	K 4	K 5	K 3

5 SHU POINTS OF THE YANG MERIDIANS & LUO, XI, YUAN POINTS

METAL Jing Well	WATER Ying Spring	WOOD Shu Stream	FIRE Jing River	EARTH He Sea	LUO	XI-CLEFT	YUAN
LI 1	LI 2	LI 3	LI 5	LI 11	LI 6	LI 7	LI 4
SJ 1	SJ 2	SJ 3	SJ 6	SJ 10	SJ 5	SJ 7	SJ 4
SI 1	SI 2	SI 3	SI 5	SI 8	SI 7	SI 6	SI 4
ST 45	ST 44	ST 43	ST 41	ST 36	ST 40	ST 34	ST 42
GB 44	GB 43	GB 41	GB 38	GB 34	GB 37	GB 36	GB 40
UB 67	UB 66	UB 65	UB 60	UB 40	UB 58	UB 63	UB 64

SIX FU ORGANS	LOWER HE SEA
STOMACH	ST 36
LARGE INTESTINE	ST 37
SMALL INTESTINE	ST 39
GALL BLADDER	GB 34
BLADDER	UB 40
SAN JIAO	UB 39

ORGAN	BACK SHU	FRONT MU
LUNG	UB 13	LU 1
PERICARDIUM	UB 14	REN 17
HEART	UB 15	REN 14
LIVER	UB 18	LIV 14
GALLBLADDER	UB 19	GB 24
SPLEEN	UB 20	LIV 13
STOMACH	UB 21	REN 12
SAN JIAO	UB 22	REN 5
KIDNEY	UB 23	GB 25
LARGE INTESTINE	UB 25	ST 25
SMALL INTESTINE	UB 27	REN 4
URINARY BLADDER	UB 28	REN 3

TISSUE	INFLUENTIAL POINT
ZANG ORGANS	LIV 13
FU ORGANS	REN 12
QI	REN 17
BLOOD	UB 17
TENDON	GB 34
PULSE/VESSELS	LU 9
BONE	UB 11
MARROW	GB 39

4 COMMAND POINTS	
Face and Mouth	LI 4
Head & Back of Neck	LU 7
Abdomen	ST 36
Back-Upper & Lower	GB 34

CONFLUENT PT.	PRIMARY CHANNEL	EXTRA CHANNEL	INDICATIONS
P 6	Pericardium	Yinwei	Heart, chest, stomach
SP 4	Spleen	Chong	
SI 3	Small Intestine	DU	Neck, shoulder, back, inner canthus
UB 62	Bladder	Yangqiao	
SJ 5	San Jiao	Yangwei	Retroauricle, cheek, outer canthus
GB 41	Gallbladder	Dai	
LU 7	Lung	Ren	Throat, chest, lungs
K 6	Kidney	Yinqiao	

EXTRA CHANNELS & COALESCENT POINTS	
EXTRA CHANNEL	COALESCENT POINTS
CHONG	Ren 1, Ren 7, ST 30, K 11-K 21
DAI	GB 26, GB 27, GB 28
YANGWEI	UB 63, GB 13-GB 21, GB 35, SI 10, SJ 15, DU 15, DU 16, ST 8
YINWEI	K 9, SP 12, SP 13, SP 15, SP 16, LIV 14, Ren 22, Ren 23
YANGQIAO	UB 1, UB 59, UB 61, UB 62, GB 29, GB 20, SI 10, LI 15, LI 16, ST 1, ST 3, ST 4, DU 16
YINQIAO	K 6, K 8, UB 1
DU	UB 12, Ren 1
REN	ST 1, DU 28

"MOTHER" & "SON" POINTS

MERIDIAN	MOTHER POINT (REINFORCING)	SON POINT (REDUCING)
LUNG	LU 9	LU 5
LARGE INTESTINE	LI 11	LI 2
STOMACH	ST 4	ST 45
SPLEEN	SP 2	SP 5
HEART	H 9	H 7
SMALL INTESTINE	SI 3	SI 8
BLADDER	UB 67	UB 65
KIDNEY	K 7	K 1
PERICARDIUM	P 9	P 7
SAN JIAO	SJ 3	SJ 10
GALLBLADDER	GB 43	GB 38
LIVER	LIV 8	LIV 2

DISTAL AND LOCAL POINT SELECTION

AREA	DISTAL POINTS	ADJACENT POINTS	LOCAL POINTS
FOREHEAD	LI 4, ST 44	DU 20	GB 14, Yintang
TEMPLE	SJ 3, SJ 5, GB 41	GB 20	Taiyang, GB 8
NAPE	SI 3, UB 60, UB 65	DU 14	UB 10, GB 10
EYE	SI 6, LIV 3, LI 4	GB 16	UB 1, ST 1, GB 20
NOSE	LU 7, ST 45, LI 4	DU 23	LI 20, Yintang
MOUTH & CHEEK	LI 4, ST 41	SI 18	ST 4, ST 6, ST 7
EAR	SJ 3, SJ 5, GB 43	GB 20	GB 2, SJ 17, SI 19
THROAT	LU 10, K 6, LI 4	UB 10	REN 23, SI 17
CHEST	P 6, ST 40	LU 1	REN 17
COSTAL REGION	SJ 6, GB 34	LIV 13	LIV 14
UPPER ABDOMEN	P 6, ST 36	ST 21	REN 12
LOWER ABDOMEN	P 6, LIV 8	ST 25	REN 4
LUMBAR REGION	UB 40, SI 3	UB 32	UB 23, UB 25
RECTUM	UB 57	UB 30	DU 1, UB 49

BIBLIOGRAPHY

O'Conner, John and Bensky, Dan, trans. **Acupuncture: A Comprehensive Text.** Seattle: Eastland Press, 1981

Xinnong, Cheng, et al. **Chinese Acupuncture and Moxibustion.** Beijing: Foreign Languages Press, 1987.

Chu, Luke S.W. et al. **Acupuncture Manual: A Western Approach.** New York: Marcel Dekker, Inc. 1979.

Qiu, Mao-Liang et al. **Chinese Acupuncture and Moxibustion.** New York: Churchill Livingstone, 1993.

Deadman, Peter and Al-Khafaji, Mazin. **A Manual of Acupuncture.** England: Journal of Chinese Medicine Publications, 1998.

NOTES

NOTES

NOTES

494

NOTES

NOTES

NOTES

NOTES

NOTES